Cosmetic Medicine and Minimally Invasive Surgery

Guest Editors

MALCOLM D. PAUL, MD
RAFFI V. HOVSEPIAN, MD
ADAM M. ROTUNDA, MD

CLINICS IN PLASTIC SURGERY

www.plasticsurgery.theclinics.com

July 2011 • Volume 38 • Number 3

SAUNDERS an imprint of ELSEVIER, Inc.

W.B. SAUNDERS COMPANY
A Division of Elsevier Inc.

1600 John F. Kennedy Boulevard • Suite 1800 • Philadelphia, Pennsylvania 19103-2899

http://www.theclinics.com

CLINICS IN PLASTIC SURGERY Volume 38, Number 3
July 2011 ISSN 0094-1298, ISBN-13: 978-1-4557-0493-4

Editor: Joanne Husovski
Developmental Editor: Teia Stone

Clinics in Plastic Surgery (ISSN 0094-1298) is published quarterly by Elsevier Inc., 360 Park Avenue South, New York, NY 10010-1710. Months of issue are January, April, July, and October. Business and Editorial Offices: 1600 John F. Kennedy Blvd., Suite 1800, Philadelphia, PA 19103-2899. Periodicals postage paid at New York, NY and additional mailing offices. Subscription prices are $411.00 per year for US individuals, $617.00 per year for US institutions, $203.00 per year for US students and residents, $467.00 per year for Canadian individuals, $721.00 per year for Canadian institutions, $530.00 per year for international individuals, $721.00 per year for international institutions, and $256.00 per year for Canadian and foreign students/residents. To receive student/resident rate, orders must be accompanied by name of affiliated institution, date of term, and the *signature* of program/residency coordinator on institution letterhead. Orders will be billed at individual rate until proof of status is received. Foreign air speed delivery is included in all *Clinics* subscription prices. All prices are subject to change without notice. **POSTMASTER:** Send address changes to *Clinics in Plastic Surgery*, Elsevier Health Sciences Division, Subscription Customer Service, 3251 Riverport Lane, Maryland Heights, MO 63043. **Customer Service: 1-800-654-2452 (US and Canada). From outside of the United States and Canada, call 314-447-8871. Fax: 314-447-8029. E-mail: JournalsCustomerService-usa@elsevier.com (for print support); JournalsOnlineSupport-usa@elsevier.com (for online support).**

Reprints. For copies of 100 or more of articles in this publication, please contact the Commercial Reprints Department, Elsevier Inc., 360 Park Avenue South, New York, New York 10010-1710. Tel.: (+1) 212-633-3812; Fax: (+1) 212-462-1935; E-mail: reprints@elsevier.com.

Clinics in Plastic Surgery is covered in *Current Contents, EMBASE/Excerpta Medica, Science Citation Index, MEDLINE/PubMed (Index Medicus), ASCA,* and *ISI/BIOMED.*

Printed and bound by CPI Group (UK) Ltd, Croydon, CR0 4YY

Transferred to Digital Print 2011

Contributors

GUEST EDITORS

MALCOLM D. PAUL, MD, FACS
Clinical Professor of Surgery, Aesthetic and
Plastic Surgery Institute, University of
California, Irvine, California

RAFFI V. HOVSEPIAN, MD
Aesthetic, Plastic and Reconstructive
Surgery, Diplomate, American Board
of Plastic Surgery; Diplomate, American
Board of Surgery; Diplomate, European
Board of Plastic Reconstructive and
Aesthetic Surgery; Diplomate, American
Board of Medical Specialties;
Assistant Clinical Professor, Division
of Plastic and Reconstructive Surgery,
University of California, Irvine, School of
Medicine, Orange; Clinical Instructor,
Aesthetic Plastic Surgery Resident
Training Rotation, Aesthetic and Plastic
Surgery Institute; Private Practice,
Beverly Hills; Newport Beach,
California

ADAM M. ROTUNDA, MD, FAAD
Diplomate, American Board of Dermatology;
Fellow, American College of Mohs Surgery;
Associate Professor, Dermatology, David
Geffen School of Medicine, University
of California, Los Angeles, California

AUTHORS

TODD V. CARTEE, MD
Total Skin and Beauty Dermatology Center,
Birmingham, Alabama

CHARBEL CHALFOUN, MD
The Plastic Surgery Group, Montclair,
New Jersey

ZOE DIANA DRAELOS, MD
Consulting Professor, Department of
Dermatology, Duke University, School
of Medicine, Durham, North Carolina

DIANE DUNCAN, MD, FACS
Private Practice, Fort Collins, Colorado

MITCHEL P. GOLDMAN, MD
Goldman, Butterwick, and Associates Cosmetic
Laser Dermatology, San Diego, California

RAFFI V. HOVSEPIAN, MD
Aesthetic, Plastic and Reconstructive
Surgery, Diplomate, American Board
of Plastic Surgery; Diplomate, American
Board of Surgery; Diplomate, European
Board of Plastic Reconstructive and
Aesthetic Surgery; Diplomate, American
Board of Medical Specialties;
Assistant Clinical Professor, Division
of Plastic and Reconstructive Surgery,
University of California, Irvine, School of
Medicine, Orange; Clinical Instructor,
Aesthetic Plastic Surgery Resident
Training Rotation, Aesthetic and Plastic
Surgery Institute; Private Practice,
Beverly Hills; Newport Beach,
California

DEREK JONES, MD
Clinical Associate Professor, Division of
Dermatology, David Geffen School of Medicine,
University of California, Los Angeles;
Founder and Director, Skin Care and Laser
Physicians of Beverly Hills, Los Angeles,
California

EUGENE K. KIM, MD
Private Practice, Beverly Hills; Assistant
Clinical Professor, Aesthetic and Plastic
Surgery Institute, University of California,
Irvine, Orange, California

GARY P. LASK, MD
Director, Dermatologic Surgery Service and
Laser Center, Division of Dermatology, David
Geffen School of Medicine at University of
California Los Angeles (UCLA), Los Angeles,
California

MARGARET W. MANN, MD
Assistant Professor of Dermatology;
Co-Director, Dermatologic and Cosmetic
Surgery, Department of Dermatology,
University of California, Irvine, California

MARK K. MARKARIAN, MD, MSPH
Plastic Surgery Resident, Division of Plastic
and Reconstructive Surgery, Saint Louis
University School of Medicine, St Louis,
Missouri

PRAKASH MATHEW
University of California, Irvine Medical School,
Irvine, California

GARY D. MONHEIT, MD
Total Skin and Beauty Dermatology Center,
Birmingham, Alabama

R. STEPHEN MULHOLLAND, MD, FRCS(C)
Plastic Surgeon, Private Practice Plastic
Surgery, SpaMedica® Clinics, Toronto,
Ontario, Canada

ANDREW A. NELSON, MD
Department of Dermatology, Tufts University
School of Medicine; South End Dermatology
and Skin Care, Boston, Massachusetts

MALCOLM D. PAUL, MD, FACS
Clinical Professor of Surgery, Aesthetic
and Plastic Surgery Institute, University
of California, Irvine, California

ANTHONY PETELIN, MD
Department of Dermatology, University of
California, Irvine, California

JENNIFER D. PETERSON, MD
Goldman, Butterwick, and Associates
Cosmetic Laser Dermatology, San Diego,
California

KENT REMINGTON, MD, FRCP(C), FACP
Director, Remington Laser Dermatology
Centre; Division of Dermatology, Foothills
Medical Centre, Calgary, Canada

ADAM M. ROTUNDA, MD, FAAD
Diplomate, American Board of Dermatology;
Fellow, American College of Mohs Surgery;
Associate Professor, Dermatology, David
Geffen School of Medicine, University
of California, Los Angeles, California

NAZANIN SAEDI, MD
Department of Dermatology, University of
California, Irvine, California

ARTHUR SWIFT, MD, FRCS(C)
Director, Westmount Institute of Plastic
Surgery; Director, Victoria Park Medical Spa;
Plastic Surgeon, Division of Plastic Surgery,
St. Mary's Hospital, McGill University,
Montreal, Quebec, Canada

CHRISTOPHER ZACHARY, MBBS, FRCP
Chairman, Department of Dermatology,
University of California, Irvine, California

Contents

The evolution of thought and process in cosmetic medicine and surgery has united specialists from various backgrounds with the goal of providing safe, reproducible techniques to improve the various elements of the aging face from within and without. The realization that the aging face is both vector and volume based has dramatically altered the approach to reversing the signs of aging. Ultimately, it was the joining of forces from multiple specialties that provided a blueprint for impressive improvement in the return of a youthful, natural look.

Minimally invasive or noninvasive procedures account for an overwhelming majority of cosmetic procedures. These procedures include botulinum toxin injections, soft tissue fillers, chemical peel, dermabrasion, and laser hair removal. This article reviews some of the principles involved in these procedures. Plastic surgeons need to be equally familiar with surgical and nonsurgical approaches to cosmetic medicine to provide a complete set of therapeutic options to their patients.

The recent availability of safe volumizing fillers has provided cosmetic physicians with the tools necessary to contour facial features non-surgically and cost-effectively. This review focuses on outlining objective parameters necessary for creating a template to maximize each individual's facial beauty. Phi relationships can be approached for all facial features and rely on the establishment of smooth ogee curves in all dimensions. Once goals have been determined and a budget established, a logical syntax is used to create an algorithm for selecting products and procedures. The methodology leads to consistent and pleasing results with a high rate of patient satisfaction.

This article discusses the role of injectable soft-tissue fillers in the aging face, and their clinical and chemical behavior. Temporary and permanent fillers are discussed, namely hyaluronic acids, calcium hydroxylapatite, poly-L-lactic acid, liquid silicone, and polymethylmethacrylate. Techniques and outcomes are presented.

This review presents skin anatomy, dermabraders, indications for dermabrasion and microdermabrasion, and dermabrasion techniques for the face, along with potential complications. Dermabrasion is a minimally invasive technique used for skin resurfacing. Its applications include treatment of rhytids, abnormal scarring, and premalignant lesions. The risks of complications are low and include pigment changes, hypertrophic scarring, and infection. Despite the introduction of newer therapies, such as lasers and chemical peels, dermabrasion remains an effective tool for physicians to combat the effects of aging without the downtime required for surgery.

The need for cosmeceutical research is ever present. This article has tried to highlight the chemistry of botanic extracts in the current marketplace and review the best research available. In some ways, more questions have been raised than answered; yet, ideas for intellectual discourse have been provided. Herein lies the physician cosmeceutical challenge.

Although the mechanism of action of botulinum toxin (BTX) has been intensively studied, many unanswered questions remain regarding the composition and clinical properties of the two formulations of BTX currently approved for cosmetic use. In the first half of this review, these questions are explored in detail, with emphasis on the most pertinent and revelatory studies in the literature. The second half delineates most of the common and some not so common uses of BTX in the face and neck, stressing important patient selection and safety considerations. Complications from neurotoxins at cosmetic doses are generally rare and usually technique dependent.

Laser technology has evolved rapidly in the last 2 decades. The theory of selective photothermolysis guides the proper selection and use of lasers to safely and effectively treat patients. This review summarizes the basic concepts and adjustable parameters for laser devices, emphasizing the importance of selective photothermolysis in clinical practice. It then covers the clinical applications of laser devices, including vascular lesions, hair removal, tattoo removal, facial rejuvenation, and fractional resurfacing. The authors intend to make the reader feel comfortable with the proper selection and application of lasers to treat their patients.

This article reviews the non-invasive and minimally invasive options for skin tightening, focusing on peer-reviewed articles and presentations and those technologies with the most proven or promising RF non-excisional skin-tightening results for excisional surgeons. RF has been the mainstay of non-invasive skin tightening and has emerged as the "cutting edge" technology in the minimally invasive skin-tightening field. Because these RF skin-tightening technologies are capital equipment purchases with a significant cost associated, this article also discusses some business issues and models that have proven to work in the plastic surgeon's office for non-invasive and minimally invasive skin-tightening technologies.

Fractional photothermolysis combines the benefits of fully ablative lasers with significantly reduced downtime and fewer complications. Skin is treated in a fractional manner, with narrow cylinders of tissue being thermally heated and normal adjacent skin left unaffected, and the fractional devices have shown effectiveness in treating a variety of conditions, especially scarring and photodamage. There are many devices that use fractional photothermolysis, and practitioners are becoming more adept at using optimal parameters to induce near CO_2 laser benefits. Fractionated lasers have become the cornerstone of a minimally invasive treatment regimen and have ushered in a new era of laser skin rejuvenation.

Cellulite affects all races, and it is estimated that 85% of women older than 20 years have some degree of cellulite. Many currently accepted cellulite therapies target deficiencies in lymphatic drainage and microvascular circulation. Devices using radiofrequency, laser, and light-based energies, alone or in combination and coupled frequently with tissue manipulation, are available for improving cellulite. Laser assisted liposuction may improve cellulite appearance. Although improvement using these devices is temporary, it may last several months. Patients who want smoother skin with less visible cellulite can undergo a series of treatments and then return for additional treatments as necessary.

With the recent US Food and Drug Administration (FDA) approval of polidocanol in the United States, there has been a resurgence of interest in sclerotherapy. Despite the popularity of laser therapy, sclerotherapy remains the gold standard for treating spider and reticular veins. Although this traditional method of treatment has been around for more than 100 years, better sclerosing agents and newer techniques have made sclerotherapy safer and more efficacious than ever before. This article is a primer for physicians interested in updating their skills in sclerotherapy. It reviews common sclerosants, sclerotherapy techniques, patient evaluation, complications, and recent advancements in sclerotherapy.

This review presents mechanisms of action and a review of the clinical applications of injections currently in development for localized fat reduction. After being received with initial enthusiasm earlier in the decade, mesotherapy and other injectable methods for fat loss (Lipodissolve, PC/DC, DC, injection lipolysis, adipolysis) have been subjects of critical scrutiny by the media and the US Food and Drug Administration. Several medications with novel detergent and lipolytic activity are in development and have demonstrated potential as minimally invasive fat reducing treatments.

Noninvasive body contouring is perhaps one of the most alluring areas of esthetic surgery today. This article discusses current noninvasive body-contouring modalities, including suction massage devices, radiofrequency energy, high-frequency focused ultrasound, cryolipolysis, and low-level light laser therapy devices. It also discusses imminent technologies awaiting approval by the Food and Drug Administration, reviews the basic science and clinical effects behind each of these existing and emerging technologies, addresses patient selection and clinical applications of each modality, and discusses the applicability and economics of providing noninvasive lipolysis services in office.

The advent of barbed sutures has been a novel and useful adjunct for the aesthetic plastic surgeon in properly selected patients. The deployment of a barbed suture minimizes the risks of cheese wiring and stress relaxation, facilitating the minimally invasive repositioning of soft tissue in the head and neck, as well as optimizing and enhancing traditionally long and potentially tedious procedures in body contouring. This article highlights the advances, advantages, and efficacy associated with the use of barbed sutures in lifting and wound closure.

Clinics in Plastic Surgery

THE CLINICS ARE AVAILABLE ONLINE!

Access your subscription at:
www.theclinics.com

Cosmetic Medicine and Surgery: A Shift in Perspective

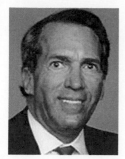
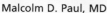

Malcolm D. Paul, MD

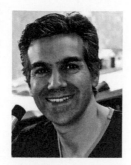

Adam M. Rotunda, MD
Guest Editors

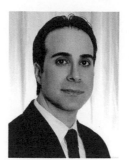

Raffi V. Hovsepian, MD

In the articles in this publication, the technologies that provide medical and surgical solutions for cosmetic indications are explored, including barbed sutures, neurotoxins, cosmeceuticals, sclerotherapy, dermabrasion, fillers, lasers, and other energy sources, including face and body contouring devices, that provide solutions that respond to a consumer demand for less aggressive solutions to the aging face and body contour deformities.

The introductory article sets the stage in depth for the content in this issue, describing the outcome of revelations of vector and volume effect on the aging face, the demand for less aggressive procedures, effects of the most recent economic downturn on industry developments and patient requests, addressing "outside-in" technologies such as peels, collagen, silicone, and topical treatments. The adoption of Botox and hyaluronic acid for use in unanticipated ways exceeding their original intended use is discussed along with laser technology and its indications for hair removal, removal of vascular lesions, tattoo removal, and, more recently, laser-based lipolysis.

Malcolm D. Paul, MD
Aesthetic and Plastic Surgery Institute
University of California, Irvine
1401 Avocado Avenue, Suite 810
Orange, CA 92660, USA

Raffi V. Hovsepian, MD
Aesthetic and Plastic Surgery Institute
University of California, Irvine
1401 Avocado Avenue, Suite 810
Orange, CA 92660, USA

Adam M. Rotunda, MD
1100 Quail Street, Suite 102
Newport Beach, CA 92660, USA

E-mail addresses:
mpaulmd@hotmail.com (M.D. Paul)
DraffiH@gmail.com (R.V. Hovsepian)
arotunda@hotmail.com (A.M. Rotunda)
www.newportskincancer.com

An Overview of Cosmetic Medicine and Surgery: Past, Present, and Future

Malcolm D. Paul, MD

KEYWORDS

- Aging face • Cosmetic surgery • Cosmetic medicine
- Soft tissue fillers

The more things change, the more they stay the same

In many disciplines including those outside medicine, the thought that there really is no change, only a realization that new things do not cause a change, has been held to be true for decades. This idea does not apply to the thought and process in reversing the signs of an aging face. Although the aging face has been treated for centuries, only recently it was recognized that the process occurred at multiple levels, from the bony structural support of the facial soft tissues and included the muscle, fat, and skin. It has been known for decades that environmental factors such as smoking, climate, and sun exposure have profound influence on the appearance of the face, and considerable energy has been devoted to informing the patient that there are ways to minimize the effect of environmental factors that accelerate facial aging and may lead to skin cancers. There are, of course, genetic influences on how and when the face ages visibly, but, at this time, the genetic forces that determine how and when the face ages cannot be modulated. A sentinel article on the "senility of the aging face" by Gonzalez-Ulloa and Flores[1] was an important attempt to understand the cause and effect of facial aging. They understood that the changes that were observed occurred at both bony and soft tissue levels. This monumental publication makes one wonder why more intellectual energy was not devoted to reversing the signs of the aging face at multiple anatomic levels rather than working solely on the skin. The early facelifting procedures had been used for decades before there was a shift in thought with regard to how and why the face ages and the understanding that merely pulling on the ptotic skin was not enough to reestablish a youthful, harmonious shape to the rejuvenated face.

ARCHITECTURE AND VOLUME: MASTER TEACHINGS

The number of available options for both medical and surgical reversal of the aging face has dramatically increased because it is now understood how and why these changes occur, and this understanding has fueled commercial interest in providing what is needed to accomplish these goals. Over the centuries, there was an understanding of what constituted a beautiful face, not only with Cleopatra but also with others (the imprint in the ruins of Persepolis in Shiraz shows all of the desired facial contours that were visible in the ancient Iranian queen). The "universal symbols of beauty" have been captured in the minds and hands of notable artists (Bill Little has repeatedly shown us how the renaissance artists

Disclosure: The author serves as Chairman of the Medical Advisory Board and receives consultant fees and stock options from Invasix, Ltd, and serves as a consultant to Angiotech, Pharmaceuticals, Inc, manufacturer of Quill SRS Barbed Sutures, and receives consultant fees.
Aesthetic and Plastic Surgery Institute, University of California, Irvine, CA, USA
E-mail address: mpaulmd@hotmail.com

Clin Plastic Surg 38 (2011) 329–334
doi:10.1016/j.cps.2011.02.004

knew what Ralph Millard called the "ideal normal"). Bill also taught that a beautiful face had to include an Ogee curve, architecturally understood, and once we saw it, we knew that Bill was correct in applying this form to the goals in facial rejuvenation.[2,3] When I looked back at the history of brow and midface lifting,[4,5] I did not appreciate that, despite the understanding of facial aging as described by Gonzalez-Ulloa and Flores in 1965, at least 75 years of facial aesthetic surgical techniques before and after this publication failed to address volume-based deficiencies. The early surgical procedures directed at repositioning ptotic facial soft tissue failed to address the volumetric loss including bone and soft tissue. These techniques were well intentioned but principally involved undermining skin and repositioning it under tension. The stretched, unnatural look was often justified by trying to convince the viewer that "my patients are happy." It was the work of Ed Terino, who, although not the first to use autologous or alloplastic implants, was the first to logically approach skeletal deficiencies with specific alloplastic implants based on his 3-dimensional understanding of facial shape.[6] His zonal analysis clearly provided an easily understandable way to address regional volume-based deficiencies. Those surgeons who understood the profound effect that volume restoration had on facial shaping clearly showed that some techniques worked better than others. The work of Hester and colleagues[7] in the 1990s directed attention at shifting the midface soft tissues vertically to augment this anatomic area and blend the lid-cheek junction. Other major contributors[8–18] also recognized the profound effect that mobilizing the ptotic midface had on facial rejuvenation. However, some of these more aggressive techniques, including the subperiosteal and extended superficial musculo-aponeurotic system approaches, carried the added risks of prolonged edema, possible neurapraxias, eyelid malposition, and, in some cases, a new look that required weeks to "look natural." As is always true in aesthetic plastic surgery, selecting the right technique for a given patient largely determines the success achieved. So, some patients do well with a given technique, others do not (understanding the negative-vector orbit taught us why vertical lifting techniques could be associated with higher morbidity, including, but limited to, lid malposition).[19] The longevity of these results was impressive, but less-aggressive means of facial rejuvenation also showed impressive longevity.[20] Vector-based correction as a sole means of reversing the signs of aging is, although well intentioned, wrong minded in light of the profound influence of the works of Lambros[20]

and Pessa and colleagues.[21,22] Loss of facial fat and absorption of skeletal support affect the shape of the face. Therefore, facial reshaping may require moving the tissues to their prior, youthful position, as well as augmenting the soft tissues, and, where indicated, augmenting the skeletal support to produce a harmonious rejuvenation. Younger patients may show significant improvement in reversing the early signs of aging by merely adding soft tissue volume and/or skeletal support without moving soft tissue. As if that were not in itself an intellectual and technical challenge, facial compartments lose fat in varying amounts.[23] Therefore, efforts can be directed at augmenting compartments to effect a change in an adjacent compartment (eg, filling the deep medial cheek fat compartment to soften the arcus marginalis and blend the lid-cheek junction). There were many early contributors to facial soft tissue augmentation with autologous fat,[24–30] who showed that fat grafts survive and the elements to ensure survival were found to be based on appropriate donor sites, graft harvesting, graft preparation, and injection of small amounts of purified fat into tension-free recipient areas.

THE ECONOMY AND AESTHETIC PROCEDURES

Whereas these techniques were widely embraced and used, patients began to demand less-aggressive procedures with shorter "down times." Although it seemed that providing a shorter pathway to enduring facial rejuvenation was not the best way to approach the aging face, the "perfect storm" occurred when economic influences on consumer spending triggered a strong interest in less-aggressive and less-expensive procedures that produced visible results with a shorter recovery period. Sure, the more aggressive option could be provided, but the economy and the interest by the public would not support traditional or more aggressive procedures. Less was not merely more; it was merely more than enough based on consumer demands. After 9/11, there was a severe downturn in the request for consultations and for aesthetic plastic surgery procedures that lasted for several weeks. I went back in time to the early part of the twentieth century and looked at the history of sentinel national and world events and how they influenced cosmetic medicine and cosmetic surgery. I found that after events such as the Great Depression and Black Monday in October, 1987, women, on average, waited no longer than 6 weeks before they began to ask for and obtain cosmetic medicine products and/or cosmetic surgery techniques to allow them to look better, and certainly, looking better was the best way to feel better. The current recession that started in 2007, but was more palpable in 2008, is the only time in more than 90 years that consumers have waited longer than 6 weeks to reenter the cosmetic medicine and cosmetic surgery markets. Concerns about job security, adequate funds for retirement, decrease in home equity, the volatility of the stock market, and so on are all factors that play into the decision to invest in looking better. The discretionary spending was more closely scrutinized and rationed, as these concerns simply would not disappear. The need to remain in the job market has encouraged many to seek cosmetic medicine and cosmetic surgery solutions to reverse the signs of the aging face and make one more competitive in the job market. Many of these consumers sought a less-expensive quick fix; however, many also understood that it would be necessary to invest more so that one could obtain panfacial rejuvenation or a result that would last longer than the time required for the deduction of funds from their savings and checking accounts.

TOPICALS FOR AGING SKIN

Techniques and products that work from the outside have been an enormous influence on reversing the signs of facial aging. These techniques would not have evolved had there not been a need both professionally and from the consumer to provide more comprehensive options for facial rejuvenation. It was the forward thinking of Fritz Barton in the 1990s who saw the need to legitimize skin care by placing their annual society meeting immediately preceding the American Society for Aesthetic Surgery Annual Meeting. This gave the Skin Care Society the platform and the validation that it needed to "convince us" that we need to pay attention what was happening on the outside as importantly as what was happening on the inside of the aging face. The aging facial skin includes both internal changes such as cellular apoptosis and genetic influences and external changes resulting from environmental influences. The aging skin is primarily related to a fragmentation in the dermal-collagen matrix, producing a visible change in the appearance of the skin, in turn becoming a major indicator of facial aging.[31] The use of chemicals for facial peeling advanced profoundly with the introduction of the Baker/Gordon phenol/croton oil peel.[32,33] Although loss of pigmentation was an issue based on the depth of the peel and the skin type, many patients were pleased with the improvement in the appearance of their skin. The environmental causes of skin aging were largely reversed by this easily administered procedure. It was decades later that Hetter[34] and Kligman and colleagues[32] provided convincing evidence that the concentration of croton oil was more important than the phenol concentration in producing the desired result, and we began to rethink how this worked and how could it be made to work better with fewer adverse side effects. "Off the shelf" filling of lines and depressions began with the introduction of bovine collagen in the 1970s. This product, although only providing a short period of correction (duration of correction determined by increasing the cross-linking), was quickly embraced by clinicians and patients and its use became widespread. Complications were few with appropriate allergy testing, and patients were mostly pleased with the temporary improvement in the appearance of facial lines and folds. Patients returned frequently for additional injections, but, of course, both patients and clinicians sought a solution to facial wrinkling and contour deformities that would be longer lasting. Permanent solutions such as the injection of medical grade silicone and other nonautologous substances were available and continually changed to allow a palette of products that had risks associated with each product. It was desirable to have a permanent correction, but often, the risk of long-term sequelae discouraged the use of permanent or semipermanent injectables, particularly in the highly litigious US market (with the notable exception of fat grafting and stem cell grafting). The introduction of topical tretinoin (vitamin A) to remove the superficially damaged skin brought enormous attention to the role that topical agents can play in facial rejuvenation.[35] A sentinel event in the evolution of skin care occurred when Obaji introduced his technique of facial peeling with modified trichloroacetic acid (TCA), adding other agents to varying percentages of TCA. Specialists from many disciplines embraced this approach to facial peeling and quickly adopted his techniques and formulas. Obagi added multiple products to his line, allowing the treatment of other skin changes that were genetic and/or environmental, including, but not limited to, the treatment of hyperpigmentation with different causes. The level of awareness of what could be done to improve the signs of aging of the skin was elevated to a new level by Obagi's pioneering work, and many clinicians began to offer various concentrations of TCA peels, as well as peels such as kojic acid peels and salicylic glycolic acid peels. The introduction of vitamin C–based cosmeceuticals[36] was another in a series of new solutions to the aging skin. There is a seemingly endless introduction of new topical preparations to improve the texture of the skin, diminish rhytids, and correct areas of hyperpigmentation or solar damage. Some are dispensed only in physicians' offices, whereas many more choices can be found in MedSpas, drug stores, retail department store outlets, or online. The public is justifiably confused, as are physicians, in knowing what to use, where, how, and when.

SERENDIPITY IN NEW MEDICAL AND SURGICAL APPROACHES

As has been true in other medical and surgical disciplines, the discovery and implementation of new pharmaceuticals and procedures may be adopted in unanticipated ways and allow benefits that were not imagined. Often, the adoption of these pharmaceutical products and procedures far exceeded the original intended use. In surgery, a prime example was the adoption of endoscopy from general surgery (laparascopic cholecystectomy) and gynecology (laparoscopy) to aesthetic plastic surgery, principally for brow lifting and midface lifting.[37–39] Based on the pioneering work in craniofacial surgery by Tessier who established the legitimacy and effectiveness of the subperiosteal plane in frontal and midface dissection,[40] long access incisions were followed by short incisions using the endoscope for visualization and for the performance of surgical maneuvers required for rejuvenation of the upper and middle one-thirds of the aging face.[41] However, the discovery by Carruthers and Carruthers[42] of the cosmetic use of botulinum toxin (for treatment of glabellar frown lines) was by far the most notable cosmetic medical adoption of a pharmaceutical agent used to treat a medical condition (benign essential blepharospasm). Listening to their story is fascinating. According to them, a patient who was being treated for benign essential blepharospasm asked for more injections. It was obvious to them that the incessant blinking had stopped. When asked why the patient wanted more injections, she reportedly stated that her frown lines had improved after the injections. What followed was the US Food and Drug Administration (FDA) approval of botulinum toxin A (Botox Cosmetic, Allergan Inc, Irvine, CA, USA) for improving the appearance of the glabellar frown lines. This single product produced and, in these difficult economic times, continues to produce incredible world-wide earnings for Allergan Inc. Consumer demand was and has remained strong because there is little or no downtime and the treatment works with minimal adverse events (even less likely as more experience was gained in the safe administration

of this toxin). There simply is no better temporary solution for the improvement in the appearance of motion-based rhytids. As expected, off-label indications became numerous (the recent FDA approval of Botox for the treatment of migraine headaches is a notable example). The economic downturn mentioned earlier would continue to encourage the use of temporary solutions that are less expensive. The introduction of hyaluronic acid allowed an off-the-shelf solution to partially fill facial lines, contour deformities, and volume deficiencies. (Hylaform Allergan Inc, Irvine, CA, USA), an early entry into the filler market was not well embraced, as it was derived from the rooster cock comb. Nonanimal based hyaluronic acid quickly took over this market and became the gold standard for filling facial lines, taking over from bovine and human collagen products. Principally it was Restylane and Perlane (QMed, Uppsala, Sweden, and Medicis Pharmaceutical Corp, Scottsdale, AZ, USA) that had control of this market in the United States. Other products emerged outside the United States and took over some of the market share. In the United States, Juvéderm Plus, Juvéderm Ultra Plus (Allergan Inc, Irvine, CA, USA), and (Prevelle Mentor, Inc, Santa Barbara, CA, USA) have taken some of the market share. Other semipermanent and permanent fillers including Radiesse (Merz Aesthetics, San Mateo, CA, USA), Sculptra (Sanofi-Aventis U.S. LLC), and (Artecoll, Pulmon Medical, Natal, South Africa) have been approved in the United States as soft tissue fillers. Many other choices are available in other countries.

LASERS AND TECH ADVANCEMENTS IN AESTHETICS

The introduction of lasers for numerous cosmetic indications did not gain substantial acceptance until the late 1990s. Originally, CO_2 lasers were introduced to ablate perioral and periocular rhytids but were soon expanded for use on the entire face.[43,44] Undesirable sequelae and complications were reported, and alternative technologies emerged (erbium and fractionated lasers).[44,45] Lasers that produce less-frequent problems, such as prolonged erythema and loss of pigmentation, have become more widely used for facial resurfacing. Lasers for the following indications are also available: hair removal, removal of vascular lesions, tattoo removal, and, more recently, laser-based lipolysis.

The market for body contouring in less-invasive and noninvasive ways has emerged as a consequence of the economic downturn, which demanded less-expensive procedures and minimal downtime. The consumer demand for body contouring solutions has emerged as the most frequently performed aesthetic plastic surgery procedure (American Society of Plastic Surgeons/American Society for Aesthetic Plastic Surgery statistics, 2008[46,47]). In many countries, men and women (and children) are increasing in their body size. Medical and surgical solutions have responded to the need to improve one's health and appearance.

The results achieved with noninvasive technologies give new meaning to "no pain/no gain," but some noninvasive platforms do provide measurable improvement in body contours. Alternative energy sources such as radiofrequency-based technologies have emerged as minimally invasive and noninvasive approaches to body contouring and skin tightening (Thermage™, Solta Medical, Hayward, CA, USA).

FACING THE FUTURE OF AESTHETIC SOLUTIONS

In the articles that follow, the technologies that provide medical and surgical solutions for cosmetic indications are explored, including barbed sutures, neurotoxins, cosmeceuticals, sclerotherapy, dermabrasion, fillers, lasers, and other energy sources including face and body contouring devices that provide solutions that respond to a consumer demand for less-aggressive solutions to the aging face and body contour deformities, both congenital and acquired. Driven by an economic downturn, corporate partners and clinicians have joined forces to provide alternatives to oftentimes more expensive solutions. However, less is still less, and even though there are visible improvements in the aging face with these techniques, in the long run, these procedures may not be more than enough. So, less-expensive procedures may actually be more expensive initially (depending on the type of procedure, who is performing it, and where it is being performed) or when a second attempt is made to reach the aesthetic goals.

When you buy quality, you only cry once

(Seen by the author on the side of a van owned by a carpet company.)

REFERENCES

1. Gonzalez-Ulloa M, Flores ES. Senility of the face: basic study to understand its causes and effects. Plast Reconstr Surg 1965;36:239.
2. Little JW. Volumetric perceptions in midfacial aging with altered priorities for rejuvenation. Plast Reconstr Surg 2000;105:252.
3. Little JW. Three-dimensional rejuvenatiion of the midface: volumetric resculpture by malar imbrication. Plast Reconstr Surg 2000;105:267.
4. Paul MD. The evolution of the browlift in aesthetic plastic surgery. Plast Reconstr Surg 2001;108(1):409.
5. Paul MD. The evolution of the midface lift in aesthetic plastic surgery. Plast Reconstr Surg 2006;117(6):1809.
6. Terino EO. Alloplastic facial contouring: surgery of the fourth plane. Aesthetic Plast Surg 1992;16:195.
7. Hester TR, Codner MA, McCord CD. Subperiosteal malar cheek lift with lower blepharoplasty. In: McCord CD, Codner MA, Hester TR, editors. Eyelid surgery: principles and techniques. Philadelphia: Lippincott-Raven; 1995. p. 210–5.
8. Ramirez OM, Maillard GG, Musolas A. The extended subperiosteal facelift: a definitive remodeling for facial rejuvenation. Plast Reconstr Surg 1991;88:227.
9. Hamra ST. Composite rhytidectomy. Plast Reconstr Surg 1992;90:1.
10. Baker DC. Lateral SMASectomy. Plast Reconstr Surg 1997;100:509.
11. Stuzin JM, Baker TJ, Gordon HL, et al. Extended SMAS dissection as an approach to midface rejuvenation. Clin Plast Surg 1995;22:295.
12. Aston SJ. FAME facelift. Presented at Aesthetic and Reconstructive Surgery of the Aging Face (live surgical demonstration of Facialplasty [FAME Technique]). New York, November 19–21, 1992.
13. Connell BF, Semalcher RA. Contemporary deep layer facial rejuvenation. Plast Reconstr Surg 1997;100:1513.
14. Paul MD. Morphologic and gender considerations in midface rejuvenation. Aesthet Surg J 2001;21:349.
15. Owsley J. Lifting the malar fat pad for correction of prominent nasolabial folds. Plast Reconstr Surg 1993;91:462.
16. Fogli AL. Orbicularis muscleplasty and facelift: a better orbital contour. Plast Reconstr Surg 1995;96:1560.
17. Byrd HS, Andochick SE. The deep temporal lift: a multi-planar lateralbrow, temporal, and upper mid-facelift. Plast Reconstr Surg 1996;97:928–37.
18. Barton FE, Kenkel JM. Direct fixation of the malar fat pad. Clin Plast Surg 1997;24:329–35.
19. Alpert BS, Baker DC, Hamra ST, et al. Identical twin face lifts with differing techniques: a 10-year follow-up. Plast Reconstr Surg 2009;123(3):1025–33 [discussion: 1034–6].
20. Lambros V. Fat injection for the aging midface. Operat Tech Plast Reconstr Surg 1998;5(2):129.
21. Pessa JE, Zadoo VP, Mutimer KL, et al. Relative maxillary retrusion as a natural sequence of aging: combining skeletal and soft tissue changes into an

integrated model of midfacial aging. Plast Reconstr
Surg 1998;102:205.

22. Rohrich JR, Pessa JE. The fat compartments of the
face: anatomy and clinical implications for cosmetic
surgery. Plast Reconstr Surg 2007;119:2219–27
[discussion: 2228–31].

23. Ellenbogen R. Free autogenous fat grafts in the face.
Combined Conference USF. San Francisco, April, 1981.

24. Ellenbogen R. Free autogenous pearl fat grafts in
the face. Hawaii: California Society of Plastic
Surgeons; April 1984.

25. Ellenbogen R. Free autogenous pearl fat grafts in
the face – a preliminary report of a rediscovered
technique. Ann Plast Surg 1986;16:3.

26. Coleman SR. The technique of periorbital lipoinfiltra-
tion. Operat Tech Plast Reconstr Surg 1994;1:120.

27. Coleman SR. Facial contouring with lipostructure.
Clin Plast Surg 1997;24:347–67.

28. Guerrero-Santos J. Fat injection of the face. Presented at Lipoplasty Society of North America. San
Diego, 1988.

29. Guerrerosantos J. Long-term outcome of autologous
fat transplantation in aesthetic facial recontouring:
sixteen years of experience with 1936 cases. Clin
Plast Surg 2000;27(4):515–43.

30. Fitzgerald R, Graivier MH, Kane M, et al. Update on
facial aging. Aesthet Surg J 2010;30(Suppl 1):11S.

31. Mosienko P, Baker TJ. Chemical peel. Clin Plast
Surg 1978;5(1):79–96.

32. Kligman AM, Baker TJ, Gordon HL. Long-term histologic follow-up of phenol face peels. Plast Reconstr
Surg 1985;75(5):652–9.

33. Hetter GP. An examination of the phenol-croton oil
peel. Part I. Dissecting the formula. Plast Reconstr
Surg 2000;105(1):227–39 [discussion: 249–51].

34. Hetter GP. An examination of the phenol-croton oil
peel. Part II. The lay peelers and their croton oil
formulas [erratum appears in Plast Reconstr Surg
2000;105(3):1083.]. Plast Reconstr Surg 2000;
105(1):240–8 [discussion: 249–51].

35. Johnson JB, Ichinose H, Obagi ZE, et al. Obagi's
modified trichloroacetic acid (TCA)-controlled

variable-depth peel: a study of clinical signs correlating with histological findings. Ann Plast Surg
1996;36(3):225–37.

36. Perricone NV. The anti-inflammatory effects of
topical vitamin C ester. Presented at the First International Symposium on Aging Skin. San Diego,
February 1997.

37. Vasconez LO. The use of an endoscope in brow lifting. A video presentation at the Annual Meeting of
the American Society of Plastic and Reconstructive
Surgeons. Washington, DC, 1992.

38. Isse NG. Endoscopic facial lift. Presented at the
Annual Meeting of the Los Angeles County Society
of Plastic Surgeons. Los Angeles, September 12,
1992.

39. Chachir A. Endoscopic subperiosteal forehead lift.
Aesthetic Plast Surg 1994;18:269.

40. Tessier P. Face lifting and frontal rhytidectomy.
1979;393.

41. Ramirez OM. Endoscopic facial rejuvenation.
Perspectives in Plast Surg 9:22, 19.

42. Carruthers A, Carruthers J. Botulinum toxin type A:
a history and current cosmetic use in the upper
face. Semin Cutan Med Surg 2001;20:71.

43. Weinstein C, Roberts TL 3rd. Aesthetic skin resurfacing with the high-energy ultrapulsed CO2 laser.
Clin Plast Surg 1997;24(2):379–405.

44. Schwartz RJ, Burns AJ, Rohrich RJ, et al. Long-term
assessment of CO2 facial laser resurfacing:
aesthetic results and complications. Plast Reconstr
Surg 1999;103(2):592–601.

45. McDaniel DH, Ash K, Lord J, et al. The erbium:YAG
laser: a review and preliminary report on resurfacing
of the face, neck, and hands. Aesthet Surg J 1997;
17(3):157–64.

46. American Society of Plastic Surgeons. 2009 Report
of the 2008 statistics: National Clearinghouse of
Plastic Surgery Statistics. Arlington Heights (IL):
2009. Available at: www.plasticsurgery.org.

47. American Society for Aesthetic Plastic Surgery. 2008
Cosmetic Surgery National Data Bank Statistics.
New York: 2009. Available at: www.surgery.org.

The Interface of Cosmetic Medicine and Surgery: Working from the Inside and the Outside

Mark K. Markarian, MD, MSPH[a],*, Raffi V. Hovsepian, MD[b,c,d]

KEYWORDS

• Cosmetic surgery • Minimally invasive • Plastic surgery

The role of noninvasive procedures as part of a thriving practice is a significant concern according to a panel on practice trends presented at The Aesthetic Meeting 2008, the annual meeting of the American Society for Aesthetic Plastic Surgery (ASAPS).[1] Two surveys[2] conducted in 2007 under the auspices of a Cosmetic Medicine Task Force formed as a joint venture between ASAPS and American Society of Plastic Surgeons (ASPS) examined consumers' attitudes and perceptions influencing their choice of plastic surgery procedures and the variety of cosmetic services offered in plastic surgery practices. Minimally invasive or noninvasive procedures, including laser and light therapies, injectables, and dermal fillers, now account for 80% of cosmetic procedures. According to the 2009 ASPS statistics, the top 5 minimally invasive procedures in 2009 were

1. BOTOX (Allergan Inc, Irvlne, CA, USA) injections (4.8 million)
2. Soft tissue fillers (1.7 million)
3. Chemical peel (1.1 million)
4. Microdermabrasion (910,000)
5. Laser hair removal (893,000).

Most consumers viewed surgical procedures as high risk, but perceived virtually no risk associated with noninvasive or minimally invasive procedures. Despite their popularity, these procedures still comprise a small part of most plastic surgeons' practices; the survey found that for 91% of surgeons, noninvasive treatments generated less than 25% of their revenue.

Plastic surgeons should remain educated and current on noninvasive or minimally invasive cosmetic surgery procedures. Patients who undergo these procedures will only develop further trust and allow the surgeon the opportunity to offer a more comprehensive set of therapeutic options. This will, in turn provide continuity of care and facilitate a successful practice.

This article provides a basic overview of the common noninvasive and minimally invasive therapies in cosmetic surgery, some areas being discussed in more detail than others. Skin care products and skin types are discussed first.

TOPICAL SKIN CARE

The modern skin care industry continues to evolve rapidly with an almost unlimited array of skin care

The authors have no actual or potential conflicts of interest, including employment, consultancies, stock ownership, honoraria, patent applications/registrations, and grants or other funding in the publication of this article.

a Division of Plastic and Reconstructive Surgery, Saint Louis University School of Medicine, 3635 Vista Avenue at Grand Boulevard, 3rd Floor North, Desloge Towers, St Louis, MO 63110-0250, USA
b Private Practice, 416 North Bedford Drive, Suite 200, Beverly Hills, CA 90210, USA
c Private Practice, 1401 Avocado Avenue, Suite 810, Newport Beach, CA 92660, USA
d Aesthetic & Plastic Surgery Institute, University of California-Irvine, Orange, CA, USA
* Corresponding author.
E-mail address: Mark_K_Markarian@yahoo.com

Clin Plastic Surg 38 (2011) 335–345
doi:10.1016/j.cps.2011.02.001

products available. Many products are categorized based on particular skin types. There are 4 parameters for characterizing facial skin types

1. Dry or oily
2. Sensitive or resistant
3. Pigmented or nonpigmented
4. Wrinkled or tight.

These 4 parameters can yield 16 different combinations, each with different skin care needs. Furthermore, each skin type may change over time in the individual (because of intrinsic or environmental causes) and thus change the subsequent management.[3]

Dry or Oily

The role of the stratum corneum (SC) is the most significant factor in the development of dry skin. In patients with dry skin the lipid bilayer of the SC is disturbed, increasing fatty acid levels and reducing ceramide layers.[4] Various extrinsic factors, including UV radiation, detergents, acetone, chlorine, and protracted water exposure or immersion, can disrupt the lipid bilayer. The maintenance of water within skin cells depends on natural moisturizing factor. Aquaporin-3 allows water transfer between the keratinocytes. Sebum, the oily secretion of the sebaceous glands, that contains wax esters, sterol esters, cholesterol, triglycerides, and squalene imparts an oily aspect to the skin and plays a significant role in acne development.[5] In normal skin, sebaceous gland–derived triglycerides are hydrolyzed to glycerol before transport to the skin surface. In sebum-deficient individuals, replacing this glycerol may be a suitable approach to alleviating skin dryness. There are numerous over-the-counter moisturizers available to help hydrate the skin, including occlusives, humectants, and emollients. Occlusives are typically oily compounds that coat the SC to impede transepidermal water loss (TEWL). Many occlusives also impart an emollient effect and are suited for treating dry skin. Examples of occlusives include petrolatum, lanolin, and propylene glycol. None of them impart long-term effects. Once the occlusives are removed from the skin, the TEWL returns to the previous level. Occlusives are usually combined with humectant ingredients because reducing the TEWL by more than 40% can increase the risk of skin maceration and subsequent bacterial infection.[6] Humectants are water soluble and can attract water from the external environment, in conditions with at least 80% humidity, as well as from the underlying skin layers. In low-humidity conditions, however, humectants may take water from the deeper

epidermis and dermis, thereby increasing the TEWL. They are thus more effective in combination with occlusives. By drawing water into the skin, humectants may cause minor swelling of the SC and yield a perception of smoother skin with fewer wrinkles. Humectant ingredients include glycerin, urea, hydroxyl acids, and lactic acid. Emollients are primarily composed of lipids and oils and are added to cosmetics to hydrate, soften, and smooth the skin. These compounds fill in the gaps between desquamating corneocytes to render a smooth surface.[7] In short, occlusives coat the SC and reduce the TEWL, humectants attract water from the outer atmosphere and hydrate the skin, and emollients soften and smooth the skin. While several expensive moisturizers contain collagen that manufacturers contend can replace the collagen lost due to aging, most of the collagen extracts have a molecular weight of 15,000 to 50,000 Da. Only substances with a molecular weight of 5000 Da or less can penetrate the SC.[6] The collagen and polypeptides in these products create a film that fills in surface irregularities but only temporarily stretches out fine skin wrinkles.

Sensitive or Resistant Skin

People with resistant skin rarely experience erythema and can use a variety of products without any significant concern for adverse reactions. However, many products are limited in their penetration of resistant skin and thus ineffective. Sensitive skin is more complex and has 4 discrete subtypes (acne, rosacea, stinging, and allergic), all sharing one common element inflammation. Patients may present with more than one subtype. Features of the acne subtype include the adherence of dead keratinocytes in the hair follicles because of elevated sebum production, clogging of the follicle, and production of a papule or pustule. Bacteria migrate into the hair follicle and trigger an inflammatory cascade. Treatment focuses on the 4 primary causal factors (1) decreasing sebum production with retinoids, oral contraceptives, or stress reduction; (2) unclogging pores with retinoids and α-hydroxy acids; (3) eliminating bacteria with antibiotics and topical care; (4) and reducing inflammation. The rosacea subtype includes prominent telangiectasias, in addition to common adolescent symptoms of facial redness, flushing, and papules. Topical treatment focuses on antiinflammatory ingredients to decrease vasodilation. The stinging subtype involves a nonallergic neural sensitivity to certain triggers. People with such a subtype should avoid topical products including those containing α-hydroxy acids, benzoic acid, lactic acid, sorbic acid, certain ammonium containing compounds, propylene glycol, urea, or vitamin C. Approximately 10% of patients with dermatologic conditions who are patch tested are allergic to at least one ingredient common in cosmetics.[8]

Pigmented or Nonpigmented Skin

The 2 general mechanisms interfering with skin pigmentation are inhibition of tyrosinase (preventing melanin formation) and blocking transfer of melanin into keratinocytes. Activation of protease-activated receptor (PAR)-2 transfers melanin to keratinocytes.[9] Soy and niacinamide block PAR-2. Tyrosinase inhibitors include vitamin C, hydroquinone, kojic acid, arbutin, mulberry extract, and licorice extract. Other mechanisms to impede pigmentation include the use of exfoliating agents (α-hydroxy acids, retinoids) and procedures (microdermabrasion) that accelerate cell turnover, preventing melanocytes from producing melanin. Sun avoidance remains the most effective method of preventing pigmentation.

Wrinkled or Tight Skin

The primary causes of extrinsic premature aging are smoking, poor nutrition, and solar exposure. Up to 80% of skin aging can be attributed to sun exposure.[10] The development of rhytides is considered the most salient manifestation of cutaneous aging. Alterations of the lower dermal layers of the skin can cause wrinkles. Few skin care products penetrate far enough. Most antiaging products and procedures are formulated or designed to salvage collagen, elastin, and hyaluronic acid. Products have been unable, however, to deliver these substances to the deep dermis in adequate amounts. Some products can stimulate the natural synthesis of these substances, that is, retinoids, vitamin C, and copper peptide can stimulate collagen production[11,12]; retinoids can augment the production of hyaluronic acid and elastin[13]; and glucosamine may improve hyaluronic acid levels.[14] Antioxidants help with wrinkle prevention by reducing inflammation and subsequent breakdown of hyaluronic acid, collagen, and elastin. Some antioxidants (used as ingredients in many topical skin care products) include green tea, vitamin C/E, ferulic acid, coenzyme Q10, silymarin, Pycnogenol, an extract from the plant Pinus pinaster, and idebenone.

SKIN CAMOUFLAGE

Skin camouflage corrects cutaneous flaws with specialized makeup preparations and techniques,

useful for patients with chronic macular conditions, such as vitiligo, melasma, rosacea, and port-wine stains.[15,16] This technique is a valuable adjunct after ablative and nonablative therapies, allowing earlier return to public activities and restoring appearance sooner after nonablative procedures. Skin camouflage can improve appearance immediately and permits surgeons to recommend and perform a greater number of surgically invasive and ablative procedures by allowing patients to reduce and more accurately schedule their expected downtime. Very few medical institutions and physician practices integrate skin camouflage into their care.

Postsurgical camouflage preparations are applied to newly epithelialized skin. These preparations are oil or cream based with pigment content up to 45% to 50%; conventional liquid makeup typically contains no more than 10% to 15% pigment. Paste makeup formulations are typically opaque and can camouflage abnormal tones that contrast with adjacent normal skin, seen with bruises, vitiligo, and port-wine stains. These preparations can also act as filler substances to fill in small indentations. A fixing spray can be used off the face to set a longer duration of use. Mineral makeup may be unsuitable early in the postoperative course of ablative procedures because the skin must be completely epithelialized, dry to the touch, and no longer require healing ointments. Mineral makeup is typically easier to apply than paste formulations and is currently the makeup of choice for erythema after chemical peels and laser resurfacing (once epithelialized), acne erythema, acne rosacea, melasma, facial lentigines, and postinflammatory hyperpigmentation.

Skin camouflage is used after planned incisional and ablative procedures and after accidental unexpected discoloration from trauma and procedures. There are 3 basic techniques for camouflaging skin defects: concealing, color correcting (neutralizing red, blue, or yellow tones to more natural tones of complimentary colors), and contouring (creating highlights and shadows to disguise swelling). These techniques cannot mask the 3-dimensional conditions such as focal edema, keloids, acne scars, and deep furrows. In preparation, patients should bring their own makeup and preoperative pictures to maximize postoperative results once the skin has completely epithelialized and sutures have been removed.

Cosmetic surgery practices commonly offer cosmeceutical and skin care products. Very few of them also offer makeup, the only remaining product that their patients may require to complete their facial grooming.

CHEMICAL PEELS

The most significant alterations resulting from chronic sun damage occur in the dermis.[17] Chemical peels can treat the most superficial aspect of the skin all the way to the deepest portion of the reticular dermis. Pretreatment evaluation includes an emphasis on history of abnormal or keloid scarring, herpes simplex virus infection, 13-*cis* retinoic acid (Accutane) therapy, prior laser resurfacing, and use of photosensitizing medications. Many physicians wait a minimum of 6 months after the last Accutane dose before performing a chemical peel. Fitzpatrick skin types III (average tanning ability) and IV (easily tan) often develop limited and transient hyperpigmentation, especially with deeper or more aggressive chemical peels. Skin types that tan even easier (Fitzpatrick skin types V and VI) should be approached with great caution because the risk of permanent pigment alteration is quite significant.

There are 3 basic types of chemical peels. Superficial peels (glycolic and salicylic acids) may penetrate to the papillary dermis. Medium-depth peels (trichloroacetic acid) reach the deep papillary and, often, superficial reticular dermis. Deep chemical peels (phenol) can penetrate into the midreticular dermis. After assessing the depth of photoaging, the proper peeling agent can be selected.

Postoperatively, patients should maintain a moist environment using a petrolatum-based emollient. Superficial peels may be followed by a medium to thick moisturizer in place of an emollient, but with frequent applications. The deeper the peel the longer the need for postoperative moisturizer use. Once reepithelialization is complete, a sunscreen is recommended as part of the moisturizing routine. Sun avoidance is essential before epithelialization. Persistent postoperative erythema can be a sign of early hypertrophic scarring, requiring a topical corticosteroid or intralesional injection if the scar begins to mature. Postinflammatory hyperpigmentation is usually transient but can be treated with bleaching agents such as hydroquinone (3%–4%).

Peeling agents are often used in combination with laser resurfacing to diminish lines demarcating the site for laser treatment. Superficial peeling agents used before laser resurfacing can reduce complications such as hyperpigmentation and may reduce the healing time.

LASER HAIR REMOVAL

Traditional methods of hair removal include shaving, bleaching, plucking, waxing, use of chemical depilatories, and electrolysis. These techniques are limited by the pain, inconvenience, and poor long-term efficacy. Only electrolysis has offered the potential for permanent hair removal, but is tedious. Several lasers and other light sources have been developed specifically to target hair follicles and rapidly treat large areas with long-term results.

Light can potentially destroy hair follicles by photothermal (by local heating), mechanical (by shockwaves or violent cavitation), and photochemical mechanisms (by generation of toxic mediators such as singlet oxygen or free radicals). Some individual laser systems are mentioned below but not discussed in detail.

Photothermal lasers include 694-nm normal-mode ruby lasers (RubyStar [Aesculap-Meditec GmBH, Jena, Germany], Sinon [WaveLight Laser Technologie AG, Erlangen, Germany]), 755-nm normal-mode alexandrite lasers (Elite [Cynosure, Chelmsford, MA, USA], GentleLASE [Candela Corporation, Wayland, MA, USA], Ultrawave II–III [Adept Medical, Rancho Santa Margarita, CA, USA], Epicare [Light Age Inc, Somerset, NJ, USA]), 800-nm pulsed diode lasers (LightSheer [Lumenis Inc, Santa Clara, CA, USA]), 1064-nm long-pulsed Nd:YAG lasers (CoolGlide [Cutera Inc, Brisbane, CA, USA], Profile [Sciton, Palo Alto, CA, USA], Cynergy [Cynosure, Chelmsford, MA, USA], Dualis [Fotona, Ljubljana, Slowenie; Petrakis Holdings Ltd, Limassol, Cyprus], Varia [CoolTouch Laser Corp, Auburn, LA, USA], Mydon [Quantel Derma GmbH, Erlangen, Germany], GentleYAG [Candela Corporation]), and 590- to 1200-nm intense-pulsed light (IPL) source lasers (Lumenis One [Lumenis, Santa Clara, CA, USA], Cynergy PL [Cynosure Inc, Westford, MA, USA], Quadra Q4 [DermaMed International Inc, Lenni, PA, USA], Estelux [Palomar, Burlington, MA, USA]). Photothermal destruction is based on the principle of selective photothermolysis. This principle predicts that selective thermal damage of a pigmented target structure will result when sufficient fluence is delivered at a specific wavelength for a required thermal relaxation time. In the visible to near infrared region, melanin is the natural chromophore for targeting hair follicles. Lasers of this wavelength are selectively absorbed by melanin in the dermis, permitting deep heating of the hair shaft, hair follicle epithelium, and heavily pigmented matrix. However, epidermal melanin competes for absorption, and epidermal injury must be minimized by selectively cooling the epidermis with various methods including cooling gels, a cooled glass chamber or sapphire window, or a pulsed cryogen spray. Ruby lasers are best indicated in light-skinned individuals with dark hairs because of the high melanin absorption at

684 nm. Higher wavelength (755 nm) alexandrite lasers penetrate the dermis deeper and deposit more energy in the dermis than ruby lasers. The risk for epidermal damage in darker skin types is thus reduced. The pulsed 800-nm diode laser is effective for removal of dark terminal hair, seen in darker skin types. The long-pulsed Nd:YAG lasers have reduced melanin absorption at their emitted wavelength of 1064 nm, requiring high fluencies to adequately damage hair. However, the poor melanin absorption is safer for darker skin types. This laser is also used for treatment of pseudofolliculitis barbae, a skin condition commonly seen in people with darker skin types. Intense-pulsed non-laser light sources used for hair reduction emit multiwavelength light and can be adjusted to specific pulse durations and delay intervals, effective for a wide range of skin types.[18–20]

Photomechanical lasers include carbon-suspension Q-switched Nd:YAG lasers and Q-switched Nd:YAG lasers. Photomechanical destruction due to small local explosions results from Q-switched laser pulses. These higher-powered short pulse width lasers target hair follicles and rapidly heat melanin. The generated photoacoustic shock waves mechanically disrupt the melanocytes in the bulb but cause incomplete follicular disruption, ineffective for long-term hair removal.

Photochemical lasers include those used in photodynamic therapy, which use light and a photosensitizer to produce a targeted photochemical reaction and therapeutic effect. Primarily used for malignant skin tumors, long-term data for their efficacy in hair removal are still needed.

An evidence-based review of laser and light sources for hair removal demonstrated partial short-term hair removal efficacy up to 6 months after treatment with the ruby, alexandrite, diode, and Nd:YAG lasers and IPL.[21] Alexandrite and diode lasers demonstrated long-term hair removal beyond 6 months. Repeated treatments improved efficacy, and there were few side effects.

NONABLATIVE REJUVENATION

Nonablative rejuvenation refers to the ability of a laser or light energy source to selectively create thermal injury to the underlying dermis with minimal effect on the epidermis.[22] Many patients prefer the minimal recovery associated with nonablative treatments, even though the final result may not be as dramatic as that obtained with laser resurfacing or a deep chemical peel. Of these devices, many cool the overlying epidermis to protect the skin from emitted energy. This effect is achieved with a cold handpiece or dynamic cryogen device delivering a cooling spray. These devices include the 532-nm laser (Versapulse [Coherent Medical Group, Palo Alto, CA, USA], Diolite [Iridex Inc, Mountain View, CA, USA]), the 585-nm pulsed dye laser, the 1064-nm Q-switched Nd:YAG laser, the 1320-nm long-pulsed Nd:YAG with coolant spray (CoolTouch Varia, CoolTouch Inc, Roseville, CA, USA), the 1450-nm diode with a coolant spray (Smoothbeam, Candela Corporation), the 1540-nm erbium (Er):glass laser (Aramis, Quantel Derma GmbH), and a broadband IPL, which emits a continuous spectrum from 515 nm to 1200 nm.

Selective absorption by chomophores including hemoglobin, collagen, and melanin, can induce neocollagenesis. Light-tissue interactions can induce collagen remodeling and other molecular events to culminate in improvement of rough texture, red and brown discoloration, and fine lines.

RADIOFREQUENCY (NONSURGICAL) TISSUE TIGHTENING

Nonablative laser and light sources provide dermal collagenesis without epidermal disruption but often require multiple treatments, can exhibit a delayed clinical effect, and can have diminished results compared with ablative laser skin resurfacing. Radiofrequency (RF) tissue tightening was developed to create deep thermal effects in the dermis, without external cutaneous wounding. In 2002, a monopolar device was developed to remodel and tighten collagen in the deeper dermis and subcutaneous tissue in order to improve lax or aging skin. Unlike traditional laser systems that generate heat by targeting specific chromophores, RF technology generates heat as a result of tissue impedance and depends on the electric properties of tissue. ThermaCool TC (Thermage Inc, Hayward, CA, USA) uses monopolar RF energy to create a uniform field of dermal and subdermal heating, whereas a contact cooling device protects the epidermis. Other devices have also been introduced for nonsurgical tissue tightening. The Polaris WR (Syneron Inc, Irvine, CA, USA) that combines bipolar RF and diode laser technologies; the Titan (Cutera Inc), a noncoherent, selectively filtered, broadband infrared light device that emits in multisecond cycles, and the GentleYag, a long-pulsed Nd:YAG laser are some examples of such devices.

Because the epidermis remains intact, postoperative care is minimal. Most patients can resume normal activities immediately. Transient mild erythema and edema typically resolves within 24 hours. Epidermal injury, although rare, can be treated with standard wound care. Clinical improvement after treatment may take weeks to months to realize.

The incidence of side effects with monopolar RF is low. Occasionally, uneven electrode contact with the skin (as a result of facial contours or patient movement during treatment) can arc the monopolar RF energy and injure the epidermis. RF overtreatment can cause dermal depressions, which may be corrected by subcision and autologous fat transfer.[23] A temporary altered sensation of treated skin has also been described.[24] Combination bipolar RF and diode lasers can cause temporary vesiculation that generally resolves without dyspigmentation or textural irregularities within 5 days.[25–27] Erythema and edema is expected after broadband infrared therapy.

ABLATIVE AND MICROABLATIVE SKIN RESURFACING

The first laser used for skin resurfacing was a continuous wave carbon-dioxide (CO_2) laser, but the excessive thermal injury can cause scarring.[28] The Er:YAG laser allows for greater cutaneous absorption by water, causing more superficial tissue ablation and finer control. However, use of this laser displays poor intraoperative hemostasis with less-impressive clinical improvement. Both lasers are effective in the treatment of sun-induced wrinkles, brown spots, and skin laxity but require a high level of operator skill to avoid complications such as scarring, dyspigmentation, lines of demarcation between treated and untreated areas, and downtime periods of a week or more with oozing and denuded skin.

CO_2 laser skin resurfacing remains the gold standard for the treatment of severely photodamaged skin. It improves rhytides, textural anomalies, dyspigmentation, and atrophic scars. However, the reepithelialization time is extended, erythema may be prolonged, and there may be a significant risk of delayed (or permanent) hypopigmentation.[29,30] Typically, the entire face as a unit because areas adjacent to treated skin have a noticeable difference in texture and pigment. Major indications are deep rhytides and atrophic scars caused by acne, trauma, or surgery. Posttreatment skin regeneration relies on the presence of skin appendages to serve as new sources of epithelium to form dermis, limiting CO_2 laser skin resurfacing to the face.

Ablative Er:YAG laser is best suited for mild to moderate rhytides, superficial pigmentation, atrophic scars, and a variety of epidermal and dermal lesions, including sebaceous hyperplasia, angiofibromas, adnexal tumors, café-au-lait macules, and xanthelasma.[31–33] Several studies have

documented its safe use in people with darker skin types.[34,35] The addition of ablative ER:YAG laser after CO_2 laser resurfacing may reducing CO_2 laser–induced necrosis and improve postoperative edema.[36] The removal of proinflammatory coagulated tissue results in less erythema and faster healing, and it does not seem to affect the clinical outcome or degree of new collagen formation.[37,38]

Recovery after CO_2 and Er:YAG laser resurfacing requires patient compliance for up to several weeks, depending on the depth of thermal injury. Topical antibiotics should not be used because of the increased risk of contact dermatitis. Occlusive dressings decrease the severity and duration of postlaser erythema, swelling, and crusting.[39,40] Patients should continue oral antibiotics and antivirals until reepithelialization is complete. Adverse effects of ablative laser resurfacing include transient erythema, edema, serous discharge, crusting, discomfort, and pruritus. Heavy ointments or occlusive dressings may cause milia, acne, and perioral dermatitis.[30,41] Hypertrophic scarring is seen more in nonfacial resurfacing such as the chin, mandible, neck, and perioral region.[32]

Fractional photothermolysis treats a small fraction of the skin at each session. Intact undamaged skin around each treated area theoretically acts as a barrier to infection and a reservoir for rapid healing.[42] This technique can be used to treatm photodamaged skin, facial rhytides, acne scars, surgical scars, melasma, and photodamaged skin. Treatment is easy with minimal downtime. Fractional photothermolysis is also safe and effective for the treatment of nonfacial areas such as the neck, chest, and extremities.[43] Redness and swelling typically last no more than 5 days. The skin may develop a bronzed appearance because of the presence of melanin-containing microepidermal necrotic debris and gradually slough off within the first week.

Each of the abovementioned treatments relies on the principles of selective photothermolysis to selectively target water-containing tissue and affect controlled tissue vaporization. Plasma skin regeneration uses pulses of ionized inert nitrogen gas to deliver heat energy directly to the skin. Unlike lasers, this technique does not rely on a specific target such as water, hemoglobin, or pigment. The nitrogen gas flushes oxygen from the treatment area, reducing charring, and the skin remains in place to act as a biological dressing on the treated area. Indications for plasma skin regeneration include mild to severe rhytides, sun damaged skin, acne scarring, and superficial benign skin lesions. Multiple low-energy treatments seem to approximate the results of treatments at higher energies, with improvement in dyspigmentation, texture, and fine lines.[11] Higher-energy treatments tend to have greater erythema because the damaged epidermis and upper dermis slough off; this erythema typically resolves in 5 to 10 days. There have been no major side effects with plasma skin regeneration.[45]

BOTULINUM TYPE A TOXIN INJECTIONS FOR COSMETIC USE

The use of botulinum toxin type A (BTX-A) for cosmesis dates to 1998 when Carruthers and Carruthers[46] noted resolution of periorbital wrinkles in patients treated with BOTOX for benign essential blepharospasm. It is now the leading cosmetic procedure as reported by the ASPS.

BTX-A interferes with acetylcholine release at the neuromuscular junction.[47] Clinically, muscle weakness becomes apparent 2 to 3 days after BTX-A injection, with complete paralysis seen after 8 to 14 days.[48] Muscles return to function approximately 2 to 5 months after injection, depending on the dose administered and the individual patient. Patients receiving mean doses of 200 U are at an increased risk for the development of neutralizing antibodies.[49] Such patients may receive injections of botulinum toxin type B but experience a diminished effect.[50]

Each vial of BOTOX contains 100 U of lyophilized BTX-A exotoxin, 0.5 mg of human albumin, and 0.9 mg of sodium chloride. The vial is kept refrigerated or frozen until reconstitution with normal saline. Alam and colleagues[51] demonstrated reduced pain on BOTOX injection when the contents were reconstituted with saline containing preservative. Another form of BTX-A, Reloxin (Ipsen, Welch, UK), is also available but is 2.4 to 4.0 times less potent.[52] Guyuron and Huddelston[53] found that a 25-U BOTOX dose was needed to achieve paralysis of the glabellar complex, lasting several months. Platysmal bands and neck wrinkles require 50 to 100 U.[54] The duration of action for BTX-A seems to lengthen to some degree in a dose-dependent manner up to a point; although, the dose is recommended to remain less than 200 U per treatment. Small "touch-ups" of 2 to 20 U can be administered 2 weeks after the initial treatment session without any apparent antibody formation. BTX-A should be avoided in patients with neuromuscular disease and is contraindicated during pregnancy, and nursing and in those with known hypersensitivity to human albumin.

Wrinkles of the upper third of the face may also be treated with filler substances and resurfacing techniques, but BTX-A is superior when used to treat dynamic rhytides. Filler substances are often used in conjunction with BTX-A, especially with lips. BTX-A also enhances and prolongs the effects of laser surfacing when used just before the procedure. The ideal patients for BTX-A injections alone are those with hyperdynamic wrinkles of the forehead, and glabella and crow's feet with limited associated pigmentary or textural changes. Patients with additional signs of photoaging may benefit from using BTX-A in combination with other therapies. Wrinkles of the lower part of the face and platysmal bands are also treated with BTX-A, but those with advanced photoaging will more likely benefit from liposuction of the neck and jowls with surgical plication of the platysma.[55]

The duration of clinical efficacy is related to several factors, including dose of BTX-A, injection technique, and individual patient variation. On average, clinical effects appear within 2 to 3 days, and remain apparent for 3 to 4 months after injection of dynamic muscles. Side effects such as diplopia and ptosis are temporary, usually resolving within 2 to 4 weeks.

SOFT TISSUE AUGMENTATION

Modern soft tissue augmentation began in 1982 with the approval of bovine collagen. Since then, soft tissue augmentation and injection of materials for cosmetic enhancement have increased considerably. Soft tissue fillers were the second most common cosmetic nonsurgical procedure in 2009. Hyaluronic acids account for the majority of the soft tissue augmentation market.

Hyaluronic acids are polysacchardeds that may be animal-derived or synthetic - each molecule consists of a repeating chain of D-glucoronic acid and N-acetyl-D-glycosamine monosaccharides. These polysaccharide chains must be crosslinked to have any tissue persistence or utility as dermal fillers. Particle size and concentration also significantly affect tissue correction. The Restylane family of products (Touch, Perlane, SubQ, and Restylane, Q-Med, Uppsala, Sweden) maintain the same hyaluronic acid concentration with variations in particle size. Other types of hyaluronic acids alter the concentration rather than the size of the gel particle. Juvederm (Allergan Inc, Irvine, CA, USA) is hyaluronic acid made with a homogenous gel rather than a particulate one.

Juvederm is typically used for injection into the mid to deep dermis for correction of moderate to severe facial wrinkles and folds (such as nasolabial folds). Other areas that are frequently treated with hyaluronic acid include the marionette lines, perioral rhytides, and lips. Bruising and swelling may follow treatment for approximately 1 week. Certain areas, such as the lips and tear troughs, may take longer to resolve.

Infection with human immunodeficiency virus is not a contraindication because many patients with lipoatrophy have been effectively treated with these molecules.[56] Botulinum toxin may be synergistic in certain areas, such as deep nasolabial creases. In the perioral and lip areas, either infraoral blocks or gingival "miniblocks" can be safely and easily used. Other areas, including the zygomatic arch and nasolabial creases, may be treated with either no or minimal anesthetic.

The nasolabial location is the most frequent area injected with hyaluronic acid. Correction of the nasolabial crease requires consideration of 3 different contributing factors-facial ptosis, local volume loss, and loss of epidermal support. The underlying cause of facial ptosis needs to be addressed. Nonsurgical methods of reversing midface descent include injections of Sculptra (Sanofi-Aventis U.S. LLC), lasers, and RF energy therapy. Local loss of deep tissue may be reversed by placement of fillers into this plane. Men with moderately deep creases require more than women and they will also tend to tolerate the thicker molecules better.

Lips are the second most popular area treated with hyalurons. The 2 main factors considered in lip augmentation are volume and definition. Injections intended to restore volume to the lip are primarily placed into the body of the lip, whereas those designed to shape them are placed at the junction of the vermilion and the surrounding epidermis. The lower lip has 2 central prominences that should be injected for an aesthetically pleasing outcome. In general, the average woman require 1 to 2 mL of product for an adequate outcome.[57]

Loss of tissue from the lateral chin and lower lateral lip may result in deep marionette lines and an angle of the mouth that is oriented inferiorly. These defects are among the most simple to correct with hyalurons and are frequently most pleasing for the patient. Adequate volume restores the corner of the mouth a horizontal neutral position and makes a significant cosmetic difference.

Perhaps more than any other area, the glabella should be approached with caution because of the risk of necrosis. Combination with botulinum toxin is synergistic.[58] Minute amounts should be introduced while watching for blanching. Toxin can be placed afterward to theoretically reduce the risk of toxin migration from introducing filler.

The periorbital area is also treated, including the tear trough and possibly crow's feet, with the associated risks of bruising and edema. Whereas botulinum toxin better treats the dynamic component, hyalurons can better treat the static component of crow's feet. In contrast to many other areas, the soft low-concentration hyalurons such as Captique (Genzyme/Inamed, Cambridge, MA,

USA) and Hylaform (Genzyme/Inamed, Cambridge, MA, USA) may be suited for this indication. Thicker products may result in bumps.

Volume restoration of the zygomatic arch can reposition the midface to a more youthful anatomically correct position and reinflate and tighten the area. The deep dermis is injected with dense material, such as Perlane, Restylane SubQ, Juvederm, and Restylane.[59]

The appearance of hands has also improved with hyaluron injection (in addition to autologous fat). Increased atrophy requires larger volumes. Areas adjacent to tendons are commonly injected. Postoperative swelling can be managed by oral steroids, diuretics, ice, or cooling agents.

Hyalurons offer a major improvement over previously approved soft tissue augmentation products such as collagen, poly lactic acid (Sculptra), silicone, and calcium hydroxyapatite (Radiesse, Merz Aesthetics, San Mateo, CA, USA). The ranges of concentrations offered, the molecule sizes available, and cross-linking variations afford the dermatologic surgeon exciting new possibilities. Collagen still retains a portion of the filler market, with minimal posttreatment bruising and its long safety record.

AUTOLOGOUS FAT TRANSPLANTATION

Structural fat grafting uses autologous fat as a long-lasting volumetric expander.[60] Some investigators have found that a variety of techniques used to collect, clean, and reinject fat do not damage the fat cells, including the presence of lidocaine.[61] Harvesting fat via manual suction produces a high yield of preadipocytes with an intact stromal cell fraction.[62] Neovascularization is necessary for transplanted fat survival, but stem cell differentiation and tissue fibrosis may also contribute to lasting augmentation.[63]

Fat should be taken from an area that benefits the patient aesthetically, has a low risk for contour irregularities, and has the greatest potential for lipogenic activity.[64] These areas often occur on the outer part of the thighs or posterior part of the waists of women and flank area of men. Fat should be extracted after tumescing with manual suction only, and then centrifuged. Small aliquots of fat are injected to keep injection pressures low during transplantation.

Further augmentation can be done in a month's time into the same or different areas. The most common complications seen with fat transfer are ecchymosis, edema, and contour irregularities.

DERMABRASION

Dermabrasion is a skin resurfacing technique that surgically abrades the epidermis with a rapidly rotating wire brush or diamond fraise.[65] This tech nique has been used for a variety of lesions, as well as facial scars secondary to acne, trauma, surgery, and varicella-zoster virus. Patient selection is key; immunosuppressed patients or patients with a propensity toward hypopigmentation or hypertrophic scarring are less likely to have optimal results. Isotretinoin use is a contraindication because of combined association with hypertrophic scars.[65] Dermabrasion has become the gold standard for resurfacing.[66]

Dermabrasion after surgical or traumatic injury interrupts the remodeling phase of wound healing. Before the first-intention wound healing process is complete, the ablative injury to the papillary and midreticular dermis superimposes secondary-intention healing mechanisms on the primary scar. Such changes include increased collagen bundle density and size parallel to the epidermal surface. Reorganization of the underlying connective tissue produces a less perceptible scar.[67] Scheduled dermabrasion of surgical and traumatic scars after 6 to 8 weeks can yield optimal results.[68]

Uncontrolled acne can result in 3 types of scars. Boxcar scars are small-diameter shallow lesions that often have an excellent response to dermabrasion alone. Icepick scars are significantly deeper (small-diameter) lesions that require punch excision before dermabrasion to obtain the best results. Rolling scars are large-diameter, atrophic, distensible, or bound-down scars that may also respond to dermabrasion. Post-Mohs' partial thickness defects can respond favorable to dermabrasion, achieving results that can be comparable to skin grafting. Dermabrasion of tattoos in the papillary dermis are successful. Deeper infiltrating pigments can be treated by lasers or surgical removal. Dermabrasion may also be used to remove residual pigment after several laser treatments.

Postoperatively, erythema after the first 2 to 3 weeks is the first sign of early scar formation and, in addition to antibiotics and antifungal medications, should be treated with topical steroids. If unresponsive, pulsed dye laser therapy can decrease scar induration and erythema.[69] Hyperpigmentation can respond to therapeutic bleaching regimens but should be started 3 to 4 weeks after dermabrasion.

SUTURE SUSPENSION LIFTS

Traditional surgical procedures for face and neck lifting are being supplanted by new noninvasive or minimally invasive techniques. Although the cosmetic benefit of these procedures may not be as dramatic, many patients are clearly willing to trade some degree of efficacy for decreased morbidity and recovery time. Use of internal suspension sutures with barbs was introduced by Sulamanidze and colleagues[70] who have generated several sutures, including Aptos Thread (KMI Inc, Anaheim, CA, USA), Isse Endo Progressive Facelift Sutures (KMI Inc, Anaheim, CA, USA), and Contour Threads (Surgical Specialties, Reading, PA, USA). Limitations include protrusion through the skin, asymmetry, poor durability of effect, and the need for subsequent suture placement.[70–73] Postoperatively, patients should limit strenuous exercise that can dislodge the tightened skin from the suture barbs. Edema may also interfere with contouring at the end of the procedure requiring the distal ends of the suture to remain exposed for final contouring several days postoperatively. Some loss of tightening is expected in nearly all patients within 3 months.

SUMMARY

The prospect of cosmetic results without the morbidity of traditional surgery is appealing. Many patients do not want the cost, risk, and downtime associated with surgical procedures, and minimally invasive and noninvasive procedures give them an alternative. These procedures have evolved as technology has advanced alongside more knowledgeable patients. We have always attempted to reduce the telltale signs of surgery, but there is now a patient-driven trend to avoid an "operated look." Like all minimally invasive rejuvenation modalities, cosmetic medicine must be incorporated into a complete patient treatment plan that addresses the desires and needs of the patient. Combination approaches, using surgical and nonsurgical modalities will usually be the best means to improve patient care.

REFERENCES

1. Singer R, Saltz R, D'Amico R, et al. Embracing the future. Program and abstracts of the Aesthetic Meeting 2008. San Diego (CA): Panel presentation; 2008.
2. D'Amico RA, Saltz R, Rohrich RJ, et al. Risks and opportunities for plastic surgeons in a widening cosmetic medicine market: future demand, consumer preferences, and trends in practitioners' services. Plast Reconstr Surg 2008;121:1787–92.
3. Baumann L. The skin type solution. New York: Bantam Dell; 2006.
4. Rawlings A, Hope J, Rogers J, et al. Skin dryness – what is it? J Invest Dermatol 1993;100:510.
5. Thiboutot D. Regulation of human sebaceous glands. J Invest Dermatol 2004;123(1):1–12.
6. Wehr RF, Krochmal L. Considerations in selecting a moisturizer. Cutis 1987;39(6):512–5.

7. Draelos Z. Moisturizers. In: Daelos Z, editor. Atlas of cosmetic dermatology. New York: Churchill Livingstone; 2000. p. 85.

8. Orton DI, Wilkinson JD. Cosmetic allergy: incidence, diagnosis, and management. Am J Clin Dermatol 2004;5(5):327–37.

9. Seiberg M, Paine C, Sharlo E, et al. Inhibition for melanosome transfer results in skin lightening. J Invest Dermatol 2000;115(2):162–7.

10. Uitto J. Understanding premature skin aging. N Engl J Med 1997;337(20):1463–5.

11. Varani J, Warner RL, Gharaee-Kermani M, et al. Vitamin A antagonizes decreased cell growth and elevated collagen-degrading matrix metalloproteinases and stimulates collagen accumulation in naturally aged human skin. J Invest Dermatol 2000;114(3):480–6.

12. Nusgens BV, Humbert P, Rougier A, et al. Topically applied vitamin C enhances the mRNA level of collagens I and III, their processing enzymes and tissue inhibitor of matrix metalloproteinase 1 in the human dermis. J Invest Dermatol 2001;116(6):853–9.

13. Margelin D, Medaisko C, Lombard D, et al. Hyaluronic acid and dermatan sulfate are selectively stimulated by retinoic acid in irradiated and nonirradiated hairless mouse skin. J Invest Dermatol 1996;106(3):505–9.

14. Matheson AJ, Perry CM. Glucosamine: a review of its use in the management of osteoarthritis. Drugs Aging 2003;20(14):1041–60.

15. Aydoglu E, Misirlioglu A, Eker G, et al. Postoperative camouflage therapy in facial aesthetic surgery. Aesthetic Plast Surg 2005;29(3):190–4.

16. Holme SA, Beattie PE, Fleming CJ. Cosmetic camouflage advice improves quality of life. Br J Dermatol 2002;147(5):946–9.

17. Steinman DA, Steinman HK. Chemical peels. In: Kaminer MS, editor. Atlas of cosmetic surgery. 2nd edition. Philadelphia: Saunders; 2009. p. 117–31.

18. Ross EV, Ladin Z, Kreindel M, et al. Theoretical considerations in laser hair removal. Dermatol Clin 1999;17:333–55.

19. Olson EA. Methods of hair removal. J Am Acad Dermatol 1999;40:143–55.

20. Liew SH, Grobbelaar AO, Gault D, et al. A preliminary report of the correlation between efficacy of treatment and melanin content of hair and the growth phases of hair at a specific site. Ann Plast Surg 1999;24:255–8.

21. Haedersdal M, Wulf JC. Evidence-based review of hair removal using lasers and light sources. J Eur Acad Dermatol Venereol 2006;20:9–20.

22. Nelson JS, Majaaron B, Kelly KM. What is nonablative photorejuvenation of human skin? Semin Cutan Med Surg 2002;21:238–50.

23. Narius RS, Tope WD, Pope K, et al. Overtreatment effects associated with a radiofrequency tissue tightening device: rare, preventable, and correctable with subcision and autologous fat transfer. Dermatol Surg 2006;32:115–24.

24. Alster TS, Tanzi E. Improvement of neck and cheek laxity with a nonablative radiofrequency device: a lifting experience. Dermatol Surg 2004;30:503–7.

25. Sadick SN, Trelles MS. Nonablative wrinkle treatment of the face and neck using a combined diode laser and radiofrequency technology. Dermatol Surg 2005;31:1695–9.

26. Doshi SN, Alster TS. Combination radiofrequency and diode laser for treatment of facial rhytides and skin laxity. J Cosmet Laser Ther 2005;7:11–5.

27. Kulick M. Evaluation of a combined laser-radiofrequency device (Polaris WR) for the nonablative treatment of facial wrinkles. J Cosmet Laser Ther 2005;7:87–92.

28. David LM, Lask GP, Glassberg E, et al. Laser abrasion for cosmetic and medical treatment of facial actinic damage. Cutis 1989;43:583–7.

29. Bernstein LJ, Kauvar AN, Grossman MC, et al. The short- and long-term side effects of carbon dioxide laser resurfacing. Dermatol Surg 1997;23:519–25.

30. Nanni CA, Alster TS. Complications of carbon dioxide laser resurfacing. An evaluation of 500 patients. Dermatol Surg 1998;24:315–20.

31. Khatri KA, Ross V, Grevelink JM, et al. Comparison of erbium: YAG and carbon dioxide lasers in resurfacing of facial rhytides. Arch Dermatol 1999;135:391–7.

32. Alster TS. Cutaneous resurfacing with CO2 and erbium:YAG lasers: preoperative, intraoperative, and postoperative considerations. Plast Reconstr Surg 1999;103:619–32.

33. Teikmeier G, Goldberg DJ. Skin resurfacing with the erbium:YAG laser. Dermatol Surg 1997;23:685–7.

34. Polnikorn N, Goldberg DJ, Suwanchinda A, et al. Erbium:YAG laser resurfacing in Asians. Dermatol Surg 1998;24:1303–7.

35. Perez MI, Bank DE, Silvers D. Skin resurfacing of the face with the Erbium:YAG laser. Dermatol Surg 1998;24(6):653–8.

36. McDaniel DH, Lord J, Ash K, et al. Combined CO2/erbium:YAG laser resurfacing of peri-oral rhytides and side-by-side comparison with carbon dioxide laser alone. Dermatol Surg 1999;25:285–90.

37. Jasin ME. Achieving superior resurfacing results with the erbium:YAG laser. Arch Facial Plast Surg 2002;4:262–6.

38. Utley DS, Koch RJ, Egbert BM. Histologic analysis of the thermal effect on epidermal and dermal structures following treatment with the superpulsed CO2 laser and the erbium:YAG laser – an in vivo study. Lasers Surg Med 1999;24:93–102.

39. Madden MR, Nolan E, Finkelstein JL, et al. Comparison of an occlusive and a semi-occlusive dressing and the effect of the wound exudates upon keratinocyte proliferation. J Trauma 1989;29:924–30.

40. Batra RS, Ort RJ, Jacob C, et al. Evaluation of a silicone occlusive dressing after laser skin resurfacing. Arch Dermatol 2001;137:1317–21.

41. Kilmer SL. Laser resurfacing complications: how to treat them and how to avoid them. Int J Aesthetic Restor Surg 1997;5:41–5.

42. Manstein D, Herron GS, Sink RK, et al. Fractional photothermolysis: a new concept for cutaneous remodeling using microscopic patterns of thermal injury. Lasers Surg Med 2004;34:426–38.

43. Geronemus RG. Fractional photothermolysis: current and future applications. Lasers Surg Med 2006;38:169–76.

44. Kilmer S, Fitzpatrick R, Bernstein E, et al. Long term follow-up on the use of plasma skin regeneration in full facial rejuvenation procedures. Lasers Surg Med 2005;36(Suppl 17):22.

45. Bogle MA, Arndt KA, Dover JS. Evaluation of plasma skin regeneration technology in low fluence full-facial rejuvenation. Arch Dermatol 2007;143:168–74.

46. Carruthers A, Carruthers J. History of the cosmetic use of botulinum A exotoxin. Dermatol Surg 1998; 24:1168–70.

47. Simpson LL. Peripheral actions of the botulinum toxins. In: Simpson LL, editor. Botulinum neurotoxin and tetanus toxin. San Diego (CA): Academic Press; 1989. p. 153–78.

48. Lange D. Systemic effects of botulinum toxin. In: Jankovic J, Hallett M, editors. Therapy with botulinum toxin. New York: Marcel Dekker; 1994. p. 109–18.

49. Goschel H, Wohlfarth K, Frevert J, et al. Botulinum A toxin therapy: neutralizing and non-neutralizing antibodies – therapeutic consequences. Exp Neurol 1997;147:96–102.

50. Moyer E, Settler P. Botulinum toxin type B: experimental and clinical experience. In: Jankovic J, Hallett M, editors. Therapy with botulinum toxin. New York: Marcel Dekker; 1994. p. 71–85.

51. Alam M, Dover J, Arndt K. Pain associated with botulinum A exotoxin reconstituted using isotonic sodium chloride with and without preservative: a double blind randomized trial. Arch Dermatol 2002;138:510–4.

52. Lowe NJ. Botulinum A toxin type A for facial rejuvenation: United States and United Kingdom perspectives. Dermatol Surg 1998;24:1216–8.

53. Guyuron B, Huddelston SW. Aesthetic indications for botulinum toxin injection. Plast Reconstr Surg 1994; 93:913–8.

54. Matarasso A, Matarasso SL, Brandt FS, et al. Botulinum A exotoxin for the management of platysma bands. Plast Reconstr Surg 1999;103:645–52.

55. Jimenez G, Spencer JM. Erbium:YAG laser resurfacing of the hands, arms, and neck. Dermatol Surg 1999;25:831–5.

56. Gooderrman M, Solish N. Use of hyaluronic acid for soft tissue augmentation of HIV-associated lipoatrophy. Dermatol Surg 2005;31:893.

57. Klein A. In search of the perfect lip. 2005. Dermatol Surg 2005;31:1599.

58. Schanz S, Schippert W, Ulmer A, et al. Arterial embolization caused by injection of hyaluronic acid (Restylane). Br J Dermatol 2002;146:928–9.

59. Lowe N, Grover R. Injectable hyaluronic acid implant for malar and mental enhancement. Dermatol Surg 2006;32:881–5.

60. Coleman SR. Facial recontouring with lipostructure. Clin Plast Surg 1997;24(2):347–67.

61. Shiffman MA, Mirrafati S. Fat transfer techniques: the effect of harvest and transfer methods on adipocyte viability and review of the literature. Dermatol Surg 2001;27(9):819–26.

62. von Heimburg D, Hemmrich K, Haydarlioglu S, et al. Comparison of viable cell yield from excised versus aspirated adipose tissue. Cells Tissues Organs 2004;178(2):87–92.

63. Yamaguchi M, Matsumoto F, Bujo H, et al. Revascularization determines volume retention and gene expression by fat grafts in mice. Exp Biol Med (Maywood) 2005;230(10):742–8.

64. Hudson DA, Lambert EV, Bloch CE. Site selection for auto-transplantation: some observations. Aesthetic Plast Surg 1990;14(3):195–7.

65. Harmon CB. Dermabrasion. In: Freedberg IM, Eisen AZ, Wolff K, et al, editors. Fitzpatrick's dermatology in general medicine, vol. 2. 6th edition. New York: McGraw-Hill Professional; 2003. p. 2536–7.

66. Rubenstein R, Roenigk HH Jr, Stegman SJ, et al. Atypical keloids after dermabrasion of patients taking isotretinoin. J Am Acad Dermatol 1986;15: 280–5.

67. Poulos E, Taylor C, Solish N. Effectiveness of dermasanding (manual dermabrasion) on the appearance of surgical scars: a prospective, randomized, blinded study. J Am Acad Dermatol 2003;14:243–51.

68. Lawrence N, Mandy S, Yarborough J, et al. History of dermabrasion. Dermatol Surg 2000;26:95–101.

69. Alster T. Laser scar revision: comparison study of 585 nm pulsed dye laser with and without intralesional corticosteroids. Dermatol Surg 2003;29:25–9.

70. Sulamanidze MA, Fournier PF, Paikidze TG, et al. Removal of facial soft tissue ptosis with special threads. Dermatol Surg 2002;28(5):365–71.

71. Sasaki GH, Cohen AT. Meloplication of the malar fat pads by percutaneous cable-suture technique for midface rejuvenation: outcome study (392 cases, 6 years' experience. Plast Reconstr Surg 2002;110: 635–54.

72. Lycka B, Bazan C, Poletti E, et al. The emerging technique of antiptosis subdermal suspension thread. Dermatol Surg 2004;30(1):41–4.

73. Silva-Siwady JG, Diaz-Garza C, Ocampo-Candiani J. A case of Aptos thread migration and partial expulsion. Dermatol Surg 2005;31(3): 356–8.

BeautiPHIcation™: A Global Approach to Facial Beauty

Arthur Swift, MD, FRCS(C)[a,b,c,*],
Kent Remington, MD, FRCP(C)[d,e]

KEYWORDS

- Beauty • Phi • Facial attractiveness
- Facial shape • Facial angles

RENAISSANCE PHYSICIANS: PURVEYORS OF BEAUTY

The Renaissance Period (1350–1550) was the rebirth transition period between the Middle Ages and the modern world, and has been described as the most productive era in mankind's history. As a cultural movement, it engulfed Europe in a revival of artistic learning based on classical sources and the development of linear perspective. Although the Renaissance saw resurgence in intellectual scientific activity, it is perhaps best known for the monumental achievements of such artistic geniuses as Leonardo Da Vinci and Michelangelo. Their influence affected and shaped the future by empowering their generation to embrace knowledge, and stood as a testament to the development of limitless skills in all the arts. These gifted Renaissance men were more than just intellectual icons: they inspired a medieval world to break free of dogmatic ideology and endeavor to develop its capabilities as fully as possible.

Da Vinci claimed, "I have offended God and mankind because my work didn't reach the quality it should have." It is time to rekindle his torch of commitment and excellence with a spark of passion and pride. We are the Renaissance artists of our time. Patients are our easels, their faces our canvas. We should strive to create beautiful works of art; to maximize each individual's natural facial beauty.

The world today is immersed in an expectation economy: aesthetic consumers do not want to look just good, they expect to look fantastic; immediately, and with little downtime. Patients always budget to look great because looking great never goes out of style even in a disruptive economy. Today's aesthetic patients realize that a youthful appearance is the best thing you can wear.

There exists a sea of sameness with a biblical flood of products, devices, and nonmedical centers, compelling aesthetic physicians to differentiate themselves through superior results. To chase lines is a guarantee of copying the competition in a race to the bottom; cosmetic specialists must separate their clinics from the monotherapist down the street by creating exceptional results through a comprehensive global approach.

The recent availability of safe volumizing fillers has provided cosmetic physicians with the tools necessary to contour facial features nonsurgically and cost-effectively. Like our Renaissance ancestors, it is incumbent on us to have a good understanding of the aesthetic goals necessary to achieve a beautiful and natural result. What should be the preferred facial volume and feature shape?

a Westmount Institute of Plastic Surgery, 4131 Sherbrooke Street West, Montreal, QC H3Z 1B7, Canada
b Victoria Park Medical Spa, 376 Victoria Avenue, Montreal, Quebec, Canada H3Z 1C3
c Division of Plastic Surgery, St. Mary's Hospital, McGill University, 3830 Lacombe Avenue, Montreal, Quebec, Canada H3T 1M5
d Remington Laser Dermatology Centre, 150-7220 Fisher Street SE, Calgary, Alberta, Canada T2H 2H8
e Foothills Medical Centre, Division of Dermatology, 1403-29 Street NW, Calgary, Alberta, Canada T2N 2T9
* Corresponding author. The Westmount Institute of Plastic Surgery, 4131 Sherbrooke Street West, Montreal, QC H3Z 1B7, Canada.
E-mail address: drswift@drarthurswift.com

Clin Plastic Surg 38 (2011) 347–377
doi:10.1016/j.cps.2011.03.012
0094-1298/11/$ – see front matter © 2011 Elsevier Inc. All rights reserved.

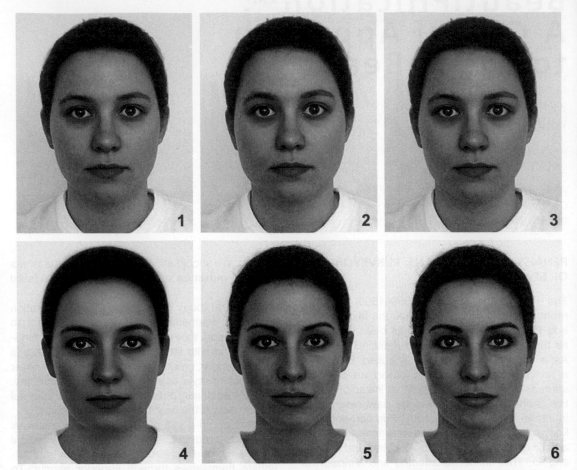

Fig. 1. Using morphing software, German researchers created gradually changing images. Images 5 and 6 consistently scored highest on the 7-point attractiveness scale when exposed to different large-volume cohorts.

What is the ideal beautiful normal for each individual face, and is there a code to unlock the patient's potential? Is it unreasonable to have lofty aesthetic goals, or should clinicians be less principled and more moderate? Thomas Paine (1737–1809), a British author who supported the American Revolution and became one of the Founding Fathers of the United States, wrote: "A thing moderately good is not as good as it ought to be. Moderation in temper is always a virtue; but moderation in principle is always a vice."

This review focuses on outlining objective parameters necessary for creating a template to maximize each individual's facial beauty. The techniques offered are the unique conceptions of the authors, experienced injectors who have applied their expertise in both aesthetic dermatology and cosmetic plastic surgery. It in no way represents the sole method to nonsurgically release the patient's facial beauty potential. The intent is to encourage aesthetic injectors to always

THE MAGNIFICENT SEVEN

I.   Facial shape (cheeks & chin)

II.   Forehead height

III. Eyebrow shape

IV. Eye size and inter-eye distance

V.   Nose shape

VI. Lips (length and height)

VII. Skin clarity/texture/color

Fig. 2. The Magnificent Seven facial features that influence our perception of facial beauty.

be result oriented, to develop methodical and comprehensive approaches to facial enhancement, and to push creativity beyond rejuvenation into the realm of beauty maximization. "The greater danger for most of us lies not in setting our aim too high and falling short; but in setting our aim too low, and achieving our mark" (Michelangelo Buonarroti).

FACIAL BEAUTY

St Thomas Aquinas, known as the angelic doctor, was one of the great philosophers of the Catholic Church in the thirteenth century. He proclaimed beauty to be "integras, proportio, et claritas": harmony, proportion, and clarity. True facial

beauty arouses the senses to an emotional level of pleasure and "evokes in the perceiver a high degree of attraction" (Stephen Marquardt).

It is essential that injection specialists have a deep understanding and a well-cultivated taste for beauty. Otherwise they would be satisfied with a low and common goal rather than the maximization of beauty potential in their patients. Although certain individuals may be endowed with an innate aesthetic sense, it can be learned, at least in part, by the ardent study of art and the constant observation of facial and body proportions and relationships.[1]

Regardless of nationality, age, or ethnic background, for the most part people universally share a sense of what is attractive.[2] When British

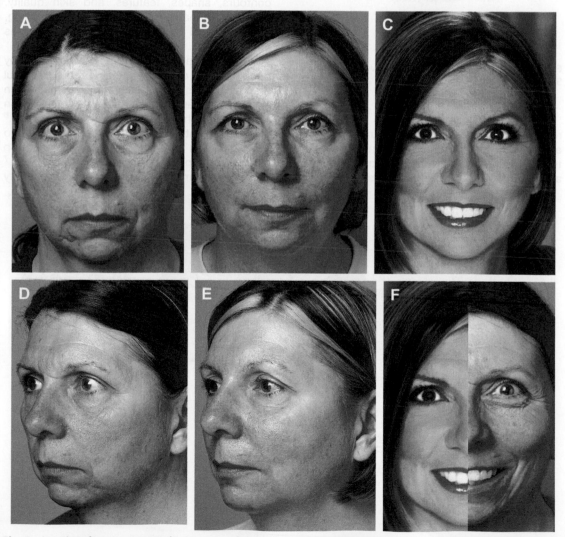

Fig. 3. (*A, D*) Before treatment. (*B, E*) After global volume restoration (HA) and neuromodulator (BTX-A). (*C*) Impact of cosmetics and hairstyle. (*F*) Hemi-face comparison, before and after treatment.

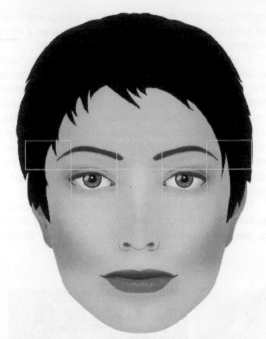

Fig. 4. Artist's rendition of an attractive face scaled to 5 eye widths across.

researchers asked women from England, China, and India to rate pictures of various Greek men, their choices were identical. When asked to select attractive faces from a diverse collection,

European White, Asian, and Latino people from a dozen countries also made the same choices.[3] Studies have shown that even babies show a sense of what is attractive: infants 3 to 6 months old gaze longer at a nice-looking face than one that is not attractive.[4]

In a large research project on facial attractiveness at several German universities, digitally composed faces were created using a specialized software algorithm based on people's perception of beauty.[5] Using a 7-point Likert scale from 1 (very unattractive) to 7 (very attractive), results proved that most people, regardless of ethnicity, seem to have similar subjective ideas about what constitutes an attractive face (**Fig. 1**). Processing attractiveness can take milliseconds; the perceiver's eyes rapidly scan the entire face while the brain analyzes contours, shapes, features, and skin quality. Contrary to patients' requests for line filling, affecting facial beauty goes far beyond wrinkles and furrows.

However, finding objective answers to why people regard one face as being more beautiful than another is not as easy as it seems. When viewing a beautiful face, the eye focuses on areas that are highlighted with pleasing shapes.[6] The angles that these features create are vital to the perception of beauty; highlights located too high or too low detract from attractiveness.[7] Review of numerous articles on facial beauty

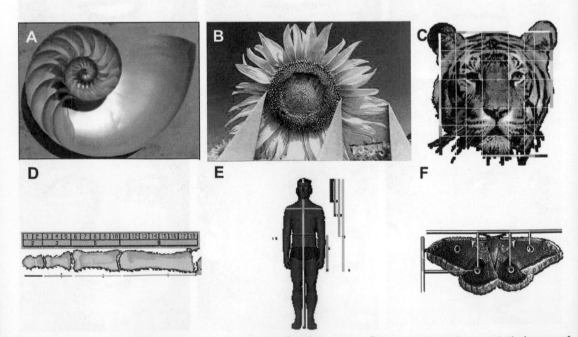

Fig. 5. The Divine Proportion in living things. (*A*) Nautilus shell. (*B*) Sunflower. (*C*) Tiger's head. (*D*) Phalanges of the hand. (*E*) Human body. (*F*) Butterfly.

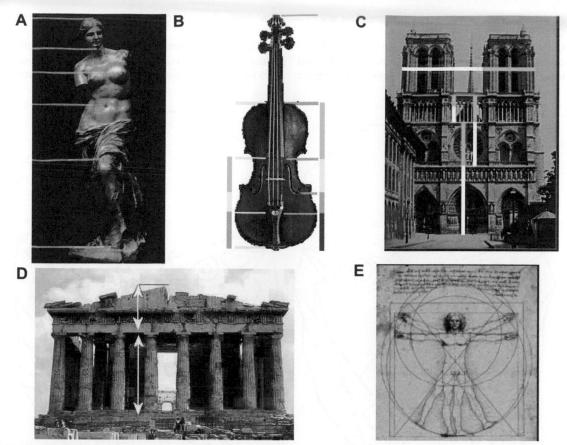

Fig. 6. The Golden Ratio in architecture, music, and art. (*A*) Venus de Milo. (*B*) Stradivarius violin. (*C*) Notre Dame Cathedral. (*D*) Parthenon. (*E*) Leonardo Da Vinci's Vitruvian Man.

identifies 7 key facial features that seem to be subconsciously assessed when determining facial beauty (**Fig. 2**). Four features of these Magnificent Seven (facial shape, eyebrow shape, nose, and lips) are amenable to injection contouring with fillers (eg, hyaluronic acids [HAs]) and neuromodulators (eg, botulinum toxin A [BTX-A]). The remaining 3 features (forehead height, eye size and intereye distance, and skin tone and texture) are beyond the domain of injection therapy. Skin clarity, texture, and color can be markedly improved with topical agents, present-day energy device technology, and judicial use of makeup; forehead height accentuated or camouflaged by hair style; and intereye distance disguised by creative shadowing when applying eye makeup. All this emphasizes the importance of working closely with skilled aestheticians and experienced hairdressers when offering patients global facial beautification (**Fig. 3**).

THE STORY OF PHI

Many Renaissance scholars and artists studied ancient Greece and Rome, attempting to recapture the spirit of these cultures in their philosophies

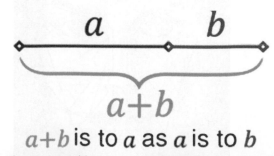

$a+b$ is to a as a is to b

Fig. 7. The Golden Section is the only point in line ab that divides line ab in a ratio of 1.618(a) to 1(b); 1(a) to 0.618(b); and 1(a) to 1.618(a+b).

and their works of art and literature. The ancient Greeks maintained that all beauty is mathematics. Leonardo Da Vinci, in his scientific search for defining ideal beauty, stated that "no human inquiry can be called science unless it pursues its path through mathematical exposition and demonstration."

The attractiveness of the female figure is often described in measured numbers (eg, 36-24-36), so why not the face? The idea of a mathematical

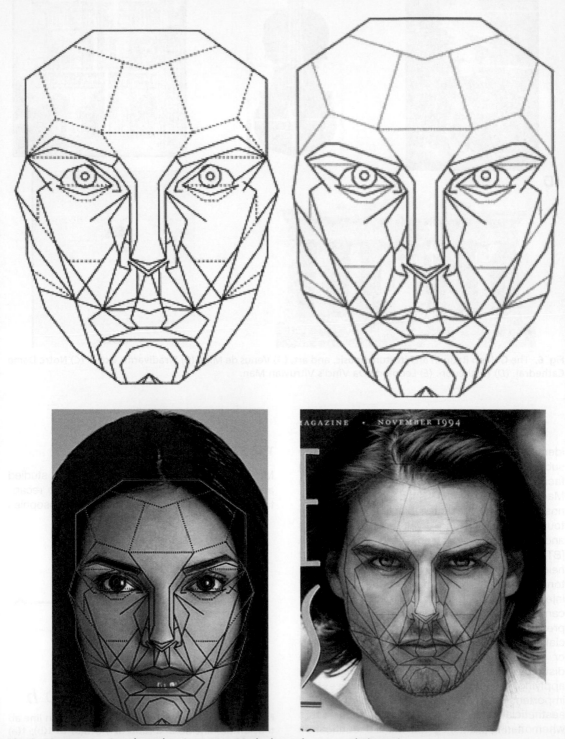

Fig. 8. Marquardt's female and male Golden Masks (www.beautyanalysis.com).

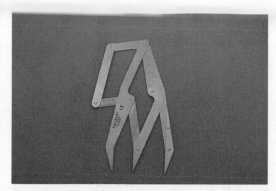

Fig. 9. Golden mean caliper. When the gauge is adjusted, the middle arm always shows the Golden Section or phi ratio point between the 2 outer arms.

code, formula, relationship, or even a number that can describe facial beauty is not a modern concept. Medieval artists were impressed by the magical number 7. For them, the perfect face was neatly divisible into horizontal sevenths: the hair the top seventh, forehead two-sevenths, nose another two-sevenths, a seventh between nose and mouth, and the final seventh from mouth to chin. Novice artists are often taught that the simplest way to approximate the relative width of facial features is to divide the face into vertical fifths, with each fifth being equal to 1 eye width (**Fig. 4**).

Only 1 mathematical relationship has been consistently and repeatedly reported to be present in beautiful things,[8] both living (**Fig. 5**) and man made (**Fig. 6**): the Golden Ratio (also known as the Divine Proportion).

The Golden Ratio is a mathematical ratio of 1.618:1, and the number 1.618 is called Phi because it was regularly used by the Greek sculptor Phidias; Phi (upper case) is 1.6180339887…, whereas phi (lower case) is 0.6180339887…, the reciprocal of Phi and also Phi minus 1. This irrational number is the only one in mathematics that, when subtracted by units (1.0), yields its own reciprocal.

Used since the time of the Egyptians, the Golden Ratio was formulated as one of Euclid's elements, one of the most beautiful and influential works of science in the history of humankind. This ratio was known to the Greeks as the Golden Section and to the Renaissance artists as the Divine Proportion. In geometry, it is a linear relation in which the smaller length is to the larger part as the larger part is to the complete line (**Fig. 7**).

Ricketts[9] noted that the golden calipers applied to the hand of man reveals that each of the phalanges of each finger is golden to the next in all 5 fingers (see **Fig. 5**D).

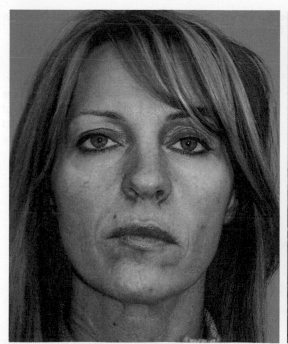
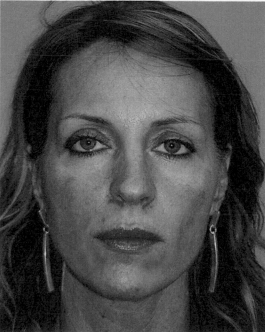

Fig. 10. Before and after BeautiPHIcation™ showing midline symmetry of lips (twins) and mild asymmetry of the left and right sides of the face (siblings).

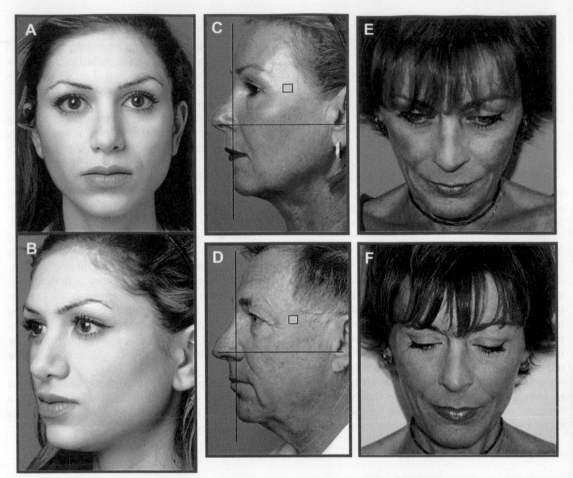

Fig. 11. Consistent clinical photography. (*A, B*) Front view and three-quarter view (tip of nose on cheek); (*C, D*) left profile showing focusing frame; (*E, F*) Towne view before and after BeautiPHIcation™.

Stephen Marquardt, a California-based Oral and Maxillofacial surgeon has conducted extensive research on human facial attractiveness.[10] His pioneering work on the mathematical construction of facial form led to his controversial[11,12] Golden Mask, derived from the Golden Ratio (**Fig. 8**). Marquardt (personal communication, 2007) maintains that the evidence shows that our perception of physical beauty is hard wired into our being and based on how closely one's features reflect phi

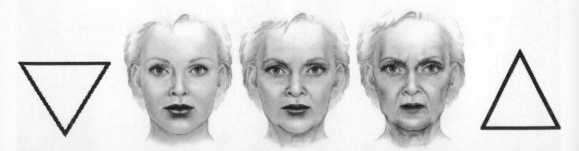

Fig. 12. The Triangle of Youth. Youth is typified by a full and wide midface. Aging results in deflation of midface structures and support, tissue deterioration, and subsequent descent of the facial envelope, causing a reversal of the triangle and facial disproportion.

Table 1
Volume loss staging in the midface

Stage 1	Stage 2	Stage 3	Stage 4
Normal	Evidence of early soft tissue ptosis or atrophy slightly visible	Visible depression or descent	Severe depression or atrophy

in their proportions. His modification of Hungerford's classic quote that "beauty is in the phi [eye] of the beholder" is convincing.

Since 2003, the authors have collaborated on a global comprehensive approach to nonsurgical facial beautification by optimizing facial volume, creating harmony, symmetry, and balance through reflation and contouring. To maintain natural results and avoid overinflation, proportions were achieved initially by the use of a golden mean caliper; a tool based on an articulated pentagon for dynamically measuring the phi ratio (**Fig. 9**). The calipers were first used by Renaissance artists to determine the divine proportions for their compositions in stone and on canvas. Golden mean calipers initially help the aesthetic injector see Phi more as a relationship than as a number. Eventually, a geometric familiarity with the Golden Ratio develops, which leads to its intuitive expression in the injection technique.

In the absence of disease, the medial canthi remain a constant cutaneous landmark with age for each individual adult face. Measuring the intercanthal distance (x) to establish the unit length on which Phi (1.618x) and phi (0.618x) are created, aesthetic goals can now be defined to maximize each patient's phi beauty potential.

FACIAL SHAPE ASSESSMENT

The single feature that matters time and again in studies on facial beauty is symmetry.[13] Many papers have discussed attractiveness in terms of 3 tenets: symmetry, balance, and harmony.[14–17] Although often referred to as the first feature of beauty, symmetry is not absolute[18]: the left and right sides of the face should be considered more as siblings than as twins. However, the 2 sides of the lips should be regarded more as twins, with balanced upper and lower vermilion show (**Fig. 10**).

It is crucial for the aesthetic injector to be fastidious about the use of consistent clinical photography. It not only is invaluable in planning treatment but also remains a vital aspect of the patient's record to document aesthetic accomplishments. Facial views should include frontal (anteroposterior [AP]), three-quarter (tip of nose in line with the outer cheek), lateral, and Towne view to highlight facial contours (**Fig. 11**). It is also beneficial for quadragenerian and older patients to provide earlier portrait photographs showing their youthful facial proportions and previously existing asymmetries.

Although dermatologic diagnoses can be made in seconds, when evaluating the aesthetic face, more time, care, and patience are warranted. Consensus guidelines point to an evolving paradigm in facial rejuvenation with a shift from the two-dimensional (2D) approach (focus on correcting dynamic facial lines) to the three-dimensional (3D) approach including loss of facial volume.[19]

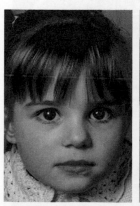 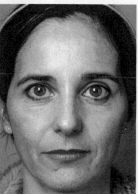 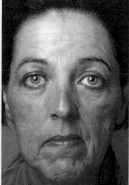 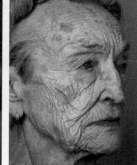

| Granddaughter | Daughter | Mother | Grandmother |

Fig. 13. The Four Ds of aging: deflation, deterioration, descent, and disproportion.

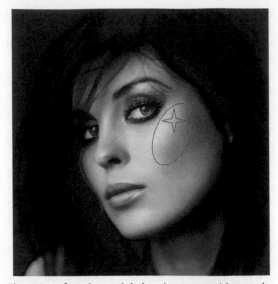

Fig. 14. A female model showing an ovoid, angular cheek mound with eccentric apex (*star*) as well as the ogee curve of the right cheek contour.

In order to create great results, aesthetic physicians must have double vision: they must be able to see the third dimension in areas of volume loss as well as seeing the end result before they begin treatment. It is important to recognize that 1 size fits none and, even though each face is similar, every face is unique.

Youth and beauty are exemplified by a full and wide midface, referred to as the Triangle of Youth (**Fig. 12**). Authoritative work on facial shape by Dr Steven Liew, an Australian plastic surgeon based in Sydney, has revealed a global standard oval facial shape that is considered attractive to people of all racial backgrounds. Liew's Universal Angle of Beauty, the angle of inclination of the vertical ramus of the mandible, is ideally measured at 9 to 12 degrees off vertical, and can be attained by either volumizing with fillers or thinning the masseter with precise botulinum toxin injections.[20]

Aging changes the 3D topography of the underlying facial structures, resulting in deflation and ptosis of the midface skin and soft tissues

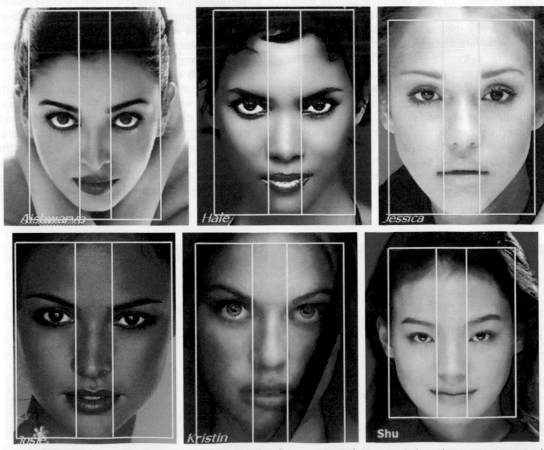

Fig. 15. Top models showing Phi facial width proportion (ie, medial canthus to medial canthus measures x; medial canthus to ipsilateral cheek apex measures 1.618x).

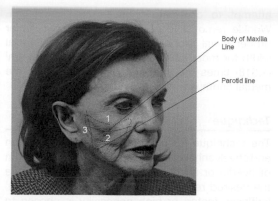

Body of Maxilla Line

Parotid line

Fig. 16. The depleted region of the right cheek is outlined (*black dashed line*). Injections overlying the body of the maxilla (zone 1 above the body of maxilla line) are placed supraperiosteally and, if necessary, subcutaneously. Depth of volume injections for zones 2 and 3 are limited to the subcutaneous plane.

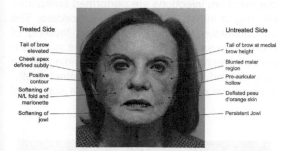

Treated Side

Tail of brow elevated
Cheek apex defined subtly
Positive contour
Softening of N/L fold and marionette
Softening of jowl

Untreated Side

Tail of brow at medial brow height
Blunted malar region
Pre-auricular hollow
Deflated peau d'orange skin
Persistent Jowl

Fig. 17. Injections of the upper midface affecting lower zones (nasolabial fold and jowl). N/L = nasolabial.

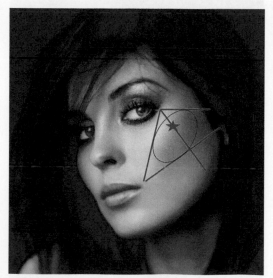

Fig. 18. BeautiPHIcation™: The oval cheek mound lies within the triangular markings (see text) with the malar apex located as depicted (*star*).

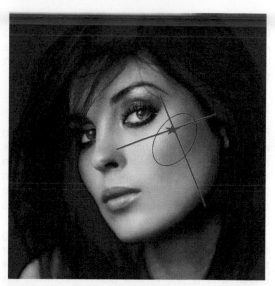

Fig. 19. BeautiPHIcation™: Cheek apex (*star*) defined by the intersection of a line drawn from the nasal alar groove to the upper tragus and a line drawn vertically down from the midpoint of the lateral orbital rim.

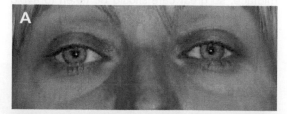

A

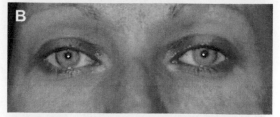

B

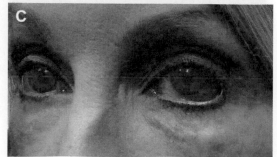

C

Fig. 20. (*A*) Tear troughs before treatment. (*B*) Appropriate tear trough correction with HA of low viscosity. (*C*) Inappropriate tear trough/infraorbital hollow treatment resulting in lower eyelid ectropion and visibility of product (HA of high viscosity).

(**Table 1**, **Fig. 13**).[21] Conventional face and brow lifting without volume replacement is unable to restore facial fullness and fails to address the issue of deteriorating facial shape secondary to soft tissue atrophy and bone resorption.

THE BEAUTI"PHI"ED CHEEK

Reasonable goals in both midface rejuvenation as well as cheek enhancement should involve adequate volume restoration and contouring in the aesthetically appropriate locations.[22,23] In 2004, Dr Wayne Carey,[24] a Canadian aesthetic dermatologist, pioneered the use of HA fillers as 3 discrete pillars to restore cheek volume.

The female cheek mound is ovoid or egg shaped, not circular, and should not extend higher than the limbus of the lower eyelid (**Fig. 14**). The cheek axis is not vertical but angled from the lateral commissure to the base of the ear helix. Most importantly, each malar prominence has a defined apex, located high on the midface, below and lateral to the lateral canthus, and eccentrically located within the cheek oval.

Proportion and harmony are paramount in the midface, so great care should be taken to avoid excessive use of filler product in this region in the attempt to obliterate lines through reinflation. Wrinkle removal is not the endpoint but rather proper facial proportion. In general, ideal facial width for most ethnicities falls approximately Phi (1.618) times the intercanthal distance from the medial canthus to the ipsilateral cheek (**Fig. 15**).

Technique

The technique for midface contour volumization and cheek enhancement should involve a minimum of needle or microcannula punctures to achieve the desired result. A filler product with a high G' (stiffness factor) or high cohesivity is chosen to maximize lifting capacity of the overlying tissue. Initial placement of the product is done vertically to create 2 to 3 pillars in the submuscular (supraperiosteal) plane. Small-gauge needles are preferred to create this tent-pole effect, with aliquots limited to no more than 0.5 mL of product per injection. Injections are performed antegrade, creating a visible lift during the procedure. The subcutaneous tent canopy requires layering of product via an angulated percutaneous microcannula (or fine needle) technique. Depending on the type of product selected for the lift effect, feathering of the cheek contour in a more superficial

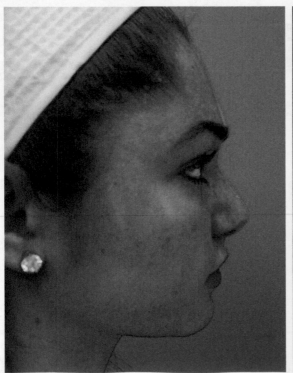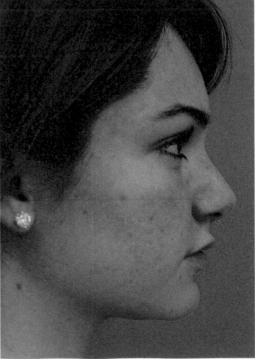

Fig. 21. BeautiPHIcation™ showing HA subgaleal injection to create gentle forehead convexity 12 degrees off vertical.

subdermal plane may be indicated using a softer (lower G') product to avoid any step-off areas. Massage with cool ultrasound gel is always performed after treatment to mold and blend the product as discerned by tactile fingertip touch rather than relying on visual observation.

A 2-step marking approach is used to create the Fabergé egg appearance to the cheek along with its eccentric apex. This process can be likened to giving the face what it wants (volume), and then giving it what it needs (the proper apogee).

Step 1: Giving the cheek what it wants (restoring the Ogee curve)

The ogee curve is an architectural shape consisting of a concave arc flowing into a convex arc, creating an S-shaped curve. In aesthetic facial surgery, the term is used to describe many facial curves, including the malar or cheekbone prominence transitioning into the midcheek hollow (see **Fig. 14**). The aim of cheek enhancement is to restore (or in some cases create) a gentle ogee curve and subtly define the zenith of the malar prominence.

Using an eyebrow pencil, the depleted and concave (negative vector) areas of the anterior cheek, malar-zygomatic, and submalar regions are marked (**Fig. 16**). The inferior border of the body of the maxilla is outlined to demarcate supraperiosteal and subcutaneous placement of product. Injections overlying the body of the maxilla are layered supraperiosteally (submuscularly) as well as subcutaneously if necessary to correct any resistant contour irregularities. Injections overlying the parotid (preauricular) region, submalar region, and lower anterior cheek are performed in the subcutaneous plane. Any preexisting irregularities in the skin are addressed by direct intradermal injection of an appropriate lower G' product. Injections are performed from superior to inferior on the face, because higher placed product influences the lower zones by lifting the adjacent inferior tissue. This effect is shown by the softening of the nasolabial fold and jowl on the treated side once the cheek mound has been restored. Often, less product is required for direct correction of whatever deformity may remain along the upper nasolabial fold triangle and prejowl sulcus (**Fig. 17**).

Step 2: Giving the cheek what it needs (the proper apogee)

Once the markings from step 1 have been wiped away and the gel massage completed, the cheek is ready for the beautiphication markings to delineate the ovoid appearance and define the cheek apex (**Fig. 18**). A line is drawn from the lateral commissure to the lateral canthus of the ipsilateral eye. This line establishes the anterior extent of the malar prominence (Hinderer line). A second line is drawn from the lateral commissure to the inferior tragus of the ipsilateral ear, denoting the lateral and inferior boundary of the malar prominence (base of the triangle). The highpoint of the cheek is marked by a horizontal line at the level of the limbus of the lower eyelid. The cheek oval is drawn within these boundaries and tangential to the lines drawn. Feathering of the edges of the oval with subcutaneous filler product is done as necessary to create a smooth, egg-shaped mound. Lastly,

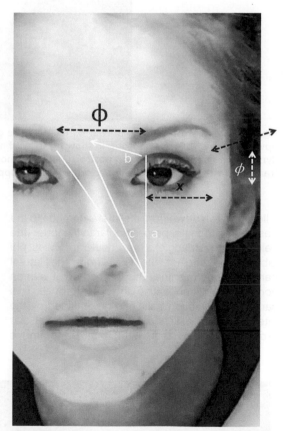

Fig. 22. The beauti"phi"ed brow. Begins vertically in line with the medial canthus (A); lies phi above the bony rim from the pupil; has a 10 to 20 degree climb from medial to lateral (B); is arched at a distance equal to the intercanthal distance (x), which is phi of the total eyebrow length (the point crossed by a line drawn from the alar base tangential to the lateral aspect of the pupil) (C); has a lateral tip higher than the medial tip; is Phi of the medial canthus in length (delineated by a line drawn from the lateral alar base through the lateral canthus (D); and has tissue fullness over the lateral supraorbital rim.

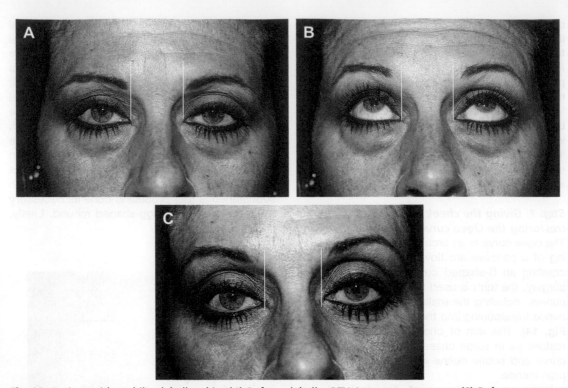

Fig. 23. Patient with mobile glabellar skin. (*A*) Before glabellar BTX-A treatment, at rest. (*B*) Before treatment, upward gaze with activated frontalis showing splay of medial brow. (*C*) Status after BTX-A browlift and glabellar dynamic line treatment showing postcorrugator chemodenervation splay of medial eyebrows. (Patient also had transconjunctival blepharoplasty performed but no upper lid surgery.)

a line is drawn down from the lateral canthus to the base of the triangle, perpendicular to the latter (the height of the triangle). The cheek apex lies phi (about one-third of the way) from the lateral canthus along this line. This defined point is in an eccentric position within the cheek oval. This same apex injection point can be obtained by the intersection of a line drawn from the nasal alar groove (phi of the nasal length) to the upper tragus

and a line drawn down vertically from the midpoint of the lateral orbital rim (**Fig. 19**). The final injection (0.25–0.5 mL of product placed on periosteum by vertical puncture) is performed at this precise point to give the cheek what it needs: a beauti"phi"ed apex. Molding and blending of this apogee is done with ultrasound gel to provide a smooth contour. Facial width can be confirmed with the Golden Ratio calipers and filler added at this

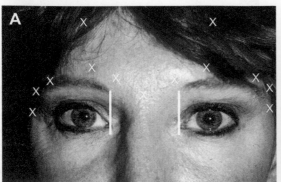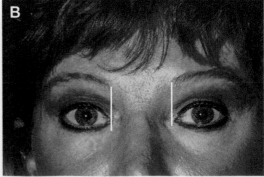

Fig. 24. (*A*) Patient with mobile glabellar skin before BTX-A treatment. (*B*) After BTX-A browlift and periorbital fractionated CO_2 resurfacing with absence of medial brow splay. Xs delineate injection points (see text).

location to idealize the facial width proportion. Each side of the face is unique, so filling volumes and depot locations vary.

Completion of the anterior ogee cheek curve by placement of low G' filler into prominent tear troughs and infraorbital and lateral orbital hollows should be reserved for experienced injectors, because these are the easiest areas to do poorly (**Fig. 20**).

Modifications for the Male Cheek

Compared with the female cheek, the male cheek has more anteromedial fullness, a broader-based malar prominence, and an apex that is more medial and subtly defined. The following modifications of the markings are noted:

The Hinderer line (anteromedial border of the cheek mound) is drawn from the lateral commissure toward the ipsilateral lateral iris, stopping at the infraorbital rim. Because of the lower jaw angle and stronger jaw, the line denoting the inferolateral border of the cheek (base of the triangle) is drawn from the lateral commissure to the base of the ipsilateral infratragal notch.

As for women, the highpoint of the cheek mound is marked by a horizontal line at the level of the limbus of the lower eyelid. The apex of the male cheek is modest and more medially located at one-third of the height of the triangle defined earlier, or one-third along a line from the lateral iris to the base of the triangle, intersecting the latter at a right angle. The ogee created should be flatter in its lower S curve (concave portion).

THE BEAUTI"PHI"ED BROW

The beautiful forehead has a gentle vertical convex ogee curve from trichion to supraorbital ridge, the height of which measures Phi of the intercanthal distance in the ideally proportioned face. A flattened or sloping brow greater than 15 degrees from vertical is often undesirable for the female forehead, and a pleasing convex appearance can be easily fashioned by the subgaleal placement of volumizing filler (**Fig. 21**). Excessive concavity of the temporal fossae is pathognomonic of advancing age, and can be restored to slight concavity or flat appearance, thus preventing the tail of the brow from disappearing around the corner.

The medial eyebrow begins vertically in line with the medial canthus and extends Phi of the intercanthal distance laterally (**Fig. 22**). An appealing female eyebrow has a 10 to 20 degree climb from medial to lateral and is arched at the phi point (approximately the junction of the medial two-thirds and outer one-third). The lateral tip should

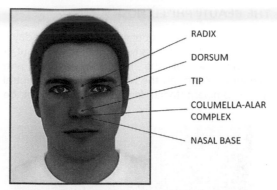

Fig. 25. Sheens' aesthetic components to the nose.

RADIX

DORSUM

TIP

COLUMELLA-ALAR COMPLEX

NASAL BASE

always be higher than the medial tip and there should be soft tissue fullness evident below the outer brow. Lateral brow location is typically 1 cm or phi above the bony rim from the pupil. Cutaneous phi landmarks of the aesthetic eyebrow are easily recognized in the clinical setting, as outlined in **Fig. 22**.

Loss of the corrugators' medial pull after chemodenervation in a glabella with mobile skin can result in excessive splay of the medial brow toward the midpupillary line because of the unopposed oblique pull of the frontalis muscles (**Fig. 23**). Concomitant treatment of the upper frontalis with small-dose neuromodulator can prevent this disturbing splaying of the medial brow (**Fig. 24**).

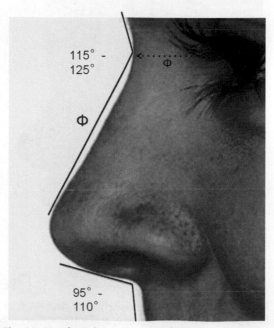

115° - 125°

Φ

Φ

95° - 110°

Fig. 26. Nasal angles and proportions (see text).

THE BEAUTI"PHI"ED NOSE

Nasal enhancement (contouring) is one of today's most sought-after cosmetic procedures, but it remains one of the most challenging and intriguing. Although the nose is the most central and prominent facial feature, it should not be dominating. It must have both a harmonious relationship and an intrinsic beauty. Nasal enhancement by injection is an art that requires the safe deposition of minute quantities of product to achieve remarkable instantaneous results. To paraphrase Winston Churchill, never in the field of nasal aesthetics was so much owed to so little.

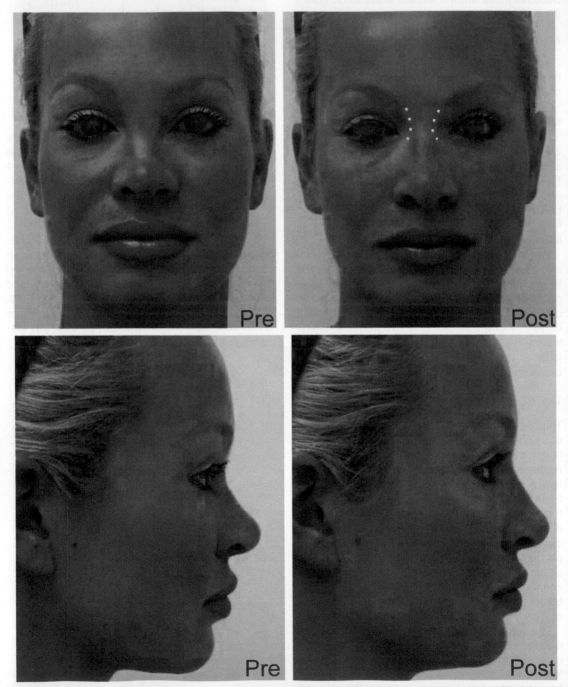

Fig. 27. Nasal dorsal enhancement only with HA filler creating the optical illusion of a narrowing of facial width (bizygomatic, transcommissure, and interpupillary measurements are identical in the photographs). Dotted lines showing divergence and concavity of radix on AP view.

A little difference in anatomy can make a big difference in appearance, both before and after filler contouring.

There are countless textbooks on rhinoplastic technique by world-renowned experts.[25-28] It would be impossible to duplicate these refined techniques with a needle and syringe; not every nose is amenable to the contouring effect of fillers within the confines of proper nasal proportion.

For aesthetic injectors to succeed at nasal enhancement, they must follow the following 4 tenets:

1. Think contour and shape of the face
2. Think skin texture and thickness
3. Think balance and proportion with other facial features

4. Always think in terms of improvement rather than perfection.

Furthermore, to achieve consistent and admirable results, the injector must respect the essential triad of anatomy, aesthetics (Phi), and sound injection principles.

Sheen and Sheen[25] described the 5 aesthetic components to the nose, which are the radix, the dorsum, the tip, the columella-alar complex, and the nasal base (**Fig. 25**).

The Radix

In women, the radix or root of the nose defines a nasofrontal angle of approximately 115 to 125 degrees (**Fig. 26**). Its height from the medial

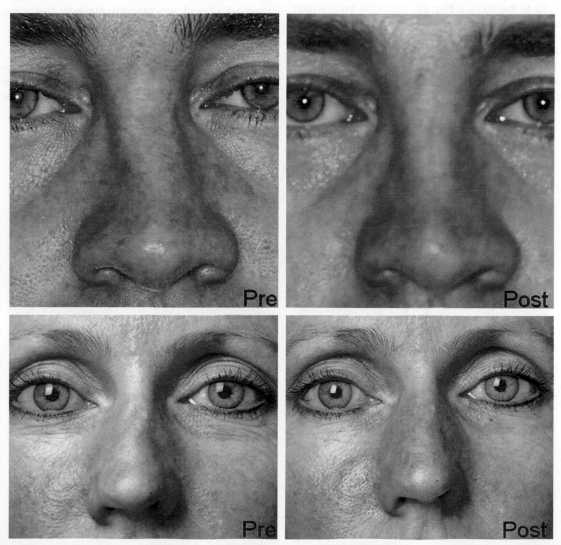

Fig. 28. HA camouflage technique of dorsal straightening (6 months after treatment).

canthus is phi of the intercanthal distance (in the order of 15–18 mm). Its location on profile is approximately at the level of the upper lid lash line in women, the superior acceptable aesthetic limit being the tarsal fold (creating a more masculine appearance).

The skin overlying this area is usually of average thickness and fairly mobile, and so the use of a product with higher G' is desirable. The radix is divergent and concave on frontal view, so the injector must not overfill this region and should pinch the corrected radix to recreate this effect (**Fig. 27**).

The Dorsum

The skin of the dorsum is thinner and more mobile than other areas of the nose. The female dorsum should lie about 2 mm under a line drawn from the radix to the tip (see **Fig. 26**). From the front, which is the view that most patients see every day in the mirror, the dorsum should be straight and no wider than phi of the intercanthal distance (**Fig. 28**). Dorsal augmentation should be done in the supraperiosteal and supraperichondrial planes, and the product used should be of higher

G' value. Use of a softer product results in decreased longevity of the result and the lateral diffusion can create a width issue for Caucasian noses.

Another interesting application of nasal injections is in the region of the nasal valve, between the upper and lower lateral cartilages (**Fig. 29**). In both the natural and postoperated state, collapse in this region can lead to tight nasal airways with resultant snoring or obstruction. External nasal strips (eg, Breathe Right™), intranasal cones (eg, Sinus Cones™), and springlike splints (eg, Breathe With Eez™) have been designed to improve airflow at this bowed area. The instillation of intradermal HA product in this region can act as an internal splint, similar to the center span of a suspension bridge, preventing collapse with inspiration (**Fig. 30**). Careful intradermal placement is critical, because product placed subdermally burdens the valve region, adding to the obstruction.

Nasal Tip

The skin of the nasal tip is thicker and more adherent than the adjacent dorsal skin, and there

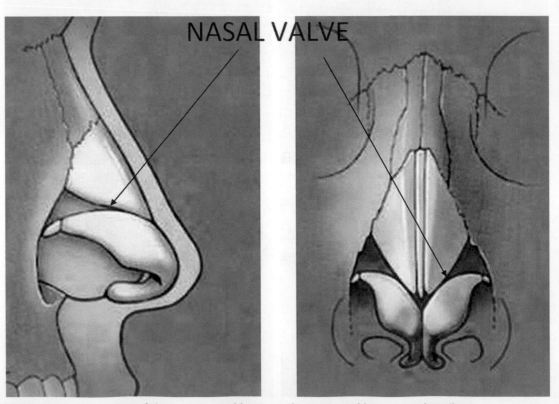

Fig. 29. Nasal valve region of the nose, located between the upper and lower lateral cartilages.

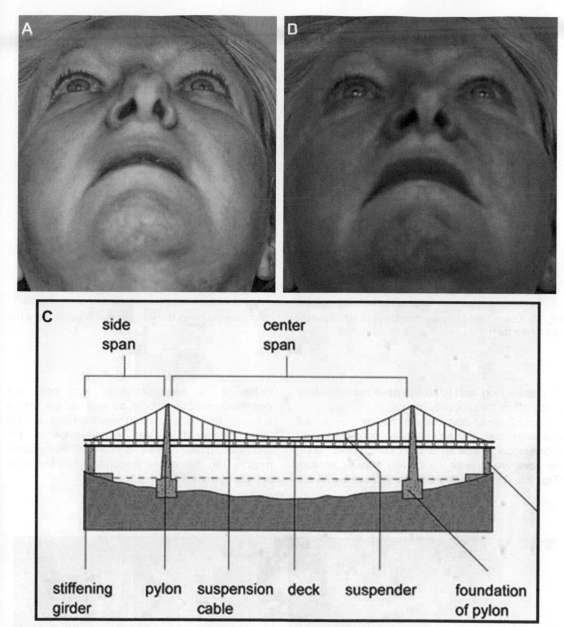

Fig. 30. (*A*) Patient with nasal valve and alar collapse during inspiration. (*B*) Patient after treatment with intradermal HA preventing airway obstruction. (*C*) Suspension bridge showing center span (see text).

is a variable amount of subcutaneous tissue. Tip height is measured at phi (0.618x) of the intercanthal distance. The beautiful nose should have 2 tip-defining points that are the most projecting aspect on profile and Phi (1.618 times the intercanthal distance) from the radix. Injections in this region should be subdermal with average G' product and designed to create symmetry and establish a domal tip light reflection (**Fig. 31**).

The nasal tip is a common site of depressed scars caused by excision/curettage of lytic skin lesions; a smooth, aesthetic contour can be reestablished by the delicate layering of HA product followed by laser resurfacing (**Fig. 32**). Because it is a watershed area for nasal circulation (especially in the postrhinoplasty patient), it is prudent for the injector to always avoid blanching of the nasal tip skin, to keep the patient 15 minutes after treatment

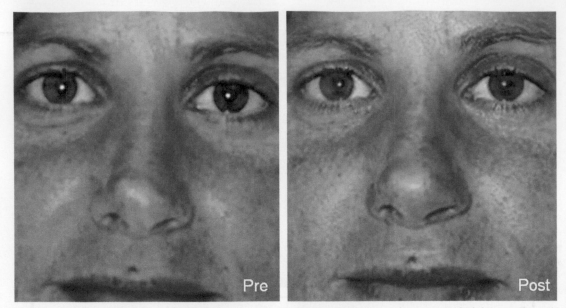

Fig. 31. Correction of tip asymmetry with HA. Tip-defining points are Phi times the intercanthal distance from the radix (see text).

for observation, and to always have hyaluronidase in the office for product erasure.

Canted nasal tips caused by anterior septal deviation can be provisionally corrected with submucosal injection of high G' product along the concave side of the curved anterior septum (**Fig. 33**). Tip elevation can be achieved with the

instillation of neuromodulator into both the depressor septae muscle as well as the dorsal component of the bilobed nasalis muscle. This latter treatment creates hyperkinesis in the untreated dilator nares portion of the nasalis muscle (**Fig. 34**) whose secondary function is to elevate the nasal tip.

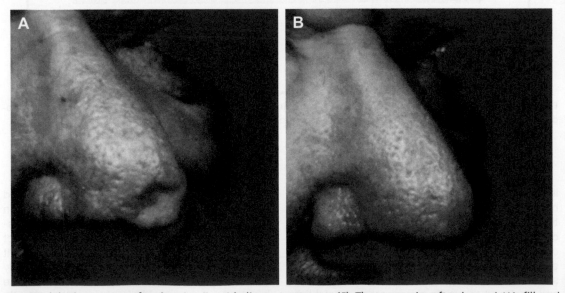

Fig. 32. (*A*) Three years after basal cell epithelioma treatment. (*B*) Three months after layered HA fill and secondary CO_2 laser treatment.

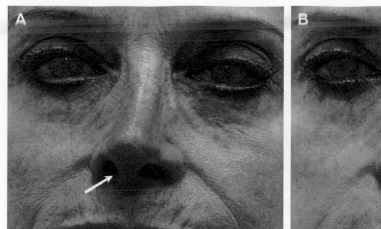
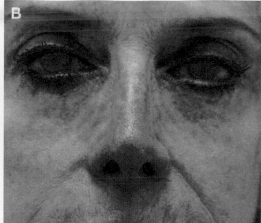

Fig. 33. Correction of a canted tip by submucosal placement of HA along the concave side of the curved anterior septum (*white arrow*). (*A*) Before treatment. (*B*) Immediately after treatment (0.4 mL).

Columella-Alar Complex

The skin of the nose is thinnest along the alar margins and columella, and shows skin-to-skin apposition. Retracted alae can be improved with the precise deposition of low G' HA between the dermal sheaths just below the leading edge of the lower lateral cartilage, making sure to maintain a symmetric gull-in-flight arc (**Fig. 35**).

Typical nasolabial angle in the female patient is around 95 to 110 degrees (see **Fig. 26**) with a 2-mm to 3-mm columellar show, which, when absent, can be created by the judicious use of higher G' product. Likewise, prominent medial crura causing a split columella can be softened in this fashion (see **Fig. 35**).

Nasal Base

Nasal base width should be approximately equal to the intercanthal distance (**Fig. 36**). In patients with mild to moderate excessive alar width, narrowing can be achieved by the deposition of high G' product on the pyriform fossa via microcannula technique (personal communication, Maurizio de Maio, 2009).

BEAUTI"PHI"ED LIPS

The stigma of the overinflated, disproportioned lip has permeated the media worldwide. The art of beautifying lips revolves around subtle enhancement and not just pure augmentation; treatment

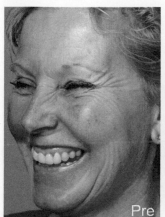
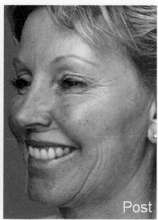
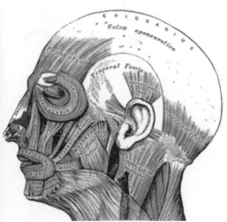

Fig. 34. Global facial treatment with neuromodulator including brow, crow's feet, glabella, gummy smile, nasalis, orbicularis oris, mentalis, and depressor anguli oris muscles. Although the depressor septae muscle was not treated, tip elevation occurred because of hyperkinesis of the dilator nares portion of the nasalis muscle (shown in figure on right).

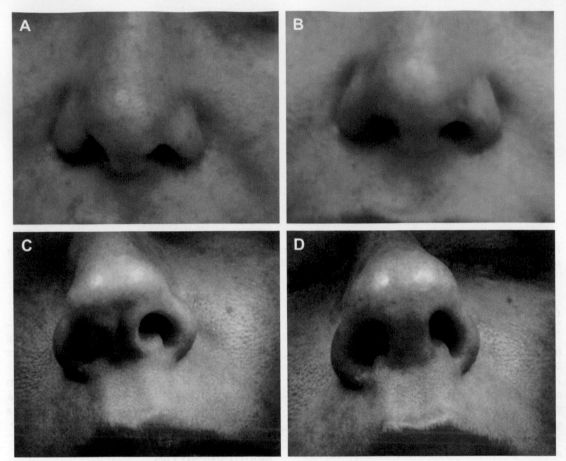

Fig. 35. Correction of retracted alae (*A*) with HA injections, maintaining the gull wing appearance (*B*). Softening of dome knuckles and split columella (*C*) with HA (*D*).

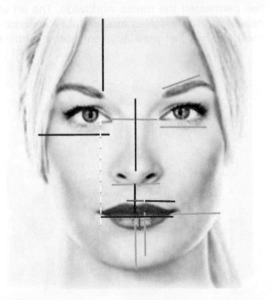

Fig. 36. Phi proportions in the face (see text). Green, x; blue, 1.618x (Phix); black, 0.618x (phix); orange, 0.382x (phi²x). Lip width of Phi correlates with a vertical line (*dotted white line*) dropped from the medial iris.

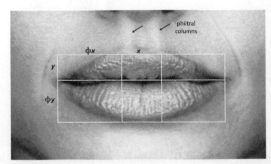

Fig. 37. Phi proportions in the lip (see text). Philtral columns are located just medial to the peaks of Cupid's bows.

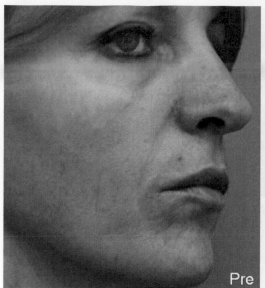 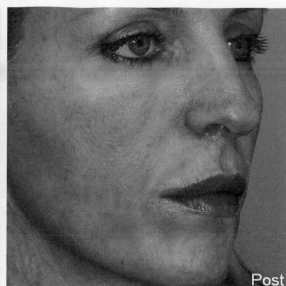

Fig. 38. Lip enhancement with HA (see text).

goals should include proper proportioning of vertical height and intercommissure width (lip length), as well as recreation of a distinct upper lip white roll.

Ideal Phi proportion (see **Fig. 36**; **Fig. 37**) for lip length maintains red vermilion show to a vertical line drawn down from the medial iris, or medial pupil in patients with prominent masseters and increased lower facial width. Vertical mucosal show in white women is also in the Phi proportion of 1 for the upper lip and 1.618 for the lower lip (Asian and African American vertical lip dimensions may approach 1:1). The ratios of the distance from Cupid's bow to Cupid's bow compared with Cupid's bow to the ipsilateral commissure is also 1/1.618. The distance between Cupid's bows is phi (0.618x) of the distance from columellar base to mid-upper lip vermilion border. The upper lip philtral columns are just inside the Cupid's bows (rather than aligned with them) in the youthful lip. Spreading and flattening of these columns with loss of upper lip pout is a common feature in the aging lip. Recreation of a lower philtral column just medial to the Cupid's bow can restore a youthful look to an aging lip. Injections are performed slowly, taking care to deposit very little product superiorly and more inferiorly where the philtral columns meet the vermilion tubercle (**Fig. 38**).

The ideal feminine youthful lower lip should be fuller but the upper lip should project more on profile by 1 to 2 mm. When enhancing the lips with fillers, the combination use of minidose neuromodulator to moderate accordion contraction of the orbicularis oris can often increase the longevity of the volume achieved.

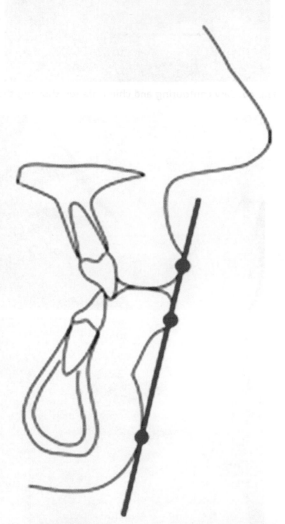

Fig. 39. Riedel plane: a line drawn tangentially through the anterior points of the lips (similar to Steiner line, which accounts for nasal projection).

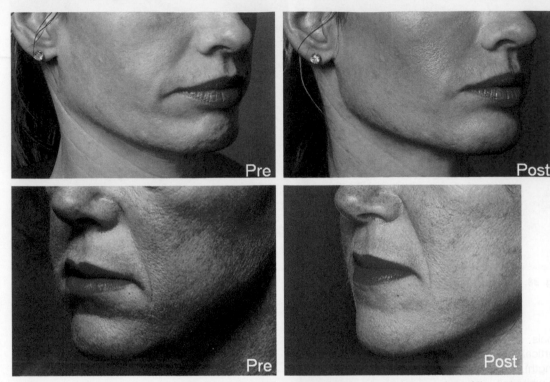

Fig. 40. Jaw contouring and chin reflation showing the synergy of neuromodulator and HA filler.

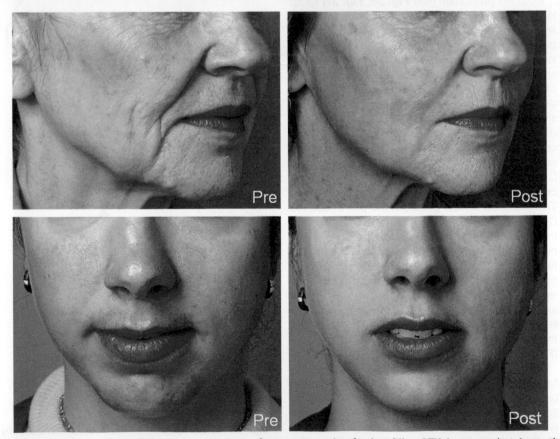

Fig. 41. Jaw contouring and chin reflation 1 year after treatment (no further filler; BTX-A repeated at 4-month intervals).

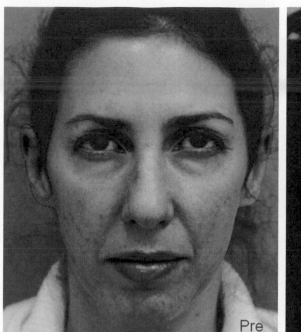
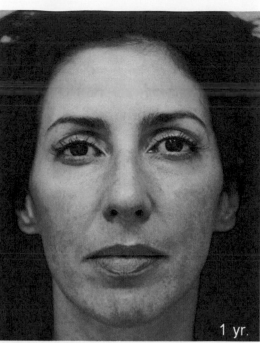

Fig. 42. BeautiPHIcation™: combination therapy result at 1 year. HA filler (midface, superior and inferior orbital rims, pyriform fossae, prejowl sulcii), panfacial neuromodulator (browlift, forehead, glabella, crow's feet, preseptal lower lids, mentalis, depressor angulae oris), microdermabrasion and ALA-aminolevulinic acid/IPL-intense pulsed light therapy, home skincare regimen. Result at 1 year (no further HA treatment; BTX-A repeated every 4 months).

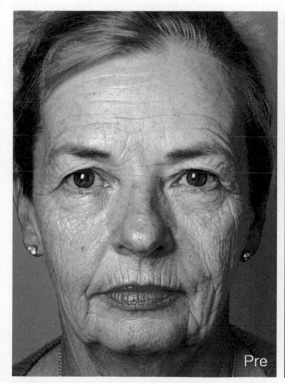
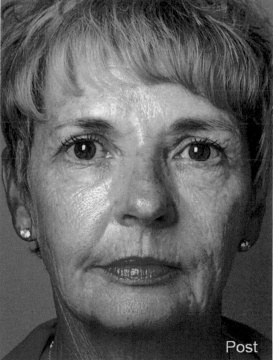

Fig. 43. BeautiPHIcation™: single-session global approach with neuromodulator (glabella, crow's feet, preseptal lower lids, depressor anguli oris, mentalis) and panfacial volume restoration (HA to glabellar creases, tear troughs, nasojugal grooves, cheeks, lateral oral commissures, marionette zones, prejowl sulci, chin, mental crease, eyebrows, postjowl sulci). Treatment followed 2 weeks later by full-face Sciton resurfacing; results shown at 4 weeks after laser treatment.

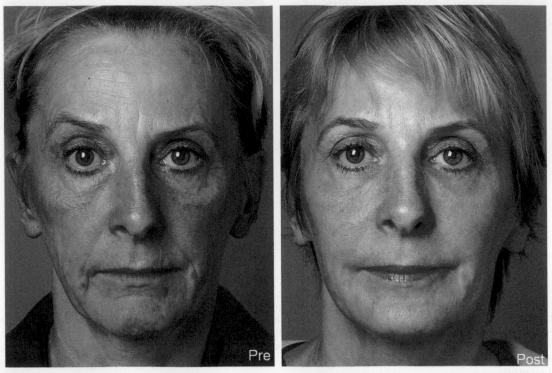

Fig. 44. BeautiPHIcation™: neuromodulator to glabella, crow's feet, preseptal lower lids, depressor anguli oris, depressor septae, nasalis, mentalis, neck (Nefertiti); HA fillers to glabellar creases, tear troughs, nasojugal grooves, cheeks, preauricular regions, eyebrows, lateral oral commissures, marionette zones, prejowl and post-jowl sulcii, chin, mental crease, and nose contouring. Result at 8 weeks.

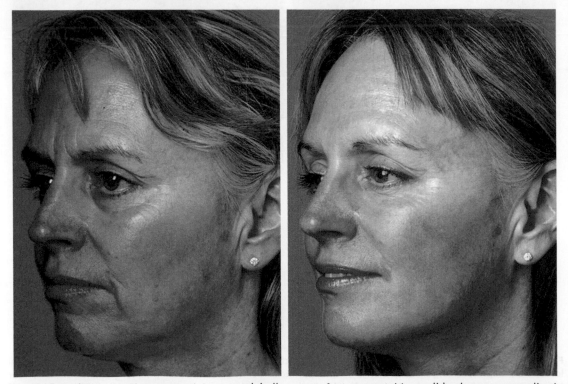

Fig. 45. BeautiPHIcation™: neuromodulator to glabella, crow's feet, preseptal lower lids, depressor anguli oris, mentalis, neck (Nefertiti); HA fillers to glabellar creases, tear troughs, nasojugal grooves, cheeks, eyebrows, lateral oral commissures, marionette zones, prejowl and postjowl sulcii, chin, and mental crease. Results at 3 months.

THE BEAUTI"PHI"ED CHIN

Chin deformities are the most common bony abnormality in the face, but even experienced injectors often focus on the prejowl sulci and overlook the opportunity to simultaneously address mild forms of microgenia and volume loss in the entire perioral region. Chin deflation and contour changes may start early, appearing sometimes in the third decade.

Many methods of analysis have been described to both classify and treat mild microgenia.[29] Just as with the other features discussed previously, the chin also follows the golden proportion in its facial relationships (see **Fig. 36**). As a general rule, anterior projection of the chin in women should be slightly behind or just at the Riedel plane, drawn tangentially through the anterior points of the upper and lower lips (**Fig. 39**).

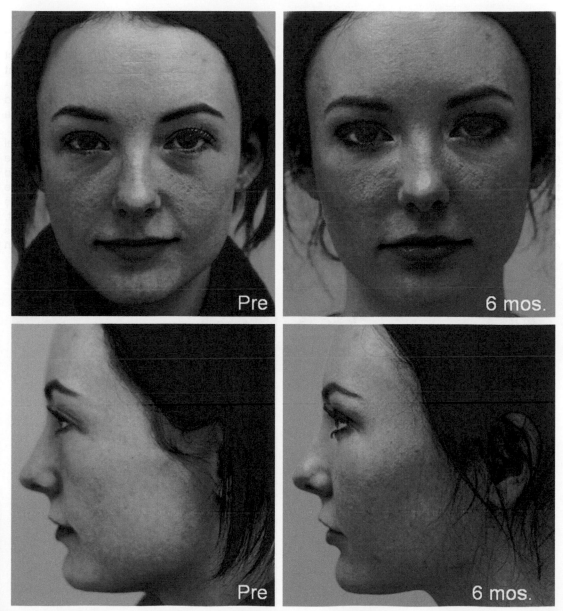

Pre

6 mos.

Pre

6 mos.

Fig. 46. BeautiPHIcation™: 6-month result with HA filler for tear troughs, lateral brows, cheek and chin enhancement.

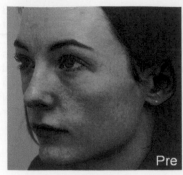
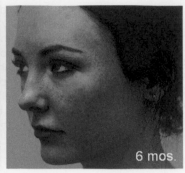
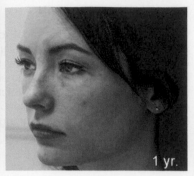

Fig. 47. BeautiPHIcation™: results at 6 months and 1 year follow-up; no additional treatment.

The chin plays a central role in facial beauty, harmony, and balance, especially through its relationship to the face in profile. The 3D aspect of projection, height, and width make the surgical planning of a genioplasty particularly difficult, whether by osteoplastic or alloplastic means. In many cases, inherent asymmetries in the region render these techniques incapable of properly addressing the underlying deformity. Surgical therapy often focuses purely on midchin projection and width with no attention paid to reflation and contouring of the lateral oral commissures, mental crease, marionette zones, and prejowl and postjowl sulcii. In perioral rejuvenation, it is not just the chin, and herein lies the distinct advantage of the physician injector skilled at percutaneous volume contouring as well as neuromodulator synergy to soften the associated apple core appearance, globally improving the entire perioral region (**Fig. 40**).

Historically the domain of the maxillofacial surgeon, chin augmentation is perfectly amenable to the physician injector using strategically placed depots of filler. Furthermore, depending on the product used and the depth of injection, it is our experience that, although not permanent, aesthetic results can last in excess of 12 months before further treatment is necessary (**Fig. 41**). In

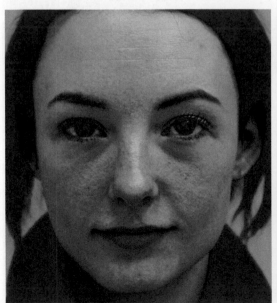
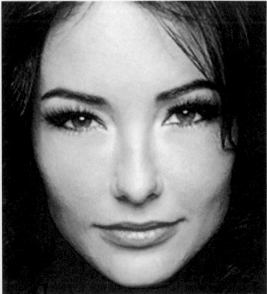

Fig. 48. BeautiPHIcation™: before and 2.5 years after treatment with makeup applied. No further filler since initial treatment except for lip enhancement.

the younger patient, maintenance of a youthful chin often requires little product, but the lateral oral commissure may require more attention because of the loss of structural support. However, the associated presence of severely altered dentoalveolar relationships is always better served by orthognathic surgery than by chin augmentation.

LEARN TO THINK IN COMBINEESE (THE LANGUAGE OF COMBINATION THERAPY)

The doctrine of BeautiPHIcation™, or any nonsurgical facial enhancement, is that it should be individualized, minimally invasive, result oriented, cost-effective, synergistic, and associated with minimal downtime, anxiety (for both the patient and physician), and pain. The art of bundling

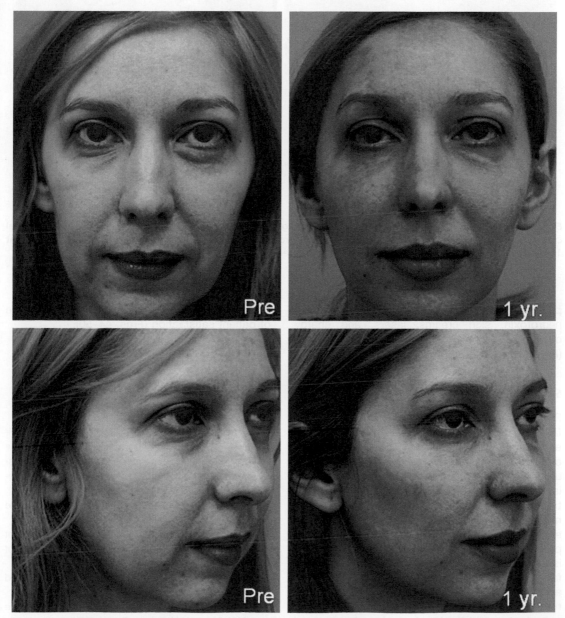

Fig. 49. BeautiPHIcation™: results at 1 year, single treatment with HA (tear troughs, cheeks, prejowl and postjowl sulcii, chin) and porcine collagen for lip phi proportion. Neuromodulator (BTX-A) given at 18-week intervals for browlift, periorbital dynamic lines, and chin.

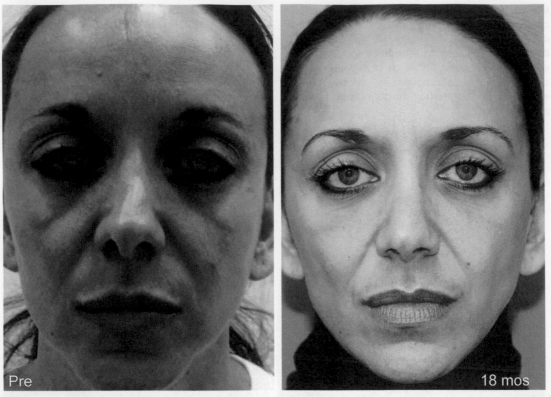

Fig. 50. BeautiPHIcation™: HA filler (cheeks, tear troughs, lateral brow, forehead, nose, prejowl sulcii, mental crease, lips, philtral columns) and neuromodulator (browlift, glabella, forehead, crow's feet, chin). Results at 18 months. Repeat treatment of BTX-A at 4-month intervals; HA enhancement of lips at 1 year.

products with procedures, of combining fillers, neurotoxin, skin creams, lasers, and energy devices, is where technology and creativity meet (**Figs. 42** and **43**).

SUMMARY

Phi Relationships can be approached for all facial features (see **Fig. 36**), and rely on the establishment of smooth ogee curves in all dimensions. As for the cheek, the use of cool ultrasound gel, which enhances proprioception, is beneficial to mold, blend, and feather all treated aesthetic zones and reveal areas that may require more attention. The point must be emphasized that having a plan and using pretreatment markings to achieve desired results is the critical element to volume restoration in the face. The aesthetic patient budgets to look great and is willing to pay for outstanding clinical results. Once goals have been determined and a budget established, a logical syntax is used to create an algorithm for selecting products and procedures. The methodology leads to

consistent and pleasing results with a high rate of patient satisfaction (**Figs. 44–50**).

REFERENCES

1. Millard DR. Principilization of plastic surgery. Boston: Lippincott Williams & Wilkins; 1987.
2. Cunningham MR, Roberts AR, Wu CH, et al. Their ideas of beauty are, on the whole, the same as ours": consistency and variability in the cross-cultural perception of female physical attractiveness. J Pers Soc Psychol 1995;68:261–79.
3. Jones D, Hill K. Criteria of facial attractiveness in five populations. Hum Nat 1993;4:271–96.
4. Langlois JH, Roggman LA, Casey RJ, et al. Infant preferences for attractive faces: rudiments of a stereotype? Dev Psychol 1987;23:363–9.
5. Available at: www.beautycheck.de/cmsms/. Accessed July, 2009.
6. Pacteau F. The symptom of beauty. Cambridge (MA): Harvard University Press; 1994.
7. Klopfer P. Sensory physiology and esthetics. Am Sci 1970;58:399.

8. Livio M. The golden ratio: the story of phi, the world's most astonishing number. New York: Broadway Books; 2002.

9. Ricketts R. The biologic significance of the divine proportion and Fibonacci series. Am J Orthod 1982;81(5):351–70.

10. Available at: www.beautyanalysis.com. Accessed July, 2009.

11. Bashour M. Is an objective measuring system for facial attractiveness possible? 2007. Available at: Dissertation.com. Accessed July, 2009.

12. Safran Ben. The mathematics of beauty: the divine proportion's effect on facial attractiveness. Providence: Brown University; 2007.

13. Rhodes G, Proffitt F, Grady JM, et al. Facial symmetry and the perception of beauty. Psychon Bull Rev 1998;5(4):659–69.

14. Brooks M, Pomiankowski A. Symmetry is in the eye of the beholder. Trends Ecol Evol 1994;9:201–2.

15. Concar D. Sex and the symmetrical body. New Sci 1995;146:40–4.

16. Enquist M, Arak A. Symmetry, beauty and evolution. Nature 1994;372:169–72.

17. Grammer K, Thornhill R. Human (*Homo sapiens*) facial attractiveness and sexual selection: the role of symmetry and averageness. J Comp Psychol 1994;108:233–42.

18. Swaddle JP, Cuthill IC. Asymmetry and human facial attractiveness: symmetry may not always be beautiful. Proceedings of the Royal Society of London: Series B. Proc Biol Sci 1995;261:111–6.

19. Carruthers J, Glogau RG, Blitzer A, et al. Advances in facial rejuvenation: botulinum toxin type a, hyaluronic acid dermal fillers, and combination therapies–consensus recommendations. Supplement to Plastic and Reconstructive Surgery. Plast Reconstr Surg 2008;121(5):5S–30S.

20. Liew S, Dart A. Non-surgical reshaping of the lower face. Aesthet Surg J 2008;28(3):251–7.

21. Raspaldo H. Volumizing effect of a new hyaluronic acid sub-dermal facial filler: a retrospective analysis based on 102 cases. J Cosmet Laser Ther 2008;10:134–42.

22. Coleman SR. Structural fat grafting. St Louis: Quality Medical Publishing; 2004.

23. Donofrio LM. Fat distribution: a morphologic study of the aging face. Dermatol Surg 2000;26:1107–12.

24. Carey W. Deep injection tri-site bolus technique. 2005. Available at: www.skinandallergynews.com. Accessed July, 2009.

25. Sheen J, Sheen A. Aesthetic rhinoplasty. 2nd edition. St Louis (MO): Quality Medical Publishing; 1997.

26. Hoefflin S. Esthetic rhinoplasty. New York: Springer-Verlag; 1998.

27. Peck G. Techniques in aesthetic rhinoplasty. New York: Gower Medical Publishing; 1984.

28. Danieal RK. Rhinoplasty, an atlas of surgical techniques. New York: Springer Science & Business; 2002.

29. Guyuron B, Michelou BJ, Willis L. Practical classification of chin deformities. Aesthetic Plast Surg 1995;19(3):257–64.

Volumizing the Face With Soft Tissue Fillers

Derek Jones, MD[a,b,*]

KEYWORDS

- Facial volumization • Facial fillers • Soft-tissue fillers
- Facial augmentation

Key Points

1. An array of injectable soft tissue fillers are now approved by the U.S. Food and Drug Administration (FDA). A complete understanding of their physicochemical properties and performance in clinical trials will aid in product selection and determining accurate volume requirements.
2. More robust fillers are used for deeper wrinkles, folds, and cheek or chin augmentation, whereas softer and less robust products, particularly hyaluronic acid (HA) products, are used for softer depressions and fine lines, periocularly, and for the lips. Often the best results occur with a combination of fillers.
3. Surgeons should use aesthetic responsibility when devising an injection treatment plan, and properly select fillers from a palate. Rather than focusing on one isolated cosmetic unit, a pan-facial approach is often best to create or restore proportion and harmony. Overvolumizing or exaggerating the proper proportions of the lips or cheeks should be avoided.

HYALURONIC ACIDS

As a person ages, the amount of HA in the skin is reduced, decreasing the skin's water-binding capacity and tissue turgor, leading to visible wrinkles and drooping skin. Degradation of HA is accelerated with sun exposure and aging. Injectable HA fillers are designed to restore the appearance of youth to the skin through replacing HA and binding water, thus reducing the appearance of sagging skin and skin folds.

Currently four HA fillers are FDA-approved: Juvederm Ultra and Ultra Plus (Allergan Inc, Irvine, CA, USA), Restylane/Perlane (Medicis, Scottsdale, AZ, USA), Prevelle Silk (Mentor, Irving, TX, USA), and Elevess (Anika Therapeutics, Woburn, MA, USA). Belotero (Merz, San Mateo, CA, USA) is expected to receive FDA approval shortly. Juvederm Voluma is currently under FDA review.

Several variables affect the performance of individual HA fillers, including the concentration of HA, degree of cross-linking, cohesivity, G' (elastic modulus), and particle size, which all interact to create the unique properties of a particular HA product. An understanding of these basic science variables will help readers differentiate among available products.

One of the most important determinants of the degree of correction obtained is the HA concentration, which is not a straightforward measurement. HAs are linear polysaccharide chains that must be chemically cross-linked to be stable in vivo. The concentration of HA, measured in milligrams per

a Division of Dermatology, David Geffen School of Medicine, University of California at Los Angeles, Los Angeles, CA, USA
b Skin Care and Laser Physicians of Beverly Hills, 9201 Sunset Boulevard #602, Los Angeles, CA 90069, USA
* Skin Care and Laser Physicians of Beverly Hills, 9201 Sunset Boulevard #602, Los Angeles, CA 90069.
E-mail address: derekjonesmd@gmail.com

Clin Plastic Surg 38 (2011) 379–390
doi:10.1016/j.cps.2011.03.011

milliliters, includes both cross-linked HA and free (non–cross-linked or soluble) HA, which is rapidly absorbed in vivo. Non–cross-linked HA is added to the various HA fillers as a lubricant to ease product flow through the needle, yet adds nothing to the final correction. It is best to think of concentration in terms of "effective HA concentration" (effective HA [EFA] = total HA – uncross-linked HA), which is a better measure of the HA that will contribute to tissue correction. The HA concentration also has important implications for long-term correction and initial reaction on injection. The hydrophilic nature of HA means that the more concentrated products will tend to imbibe more water, and thus have more tissue swelling after injection. After steady state equilibrium is reached with the surrounding tissue, more concentrated products will maintain more swelling and have more fullness in the area injected. Prevelle Silk, Restylane, Belotero, Juvederm, and Elevess contain 5.5, 20, 22, 24, and 28 mg/mL of HA, respectively.

When a dermal filler is implanted into or under the skin, the skin's natural elasticity or tension will tend to flatten out the implant, reducing the initial desired correction. The force of the filler that opposes and resists this tension determines the "lift capacity" of a dermal filler. Although complicated and multifactorial, lift capacity is partly directly related to two material properties of the HA gel, namely the elastic (also known as storage) modulus or G' (pronounced G-prime), and cohesivity. The lift capacity of an HA filler increases with higher values of both G' and cohesivity. G' is measured through placing a specific HA product between two metal plates (a parallel plate rheometer). The amount of resistance encountered by the top plate as it slides over the gel determines the G' for that gel and is affected by the degree of cross-linking between the chains, total HA concentration, and particle size and shape. More heavily cross-linked products tend to be stiffer and have a higher G', and are more difficult to push through a needle.[1–3] Often, HA products with a high G' will have higher amounts of free HA to serve as a lubricant and ease the product flow through small needles. Cohesivity, on the other hand, is related to a specific HA gel's ability to retain its shape on injection. A higher cohesivity value represents a higher resistance to deformation of the product. Of the products currently available in the United States, Prevelle Silk has the lowest concentration and lift capacity. Restylane, Juvederm, and Belotero products have a similar HA concentration and similar lift capacities, although the Restylane family, compared with the Juvederm family, relies on a higher G' to achieve lift, whereas Juvederm relies on higher cohesivity.

During manufacturing, HA gels are produced in large gelatinous blocks of cross-linked material. Once the gel blocks are manufactured, they must be reduced in size to pass through a syringe and needle. Pushing the gel block through a "screen" mechanism produces Restylane and Perlane, so that the final particles are of a similar size with standardized shapes. It has been hypothesized that the larger particles found in Perlane have a smaller surface to volume ratio that conveys longer duration of correction because of resistance to enzymatic breakdown by hyaluronidase. However, contradicting this is the fact that both Restylane and Perlane (which has larger-sized particles) have the same duration of correction in the nasolabial crease.[4] This property is believed to be from the porous nature of the particles that negates the surface area effects. A second way of sizing the gel block is *homogenization*, which is used for the Juvederm family of products.[1] Homogenization results in particles that are variable in size, and is partially responsible for the lower G' and extrusion force of the products. Belotero relies on a cohesive polydensified matrix that contains zones of HA that have different degrees of cross-linking, which results in a continuous gel that does not undergo particle formation before injection.

The most important aspect of injectable HAs is how they behave clinically. Prevelle Silk is a 5.5-mg/mL HA particle gel containing lidocaine, which decreases pain on injection. Compared with Restylane and Juvederm, it contains a much lower concentration of HA and is considered a "softer" HA filler with less lift capacity, and has an average duration of correction of approximately 3 months.[4] Because it is maximally saturated with water, it undergoes little swelling on injection, which limits edema, redness, and bruising. It is a niche filler for finer lines and for patients who desire a minimum of downtime and are willing to sacrifice duration of correction.

The pivotal FDA trials and extended-duration trials for Restylane, Juvederm, and Belotero all have produced similar data. Despite differences in G', cohesivity, concentration, cross-linking, and amounts of free HA, all three products seem to be capable of producing a similar result in the nasolabial fold (NLF). Specifically, randomized, split-face, double-blinded trials comparing each product with Zyplast collagen show that each product is superior to Zyplast at 6 months.[5–7] Furthermore, each of these fillers seems to be capable of achieving corrections that persist for up to a year or longer, particularly after repeat treatment. Extended-duration studies using repeat treatment with each product show that when given 6 months or more after initial optimal correction, less product is required to maintain optimal correction and that duration of correction becomes progressively longer with each retreatment.[8–10] This finding may be because of accumulation of product or HAs ability to produce neocollagenesis on fibroblast stretching. Proponents of Juvederm posit that the gel is smoother and more cohesive, with less swelling on injection, particularly in the lips. Proponents of Belotero cite histologic studies to argue that injection with Belotero results in a more even distribution of HA within the dermis and less inflammation on injection, resulting in less edema and redness, and that it is a product that performs well in fine lines without producing a Tyndall effect. These claims remain to be proven in well-designed head-to-head clinical trials comparing each product directly. Juvederm and Restylane are now available with admixed lidocaine, which has been proven to significantly reduce pain on injection.

Elevess is a 28-mg/mL HA filler that contains admixed lidocaine. It also contains sodium metabisulfite as an antioxidant and is contraindicated in patients with sulfite allergies. The FDA pivotal trial was a prospective, randomized, double-blinded, multicenter study comparing Cosmoplast with Elevess.[4] Results proved that, compared with Cosmoplast, less Elevess was required to achieve optimal correction. Compared with Cosmoplast, Elevess showed a statistically significant greater improvement in correction at 4 months but not at 6 months. Adverse events were similar, except that more bruising and swelling occurred with Elevess than with Cosmoplast. Anecdotal reports suggested that inflammatory reactions might be more common with Elevess, which may be because of its high concentration and cross-linking.

All currently FDA-approved HAs have only been studied in NLFs, and carry the specific indication on package inserts that they are approved for dermal injection for correction of moderate to severe facial wrinkles and folds, such as NLFs. Although not specifically FDA-approved, available HAs have been studied off-label for correction of glabellar rhytides, oral commissures (meilolabial folds), lips, mid-face volumizing, infraorbital or nasojugal grooves (tear troughs), and augmentation of the dorsal hand.[4]

Many signs of aging are caused by loss of subcutaneous fat in the malar and submalar cheek regions. Fillers, including HAs, may successfully volumize this area when injected appropriately. Juvederm Voluma is a newer category of injectable HA intended for midface volumizing when a high lift capacity and larger volumes are required. It incorporates HA that is of lower molecular weight (representing shorter chain lengths of HA), which allows for more effective cross-linking and results in a more viscous product with a robust lift capacity. Voluma is approved for use in Europe, Canada, and Australia. It is not yet FDA-approved, although FDA studies are underway. It is a 20-mg/mL HA of streptococcal origin with a higher lift capacity. It has a lower molecular weight and a higher cross-linking ratio than other available HAs. It will be indicated for subcutaneous/supraperiosteal injection for facial volumizing and contouring (**Figs. 1** and **2**).

Fillers must be injected in the subcutaneous or supraperiosteal plane when volumizing the midface. Intradermal or too-superficial injection may create persistent dermal contour irregularities. A recent study performed by Raspaldo[11] assessed effectiveness and safety of Voluma in maintaining increased volume in the malar area for up to 18 months posttreatment. Retrospective record data were analyzed for 102 patients (93 women, 9 men; mean age, 51.27 years) who received Voluma injected into the midface. All patients were assessed at baseline and 1 month, and 6 to 18 months postinjection. The Investigator Global Aesthetic Improvement assessment after 1 month and 6 to 18 months showed that most patients were "much" or "very much" improved. Investigator volume loss assessment confirmed that most patients were either stage 1 or 2 (normal or slight mid-facial atrophy) at 1 month posttreatment, which was maintained at 6 to 18 months. Patient efficacy assessment was "very good" or "good" in most cases. The study concluded that Voluma provides aesthetic improvements according to investigator and patient assessment for up to 18 months posttreatment, with an excellent safety profile. Other studies have also documented excellent results with Voluma for age-related and HIV-related mid-facial lipoatrophy.[12–15]

The safety profiles of currently FDA-approved HA fillers are good. The most common procedure- or device-related events are injection-site erythema, swelling, pain, and bruising, which all usually resolve within a few days. More serious complications can sometimes occur, but most can be avoided with appropriate injection techniques. Inappropriate and superficial placement are among the most frequent reasons for patient dissatisfaction. Too-superficial placement of HA in the dermis can result in a Tyndall effect, which is a blue discoloration caused by the refraction of light from the clear gel visible superficially in the skin. To avoid superficial injection, the metal barrel

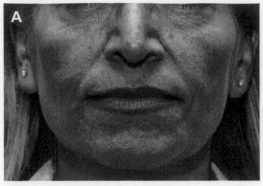
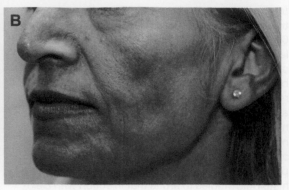

Fig. 1. (*A, B*) Before Voluma. (*Courtesy of* Nowell Solish, MD.)

of the needle should not be visible through the skin in the plane of injection when injecting in a linear fashion.

True hypersensitivity to injectable HA is rare, and occurring approximately 1 in 5000 cases. Infection is also uncommon and can usually be managed with either antibiotics or antivirals, depending on the clinical features. Injection of HA into the perioral area can potentiate recurrence of herpes simplex virus (HSV), and patients prone to recurrent perioral HSV should receive appropriate antiviral prophylaxis before treatment. The most worrisome complication is cutaneous necrosis, which is most commonly caused by occlusion of vascular structures through inadvertent injection of HA intravascularly, or through sidewall compression of vascular structures from overvolumizing of the surrounding soft tissue. The supratrochlear artery in the glabellar area and the angular artery in the superior NLF are particularly susceptible, and these areas should be considered high risk. The injecting physician should have masterful knowledge of vascular structures in areas of injection (**Fig. 3**). A protocol to treat the full spectrum of cutaneous necrosis was recently reviewed by Hirsch and colleagues.[16]

Because of the reversibility of HA, complications from these fillers can be easily corrected. The use of ovine testicular hyaluronidase (Vitrase) can dissolve injected HA, which is highly useful if the product is misplaced,[17] if a complication occurs postinjection (eg, vascular occlusion, delayed granulomatous reactions)[17] or if there is impending vascular necrosis.[16] A recent in vitro study proves that more hyaluronidase is required to dissolve Juvederm than Restylane.[18] In the author's experience, 10 units of hyaluronidase per 0.1 mL of Juvederm or 5 units per 0.1 mL of Restylane to be dissolved is the most appropriate dose (**Fig. 4**). The need for the greater amount of hyaluronidase for Juvederm is probably because the product is more highly cross-linked and the randomly shaped particles are more cohesive.

CALCIUM HYDROXYLAPATITE

Calcium hydroxylapatite (CaHA), marketed as Radiesse (Merz/BioForm, San Mateo, CA, USA) is a normal component of human bone and teeth and has been used as implant or coating material in dentistry and other therapeutic areas for more than 20 years. The filler is composed of CaHA

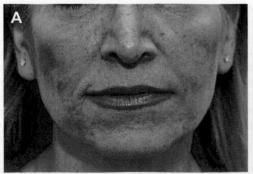
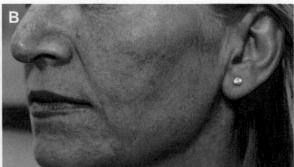

Fig. 2. (*A, B*) After Voluma. (*Courtesy of* Nowell Solish, MD.)

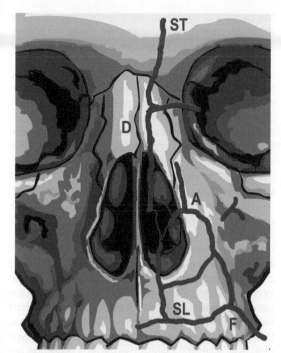

Fig. 3. Facial arteries and their anastomoses. A, angular artery; D, dorsal nasal artery; F, facial artery; SL, superior labial artery; ST, supratrochlear artery.

microspheres (25–45 μm) suspended in an aqueous carboxymethylcellulose gel carrier. As the gel is phagocytized, the process of neocollagenesis begins in and around the microspheres, stimulating the gradual growth of the patient's own collagen.[19] The spherical CaHA particles are gradually broken down and degraded via normal metabolic processes, and eliminated as calcium and phosphate ions through the urinary system. The proliferation of collagen along with the slow breakdown of the CaHA is understood to account for the

product's prolonged effects lasting a year or more.[20] It is approved for the treatment of moderate to severe wrinkles and folds, including NLFs, and correction of HIV-associated facial lipoatrophy. It is also indicated for vocal fold insufficiency, oral/maxillofacial defects, and radiographic tissue marking. Off-label facial uses also include correction of marionette lines and oral commissures, the prejowl sulcus, midface volume loss, dorsal nasal deformities, and chin augmentation. CaHA is not appropriate for use in the lips. Skin testing is not required.

CaHA was compared with a human collagen product in a United States pivotal trial of 117 subjects with moderate to severe NLFs. These patients were randomized to receive CaHA on one side of the face and an existing human collagen product (Cosmoplast, Inamed, Santa Barbara, CA, USA) on the other. CaHA provided significantly longer correction than human collagen, with 94.6% of folds graded improved, much improved, or very much improved, compared with 2.7% for human collagen. The adverse event profile was similar to that of human collagen.[21] Adverse events were limited to erythema, edema, and ecchymosis. Edema and bruising were more common on the CaHA-treated sides than those treated with human collagen ($P<.0001$). Edema and bruising lasted approximately 1 week after any injection, and the average duration for erythema was 2 to 3 weeks, with no significant difference between the materials. One nongranulomatous nodule was observed with CaHA versus three with human collagen. All adverse events resolved without sequelae. Another found longer-lasting results and increased satisfaction with CaHA compared with two HA products.[22]

A recent study examined whether the addition of anesthetic agents (such as lidocaine) to prefilled

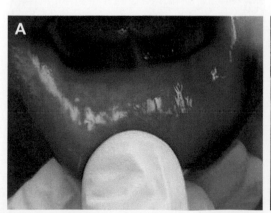

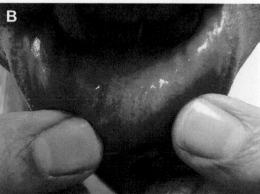

Fig. 4. (A) Before Vitrase. (B) After 10 units Vitrase injected to dissolve an estimated 0.1-mL mucosal nodule secondary to Juvederm Ultra.

CaHA syringes might provide sufficient anesthetic prophylaxis to reduce the need for conventional nerve blocks. The study showed that lidocaine can be added to CaHA syringes safely without harmful changes in the physical properties of the original soft tissue filler.[23] Admixing lidocaine into CaHA at treatment was recently FDA-approved and is described on the package insert.

Radiographic studies have found that CaHA is not consistently evident on x-ray but is clearly visible on CT scans. However, CaHA is unlikely to be confused with usual abnormal and normal radiographic findings. Although usually visible on CT scans, its appearance is distinct from surrounding bony structures, does not obscure underlying structures, and does not interfere with normal analysis.[24]

CaHA should be injected in small amounts in a retrograde fashion into the immediate subcutaneous plane or epiperiosteal plane, using a linear retrograde tunneling technique. Crosshatched linear threading may be also used. Overcorrection should be avoided. The nondominant index finger should be used to guide the needle, and the thumb and forefinger used to mold the product and remove any contour irregularities. CaHA should be injected very slowly in long, linear microthreads of approximately 0.05 mL per pass. Extreme caution should be taken when injecting into the subdermal plane around the superior NLF, where the angular artery and branches are present. Occlusion of this vessel can occur via external compression from CaHA or through injection of CaHA directly into the lumen of the vessel, creating embolic ischemia and tissue necrosis of

the nasal alar region along the distribution of the angular arteries or its branches. Reports of alar vascular necrosis have been reported to the author, and the superior NLF should be considered a high risk area not only for CaHA but also for all injectable fillers. Care should also be taken not to inject CaHA epiperiosteally near the infraorbital nerve, because cases of prolonged anesthesia and paresthesia in the distribution of the infraorbital nerve have occurred with this approach.

CaHA is an excellent cheek, midface, and chin volumizer (**Fig. 5**). It is particularly important to use a sufficient volume of CaHA to treat HIV-related lipoatrophy and more advanced stages of facial lipoatrophy associated with age or lean body mass. Although previous studies have shown different efficacy end points, such as photographic documentation of global improvement and change in mean skin thickness using ultrasound or skin calipers, treatment of HIV facial lipoatrophy often falls short of optimal correction in clinical practice. In a recent study on CaHA for HIV facial lipoatrophy, the authors defined optimal correction as "very much improved" on the Global Aesthetic Improvement Score (GAIS) scale (indicating a touch up is not required) and sought to determine the volume necessary to achieve optimal correction. Using a mean cumulative volume of 13.4 mL of CaHA, 80% of patients in this study achieved the top GAIS score of "very much improved" at 3 months and 59% did so at 6 months, compared with 26% at 3 months and 7% at 6 months in a similar study that used only a mean cumulative volume of 8.4 mL of CaHA.[25,26]

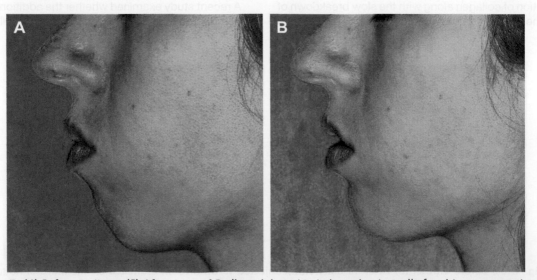

Fig. 5. (*A*) Before Radiesse. (*B*) After 1-mL of Radiesse injected in bolus epiperiosteally for chin augmentation.

POLY-L-LACTIC ACID

Poly-L-lactic acid (PLA) is a synthetic polymer that is biodegradable and resorbable. Injectable PLA (Sculptra, Sanofi-Aventis U.S. LLC) consists of microparticles of PLA in a sodium carboxymethyl-cellulose gel. The filler must be reconstituted with sterile water before administration. No skin test is required. The FDA approved PLA in 2004 for the treatment of HIV-related facial lipoatrophy. More recently it was FDA-approved for use in immuno-competent people as a treatment for deep NLFs and facial wrinkles.

PLA is administered into the subcutaneous plane. There, the suspension of reconstituted PLA provides mechanical correction and filling. Immediate volumizing is mostly from fluid, which becomes absorbed over a few days. Over weeks to months, the PLA microparticles are gradually degraded, while treated areas undergo subtle volume expansion via neocollagenesis as the host tissue responds to the PLA.[27] Monthly injections of one to two vials into the subcutis over many treatments (four to six is usual) often restore subcutaneous volume (**Fig. 6**). Correction of subcutaneous fat loss often lasts for 12 to 24 months. After this time, patients will often seek re-injection. In the author's experience, PLA is often not successful in treating more advanced cases of HIV-associated facial lipoatrophy.

PLA was initially approved through a fast-track process—an accelerated review procedure often used for HIV drugs. Efficacy and safety data for the approval were derived from physician-sponsored Investigational Device Exemption studies in the United States[28] and the European VEGA study. The VEGA study followed up 50 patients treated with PLA for 96 weeks.[29] Patients with HIV-associated facial lipoatrophy received four sets of injections: on day 0, and then every 2 weeks for 6 weeks. Patients were evaluated using clinical examination, facial ultrasonography, and photography. At entry, the median facial fat thickness was 0 mm. The median total cutaneous thickness increased significantly from baseline (up to 7.2 mm at weeks 48 and 72). By week 96, the median total thickness was 6.8 mm. No significant adverse events were observed. In 22 (44%) patients, palpable but nonvisible subcutaneous nodules were observed, which tended to resolve spontaneously with time. The study did not use ratings of pretreatment and posttreatment photographs by experienced physicians not performing the treatment to measure whether optimal correction with complete restoration of cheek contours was achieved.

PLA was approved for aesthetic use in 2009, based on the results of a randomized, evaluator-blinded, parallel group, multicenter trial of 233 immunocompetent patients using a 5-mL dilution per vial, a 2-hour hydration time, and a deep dermal grid pattern injection technique to place product in the NLF in multiple treatment sessions (up to 4 total) placed 3 weeks apart.[30] Collagen was used as the comparator in the contralateral NLF. Sculptra Aesthetic showed better improvement over the collagen control, with a statistically significant improvement from baseline in the Wrinkle Assessment Score at the 13-month follow-up and at all time points after week 3. The mean cumulative volume and number of Sculptra treatments required to reach optimal correction

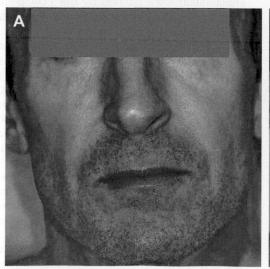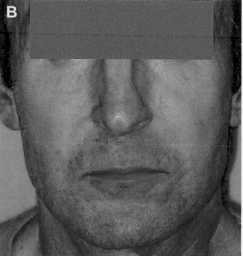

Fig. 6. (*A*) Before PLA. (*B*) After five treatments with PLA (10 vials) over 4 months.

for one NLF was 11.7 mL (5-mL dilution per vial) over 3.2 treatment sessions, whereas the mean cumulative volume and number of collagen treatments required to reach optimal correction for one NLF was 6.2 mL over 2.6 treatments. The results also show that Sculptra Aesthetic is associated with a gradual improvement of the NLF, with a time to peak correction of 192.7 days. During the extension phase study (19 and 25 months follow-up), most patients treated with Sculptra Aesthetic continued to show improvements in the Wrinkle Assessment Score without retreatment.[31] The adverse event profiles of the two products were considered similar, although in the controlled phase study of 0 to 13 months, 17.2% of patients treated with Sculptra Aesthetic experienced nodules or papules compared with 12.8% in the Cosmoplast control group. The mean onset of nodules and papules in the Sculptra Aesthetic treatment group was 209 and 159 days, respectively, and the mean duration was 180 and 176 days, respectively. Most nodules and papules resolved spontaneously (Sculptra Aesthetic Package Insert, July 2009). One patient in the Sculptra group required intralesional cortisone to resolve a nodule.

In addition to the adverse events in the VEGA study, persistent granulomatous reactions have been observed.[32] PLA should be injected into the subdermal plane, not into the dermis, to limit the likelihood of nodule and papule development. Red, palpable, persistent dermal nodules may occur with intradermal injection. Dermal defects are better treated with an HA filler. In the author's experience, a linear retrograde technique, with a crosshatching approach, should be used with a 25-gauge, 1- or 2-in needle. Smaller-bore needles tend to become easily clogged. Practitioners should use 1-mL tuberculin syringes, and shake the solution well first before transferring to the syringe and then again immediately before injection. The 25-gauge needle entry site may be anesthetized with small intradermal injections of 1% lidocaine with epinephrine through a 30-gauge needle, resulting in tolerable injections. Intravascular injection should be avoided; the angular artery runs in the immediate subdermal plane in the area of the superior NLF. Injection of the parotid duct, which overlies the buccinator muscle in the lateral cheek, should also be avoided. Outlining the treatment area before injection is also helpful. The treated area must not extend above the inferior orbital rim. To prevent contour irregularity and visible or palpable nodules, the product must be injected epiperiosteally in small amounts in the infraorbital area, deep to the muscle layer, using a serial puncture technique. However, care should

be taken not to inject epiperiosteally at the infraorbital foramen, which is positioned in the mid-pupillary line approximately 1 cm inferior to the lower orbital rim. Patients should also be made aware that the immediate posttreatment appearance will fade within 2 to 4 days. This instantaneous effect is caused by fluid from the filler, which produces edema on injection. Optimal augmentation will become apparent after multiple treatments at 3- to 4-week intervals, as new collagen is regenerated.[27] The reconstituted vial should be shaken vigorously immediately before transfer into the syringe, because settling of the product in the syringe may lead to uneven application and contribute to nodule formation.[27] Patients should be instructed to frequently massage the treated area in the days to weeks after the procedure to prevent the formation of uneven or lumpy fibroplasia. Some advocate the "rule of 5s," whereby the patient massages the area for 5 minutes, 5 times daily, for 5 days after the injection.

PLA's effect is subtle, and many treatments may be required to reach optimal correction. Duration is generally 1 to 2 years.

PERMANENT FILLERS
Liquid Silicone

Liquid injectable silicone (LIS) was first used as an injectable filler in the 1950s. Before collagen injectable fillers became available in the early 1980s, LIS was the preferred injectable filler. No standardized FDA-approved product existed and many products of varying purity were injected often in large bolus form, which led to frequent product migration and foreign body reactions. Subsequently, in the early 1990s, all forms of silicone for cosmetic implantation were banned by the FDA because of possible toxicity and systemic reactions related to LIS and silicone breast implants.

In the late 1990s, after the FDA resolved safety issues regarding implantable and LIS, two new forms of highly purified LIS were approved (Silikon-1000 and Adatosil-5000) for use as intraocular implants to tamponade retinal detachment. Although this use is the only official indication for LIS, the FDA Modernization Act of 1997 makes off-label uses legal, provided that the physician or drug manufacturer does not advertise the use. LIS is now used off-label for soft-tissue augmentation. Silikon-1000 has a lower viscosity and is the most suitable for injectable soft tissue augmentation, because it is easier to inject through smaller-gauge needles.

Current opinion on LIS is polarized between opponents and advocates. Opponents argue that despite use of proper technique and products, serious adverse events are common and unpredictable. Proponents rely on a wealth of anecdotal data to argue that LIS is safe and effective as long as three rules are followed:

1. Highly purified FDA-approved LIS is used.
2. Microdroplet serial puncture technique (defined as 0.01 mL per injection site injected into the subdermal plane) is used.
3. Small volumes (0.5 mL for smaller defects and up to 2 mL for larger areas of atrophy) are used at each session, with multiple sessions staged at monthly intervals or longer.

After LIS is injected, a capsule of new collagen develops to encircle each microdroplet of silicone. This process continues for approximately 3 months, during which time the collagen capsule adds volume to the augmentation of the LIS microdroplet. The collagen also holds the droplets in place to prevent migration. Although LIS is used off-label for many indications, the author believes that LIS should not be routinely used for the average cosmetic patient until longer-term studies with current products resolve some of the controversy regarding long-term safety and efficacy. However, for the unique and disfiguring defects associated with HIV facial lipoatrophy and serious acne scarring, LIS produces cosmetically superior and more durable results than currently available less-permanent options.

LIS has been shown to be an excellent choice for HIV-associated facial lipoatrophy (**Fig. 7**). In one trial, highly purified 1000-cSt silicone oil was studied among 77 patients to determine the number of treatments, amount of silicone, and time required to reach complete correction. Patients received 2 mL of Silikon 1000 at monthly

intervals using the microdroplet technique until optimal correction was achieved. The researchers elucidated two important findings: that all three of these parameters were directly related to the initial severity of lipoatrophy, and that highly purified 1000-cSt silicon oil is a safe and effective treatment option for HIV-associated lipoatrophy.[33]

More recently, the author reported on 135 patients followed up for 5 years and beyond after treatment with highly purified LIS for HIV-associated facial lipoatrophy,[34] and concluded that LIS is a safe and effective long-term treatment option for HIV-associated facial lipoatrophy. Once optimal correction is achieved, a subset of patients will experience progressive facial lipoatrophy and require touch-up treatment, but the number of treatments and amount of filler required to maintain optimal correction is less than what is expected with less-permanent treatment options. Of the 135 patients, 4 experienced late-onset firm localized subcutaneous induration, which was generally palpable but not visible and considered moderate in severity. All experienced complete response to intralesional triamcinolone and oral minocycline. The specific histories of each patient support a bacterial and immunologic basis for these reactions.

Using the microdroplet, multiple-injection technique, Barnett and Barnett[35] had success with injections of LIS for acne scars, which lasted over follow-up periods of 10, 15, and 30 years.

Clinicians should inject only highly purified FDA-approved LIS, such as Silikon-1000, using the microdroplet serial puncture technique ($\leq$0.01 mL injected through a 27-gauge needle into the immediate subdermal plane at 2- to 4-mm intervals). Intradermal injections should be avoided, because these may create intradermal

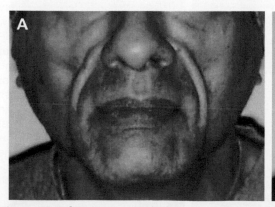
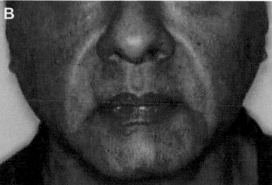

Fig. 7. (*A*) Before LIS for HIV facial lipoatrophy. (*A, B*) 5 years after correction with more than 30 mL of highly purified LIS, applied in 2-mL increments over multiple monthly sessions with microdroplet serial puncture technique.

papules.[36] However, intradermal injections may be used for atrophic dermal acne scars, using 0.001-mL microdroplets. Very small amounts of LIS should be injected at monthly intervals, or longer. The immediate goal is undercorrection. Optimal correction occurs slowly as fibroplasia develops around the microdroplets, creating further tissue augmentation and anchoring each microdroplet into place.

POLYMETHYLMETHACRYLATE

Injectable polymethylmethacrylate (PMMA) (Artefill, Suneva, San Diego, California) is a suspension of 20% PMMA smooth microspheres in 80% bovine collagen. Artefill is the product of third-generation PMMA microsphere technology. Previous generations include Arteplast (used in Germany from 1989–1994) and Artecoll (used worldwide, except in the United States and Japan, from 1994–2006). Artefill represents a third-generation product containing fewer nanoparticles (<20 μm), which were thought to be associated with granulomatous reactions observed with previous generations. Artefill was approved by the FDA in 2006 for the correction of NLFs (**Fig. 8**).

After PMMA is injected, the collagen vehicle is absorbed within 1 to 3 months. Afterward, new collagen is deposited by the host to encapsulate and engulf the remaining estimated 6 million PMMA particles in 1 mL of Artefill. This process contributes to tissue augmentation through fibroplasia. Although the collagen is absorbed, the PMMA is permanent and not reabsorbed. Injectable PMMA is indicated for NLFs. It is also used off-label for glabellar frown lines, radial lip lines, and mouth corners. Injectable PMMA is contraindicated for use in patients with a positive result to the required Artefill skin test, severe allergies (as indicated by a history of anaphylaxis or multiple severe allergies), known lidocaine hypersensitivity, a history of allergies to bovine collagen products, and known susceptibility to keloid or hypertrophic scarring. The product should not be used for lip augmentation.

The pivotal clinical trial for Artefill was a controlled, randomized, prospective, double-masked trial of 251 patients at eight centers in the United States. Patients received either Artefill or bovine collagen dermal filler (control). Efficacy was rated by masked observers using a photographic Facial Fold Assessment Scale. At 6 months, the study showed a significant improvement in NLFs in patients treated with Artefill compared with the control group (P<.001). A subset of patients observed at 12 months all showed persistent wrinkle correction.[37] A subgroup of 69 patients returned for follow-up 4 to 5 years later, at which time Investigator Facial Fold Assessment ratings were improved from baseline by 1.67 points (P<.001). Nearly all subjects (95.5%) reported that they were at least somewhat satisfied, and 81.8% reported that they were either satisfied or very satisfied.[38] Five patients reported six late adverse events that occurred from 2 to 5 years after the initial injection. Of these, four were mild cases of lumpiness, and two were severe. The total number of late adverse events was 6 of 272 (2.2%) wrinkles injected. Granulomatous reactions (manifested by inflamed red nodules) may be treated with intralesional cortisone combined with antibiotic therapy.

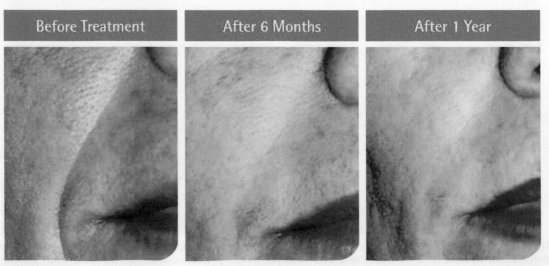

Before Treatment   **After 6 Months**   **After 1 Year**

Fig. 8. Artefill.

Injectable PMMA is placed into the dermal–subcutaneous junction or deeper using the tunneling or linear threading technique with a 26-gauge, 5/8-in needle. Overcorrection is not recommended. Superficial injection, which can cause permanent skin surface texture or color impairment, should be avoided.

Patients should be evaluated 4 to 6 weeks after injection to determine the need for further treatments. Optimal correction usually requires two to three treatments, and touch-up implantations should be at intervals of at least 2 weeks or longer, depending on the amount of implant used, the site of placement, and the dynamics of the corrected sites.

Success with Artefill was also recently described in atrophic acne scars, HIV-associated lipoatrophy, and malar augmentation.[39–41]

REFERENCES

1. Tezel A, Fredrickson GH. The science of hyaluronic acid dermal fillers. J Cosmet Laser Ther 2008; 10(1):35–42.
2. Falcone SJ, Berg RA. Crosslinked hyaluronic acid dermal fillers: a comparison of rheological properties. J Biomed Mater Res A 2008;87(1):264–71.
3. Collins MN, Birkinshaw C. Physical properties of cross-linked hyaluronic acid hydrogels. J Mater Sci Mater Med 2008;19(11):3335–434.
4. Jones D, Flynn T. Hyaluronic acids: clinical applications. In: Jones D, editor. Injectable fillers: principles and practice. Chichester (UK): Wiley-Blackwell; 2010. p. 158–74.
5. Narins RS, Brandt F, Leyden J, et al. A randomized, double-blind, multicenter comparison of the efficacy and tolerability of Restylane versus Zyplast for the correction of nasolabial folds. Dermatol Surg 2003; 29(6):588–95.
6. Baumann L, Lupo M, Monheit G, et al. Comparison of smooth-gel hyaluronic acid dermal fillers with cross-linked bovine collagen: a multicenter, double-masked, randomized, within-subject study. Dermatol Surg 2007;33(Suppl 2):S128–35.
7. Narins R, Coleman W, Donofrio L, et al. Nonanimal sourced hyaluronic acid-based dermal filler using a cohesive polydensified matrix technology is superior to bovine collagen in the correction of moderate to severe nasolabial folds: results from a 6-month, randomized, blinded, controlled, multicenter study. Dermatol Surg 2010;36(1):730–40.
8. Narins RS, Brandt FS, Baldwin EK. Persistence and improvement of nasolabial fold correction with nonanimal-stabilized hyaluronic acid 100,000 gel particles/mL filler on two retreatment schedules: results up to 18 months on two retreatment schedules. Dermatol Surg 2008;34(Suppl 1):S2–8.
9. Smith S, Jones D, Thomas J, et al. Duration of correction following repeat treatment with Juvederm hyaluronic acid fillers. Arch Dermatol Res 2010;302: 757–62.
10. Narins R, Coleman W, Donofrio L, et al. Improvement in moderate to severe nasolabial folds with a cross-linked non-animal stabilized hyaluronic acid filler utilizing a cohesive polydensified matrix technology (CPMHA): results from an open-label extension trial. Dermatol Surg 2010;36:730–40.
11. Raspaldo H. Volumizing effect of a new hyaluronic acid sub-dermal facial filler: a retrospective analysis based on 102 cases. J Cosmet Laser Ther 2008; 10(3):134–42.
12. Bechara F, Gambichler T, Brockmeyer N, et al. Hyaluronic acid new formulation: experience in HIV-associated facial lipoatrophy. Dermatology 2008; 217:244–9.
13. Hoffman K. Volumizing effects of a smooth, highly cohesive, viscous 20-mg/mL hyaluronic acid volumizing filler: prospective European study. BMC Dermatol 2009;9:9.
14. Carruthers J, Carruthers A. Volumizing with a 20 mg/mL smooth, highly cohesive, viscous hyaluronic acid filler and its role in facial rejuvenation therapy. Dermatol Surg 2010;36(3):1886–92.
15. Jones DA. New option for facial volume: volumizing with a 20 mg/mL smooth, highly cohesive, viscous hyaluronic acid filler and its role in facial rejuvenation therapy. Dermatol Surg 2010;36(3):1893–4.
16. Hirsch R, Carruthers J, Cohen J. Successful management of an unusual presentation of impending necrosis following a hyaluronic acid injection embolus and a proposed algorithm for management with hyaluronidase. Dermatol Surg 2007;33(3):357–60.
17. Brody HJ. Use of hyaluronidase in the treatment of granulomatous hyaluronic acid reactions or unwanted hyaluronic acid misplacement. Dermatol Surg 2005;31(8):893–7.
18. Jones D, Tezel A, Borrell M. In vitro resistance to degradation of hyaluronic acid fillers by ovine testicular hyaluronidase. Dermatol Surg 2010;36(1):804–9.
19. Coleman KM, Voights R, DeVore DP, et al. Neocollagenesis after injection of calcium hydroxylapatite composition in a canine model. Dermatol Surg 2008;34:S53–5.
20. Berlin AL, Hussain M, Goldberg DJ. Calcium hydroxylapatite filler for facial rejuvenation: a histologic and immunohistochemical analysis. Dermatol Surg 2008;34:S64–7.
21. Smith S, Busso M, McClaren M, et al. A randomized, bilateral, prospective comparison of calcium hydroxylapatite microspheres versus human-based collagen for the correction of nasolabial folds. Dermatol Surg 2007;33:S112–21.
22. Moers-Carpi M, Vogt S, Santos BM, et al. A multicenter, randomized trial comparing calcium

hydroxylapatite to two hyaluronic acids for treatment of nasolabial folds. Dermatol Surg 2007;33:S144–51.

23. Busso M, Voigts R. An investigation of changes in physical properties of injectable calcium hydroxylapatite in a carrier gel when mixed with lidocaine and with lidocaine/epinephrine. Dermatol Surg 2008;34:S16–23.

24. Carruthers A, Liebeskind M, Carruthers J, et al. Radiographic and computed tomographic studies of calcium hydroxylapatite for treatment of HIV-associated facial lipoatrophy and correction of nasolabial folds. Dermatol Surg 2008;34:S78–84.

25. Carruthers A, Carruthers J. Evaluation of injectable calcium hydroxylapatite for the treatment of facial lipoatrophy associated with human immunodeficiency virus. Dermatol Surg 2008;34:1486–99.

26. Silvers SL, Eviatar JA, Eschavez MI, et al. Prospective, open-label, 18-month trial of calcium hydroxylapatite (Radiesse) for facial soft-tissue augmentation in patients with human immunodeficiency virus-associated lipoatrophy: one year durability. Plast Reconstr Surg 2006;118:34S–45S.

27. Jones D, Vleggaar D. Technique for injecting poly-L-lactic acid. J Drugs Dermatol 2007;6:S13–7.

28. Mest DR, Humble G. Safety and efficacy of poly-l-lactic acid injections in persons with HIV-associated facial lipoatrophy. The US experience. Dermatol Surg 2006;32:1336–45.

29. Valantin MA, Aubron-Olivier C, Ghosn J, et al. Polylactic acid implants (New-Fill) to correct facial lipoatrophy in HIV-infected patients: results of the open-label study VEGA. AIDS 2003;17:2471–7.

30. Narins R, Bauman L, Brandt F, et al. A randomized study of the efficacy and safety of injectable poly-l-lactic acid versus human-based collagen implant in the treatment of nasolabial fold wrinkles. J Am Acad Dermatol 2010;62:448–62.

31. Sculptra aesthetic [package insert]. Bridgewater (NJ): Dermik Laboratories; 2009.

32. Wildemore JK, Jones DH. Persistent granulomatous inflammatory response induced by injectable poly-L-lactic acid for HIV lipoatrophy. Dermatol Surg 2006;32:1407–9.

33. Jones D, Carruthers A, Orentreich D, et al. Highly purified 1000-cST silicon oil for treatment of human immunodeficiency virus-associated facial lipoatrophy: an open pilot trial. Dermatol Surg 2004;30:1279–86.

34. Jones DA. Report of 135 patients with 5 year and beyond follow up after treatment with highly purified liquid injectable silicone (LIS) for HIV associated facial lipoatrophy (HIV FLA). Presented at: American Society for Dermatologic Surgery Annual Meeting. Chicago (IL), October 24, 2010.

35. Barnett JG, Barnett GR. Treatment of acne scars with liquid silicone injections: 30-year perspective. Dermatol Surg 2005;31:1542–9.

36. Jones D. HIV facial lipoatrophy: causes and treatment options. Dermatol Surg 2005;31:1519–29.

37. Cohen SR, Holmes RE. Artecoll: a long-lasting injectable wrinkle filler material: report of a controlled, randomized, multicenter clinical trial of 251 subjects. Plast Reconstr Surg 2004;114:964–76.

38. Cohen SR, Berner CF, Busso M, et al. Artefill: a long-lasting injectable wrinkle filler material—summary of the U.S. Food and Drug Administration trials and a progress report on 4- to 5-year outcomes. Plast Reconstr Surg 2006;118(35):64S–76S.

39. Epstein R, Spencer JM. Correction of atrophic scars with Artefill: an open-label pilot study. J Drugs Dermatol 2010;9(9):1062–4.

40. Eviatar J, Barbarino S. Artefill: a long lasting filler used to treat HIV lipoatrophy. Presented at: 26th Annual Scientific Meeting of the American Academy of Cosmetic Surgery, Orlando (FL), January 12–16, 2010.

41. Mills D, Hurwitz D, Mosser S, et al. A pilot study to evaluate the local volumizing effects of a long-lasting PMMA filler. Two-month data. Presented at: 2nd American Brazilian Aesthetic Meeting (ABAM) and the 24th Annual Virgin Islands Workshop in Plastic Surgery. 2010.

Dermabrasion

Eugene K. Kim, MD[a,b,*], Raffi V. Hovsepian, MD[c,d,e],
Prakash Mathew[f], Malcolm D. Paul, MD[g]

KEYWORDS

- Dermabrasion • Microdermabrasion • Rhytids
- Wrinkles • Photoaging • Noninvasive • Scar revision

Key Points

- There has been a 70% increase in minimally invasive cosmetic procedures and a 50% increase in dermabrasions over the past decade.

- Dermabrasion is a minimally-invasive, low-risk technique for skin resurfacing.

- Dermabrasion is indicated for the treatment of superficial and moderate depth wrinkles in the perioral area.

- Dermabrasion may be more effective than chemical peels and laser therapy for certain skin conditions.

The past decade has seen a dramatic rise in the number of minimally invasive cosmetic procedures performed. In 2009, 12.5 million cosmetic procedures were performed by American Board of Medical Specialties board-certified physicians, an increase of almost 70% from 2000.[1] These minimally invasive procedures have provided the public an alternative to surgery that can improve aesthetic appearances and combat the effects of aging. The popularity of these procedures can be attributed to lower costs as well as less time for recovery and healing.

Dermabrasion is a skin-resurfacing technique that has been around since the 1930s. Kromeyer first treated skin complaints with a rotating burr or rasp after freezing the skin with carbon dioxide snow or ether spray.[2] Its use was expanded to traumatic tattoo removal when Iverson successfully used sandpaper to remove debris from the face in 1947.[3] Over the past 50 years, dermabrasion has also been used for many other problems, including wrinkling, scar revision, and the treatment of precancerous lesions.

A 50% increase in the number of dermabrasion procedures was seen in the past 10 years. However, the popularity of this technique has recently declined with the advent of other resurfacing treatments. Chemical peels and laser therapies have become increasingly popular to address similar problems that are treated by dermabrasion. However, dermabrasion can still be a more effective tool to treat severe or deeper problems of the skin.

ANATOMY OF THE SKIN

Comprising 16% of the total body weight, the skin is the largest organ system and plays a key role as an immunologic barrier and in the maintenance of homeostasis. Considering how insults to the

---

[a] Private Practice, 436 North Bedford Drive, Suite 305, Beverly Hills, CA 90210, USA
[b] Aesthetic and Plastic Surgery Institute, University of California-Irvine, 200 South Manchester Avenue, Suite 650, Orange, CA, USA
[c] Private Practice, 416 North Bedford Drive, Suite 200, Beverly Hills, CA 90210, USA
[d] Private Practice, 1401 Avocado Avenue, Suite 810, Newport Beach, CA 92660, USA
[e] Aesthetic and Plastic Surgery Institute, University of California-Irvine, Orange, CA, USA
[f] University of California-Irvine Medical School, 836 Health Sciences Road, Irvine, CA 92697, USA
[g] Aesthetic and Plastic Surgery Institute, University of California, Irvine, CA, USA
* Corresponding author. 436 North Bedford Drive, Suite 305, Beverly Hills, CA 90210.
E-mail address: eugene@ekimplasticsurgery.com

Clin Plastic Surg 38 (2011) 391–395
doi:10.1016/j.cps.2011.05.001
0094-1298/11/$ – see front matter © 2011 Elsevier Inc. All rights reserved

integumentary system serve as a nidus for many serious systemic infections, a thorough understanding of skin anatomy is necessary in order for the physician to safely treat disorders of the skin.

The skin is functionally divided into 2 layers: the epidermis and the dermis. The epidermis is composed of epithelium and can be further subdivided into 5 layers: the stratum corneum, stratum lucidum, stratum granulosum, stratum spinosum, and the stratum basale (germinativum). As the most superficial layer, the stratum corneum is composed of multiple layers of keratinocytes that are continually lost and regenerated. This layer is targeted during mechanical or chemical exfoliation. The stratum lucidum, found mainly in the palms of the hand and soles of the feet, contains a dense layer of keratin filaments that provides additional structural support. The stratum granulosum contains membrane-coating granules whose lipid-rich contents create a waterproof barrier for the skin. The stratum spinosum is the thickest layer of the epidermis and is characterized by the presence of multiple spiny cells rich in cytokeratin. The stratum basale contains the mitotically active cuboidal cells that generate the cells composing all other layers of the epidermis.

The connective tissue dermis forms 2 layers: the papillary layer and the reticular layer. The loose papillary layer is located directly beneath the stratum basale of the epidermis and houses the capillary network supplying the integument as well as the nerve endings critical to touch sensation. The markedly thicker reticular layer contains densely packed collagen that accounts for the skin's great tensile strength. It also serves as the foundation for hair follicles as well as sweat and sebaceous glands.[4]

DERMABRADERS

Many dermabraders are available for skin resurfacing (**Fig. 1**). Most are handheld devices that are attached to a control unit that regulates the speed of the endpiece (**Fig. 2**). These handpieces may be driven by pneumatic or electric motors. The operator is able to control the dermabrader with a foot pedal. Typically, the speed ranges from 10,000 to 85,000 revolutions per minute

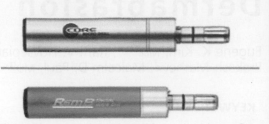

Fig. 2. Micro drill. (*Courtesy of* Stryker, Inc., Kalamazoo, MI; with permission.)

(RPM); however, most operators control the dermabrader at 12,000 to 15,000 RPM.

The burrs come in many different sizes, shapes, and levels of coarseness. The most common endpieces used include diamond fraises, serrated wheels, or wire brushes. The operator chooses the tip based on the area needing dermabrasion and the desired depth of penetration. During the procedure, the dermabrader must be kept in constant motion across the skin with a gentle application of pressure. The amount of pressure applied and the selected speed are the 2 most important factors in determining the end results.

INDICATIONS

Dermabrasion has many applications as a skin-resurfacing technique and is commonly used for the treatment of fine perioral rhytids and fine wrinkles found in other regions of the face. Rhinophyma is another disease of the face often treated with dermabrasion. It is characterized by granulomatous infiltration of the nose, making it appear large and bulbous. With dermabrasion, the nose is debulked and rapid reepithelialization follows. Dermabrasion may also be used to revise scars from trauma, skin grafts, acne, and surgical incisions.

Premalignant and superficial malignant lesions of the skin can sometimes be treated with dermabrasion. Actinic keratoses, basal cell carcinomas, and squamous cell carcinomas have all been treated with success using skin-resurfacing techniques. However, treatment of malignant lesions using dermabrasion should be used cautiously because of the inability to accurately stage the tumor and determine clear margins.

PREOPERATIVE WORKUP

A thorough history and physical is performed at the initial consultation. Any pertinent medical history must be noted, including any bleeding disorders and history of rashes or cold sores. Patients who have had prior outbreaks of herpes simplex virus may require prophylactic antiviral medications, such as acyclovir.

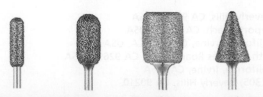

Fig. 1. Dermabraders. (*Courtesy of* Stryker, Inc., Kalamazoo, MI; with permission.)

Physicians should obtain medication lists to ensure that patients are not taking drugs that may lead to complications or compromise wound healing. If medically feasible, blood thinners and any medications that cause hyperpigmentation should be discontinued preoperatively. Isotretinoin (Accutane), a drug used to treat severe acne, may delay wound healing and cause hypertrophic scarring or keloid formation and, therefore, should be stopped at least 6 months to 1 year before undergoing the procedure. However, dermabrasion treatment during active acne may increase the risk of infection postoperatively and is a relative contraindication.

Dermabrasion can be performed on patients of varying ages. It is important to recognize the skin types of the patients and determine their Fitzpatrick skin type (**Table 1**). Those with dark complexions may experience permanent pigment changes following dermabrasion and, therefore, are not ideal candidates for the procedure. In addition, during the physical examination the skin on the entire body is surveyed for any evidence of keloids or hypertrophic scars that would discourage the use of dermabrasion.

The area that is to be treated by dermabrasion is closely examined. Patients must be informed of the limitations of the procedure and must have realistic expectations. Dermabrasion is more suitable for fine wrinkles and may not completely eradicate all imperfections, especially the deeper, coarse ones.

A few weeks before the performance of dermabrasion, patients can be pretreated with tretinoin (Retin-A). This medication promotes wound healing by increasing collagen formation. For patients at risk of hyperpigmentation postoperatively, hydroquinone, a bleaching agent, may be prescribed before the procedure.

PROCEDURE

Dermabrasion is commonly performed in office-based procedure rooms, surgery centers, and occasionally in the hospital. It is done under local anesthesia with the option of sedation or general anesthesia. Regional blocks are effective and additional topical anesthetics may be used to freeze the skin. If sedation or general anesthesia is used, patients must be monitored appropriately. The surgical team must wear appropriate sterile attire, including a mask with a facial shield. Protection from blood exposure and aerosolized particles during the procedure is important, especially when treating patients with a history of HIV or hepatitis.

The area to be dermabraded is marked and may be divided into sections when dealing with large surface areas to ensure uniformity. The appropriate diamond fraise tip or wire brush is chosen and attached to the handpiece. The skin is held taut with one hand or held by an assistant, and the dermabrader is moved across the skin with constant, gentle pressure. A back-and-forth motion is used for the diamond fraise tip, but the wire brush is moved in one direction (**Fig. 3**).[5]

The borders of the treated area are feathered to prevent any noticeable transitions. The depth of skin that is dermabraded is one of the most important factors that will determine the outcome. No bleeding is seen while treating the epidermis because of the lack of vasculature. Punctate bleeding is visualized when entering the papillary dermis. The papillary-reticular junction is the ideal endpoint of dermabrasion and is identified by increased, confluent bleeding. Dermabrasion beyond the reticular dermis can lead to significant scarring.

POSTOPERATIVE CARE

Immediately following the procedure, saline-soaked gauze moistened with dilute epinephrine may be temporarily placed on the open wounds to achieve hemostasis. A moist environment is necessary to promote wound healing. Multiple petroleum-based products are available to maintain a moist environment and prevent desiccation, such as Aquaphor (Beiersdorf Inc, Hamburg, Germany) and Xeroform gauze (Kendall Inc, Mansfield, MA, USA). The wound is cleansed daily and ointment is reapplied as necessary. Reepithelialization is completed 7 to 14 days following the procedure.

Patients should minimize sun exposure or wear appropriate sunblock for 6 to 12 months following the procedure to avoid hyperpigmentation. Hydroquinone may be used to treat any hyperpigmentation seen after dermabrasion. Residual erythema and edema should be expected to last 1 to 2 months and nonallergenic makeup is worn during that time. Recovery from dermabrasion usually lasts 2 to 4 weeks. Patients are able to return to work within 2

Table 1	
Fitzpatrick skin type classification	
Type	Reaction to Sun
I	Always burns, never tans
II	Usually burns, tans with difficulty
III	Sometimes burns, average tan
IV	Rarely burns, tans easily
V	Very rarely burns, tans very easily
VI	Never burns, tans very easily

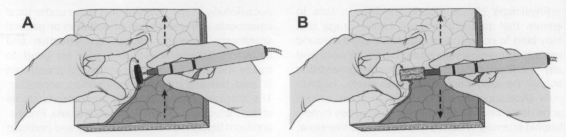

Fig. 3. (*A*) The wire brush is moved in a single direction during dermabrasion. (*B*) The diamond-fraise tip is used in a back-and-forth motion. (*From* AlKhawam BA. Dermabrasion and microdermabrasion. Facial Plast Surg 2009;25(5):307; with permission.)

weeks; however, they are advised to avoid strenuous activities and exercise for 4 to 6 weeks.

COMPLICATIONS

Although dermabrasion is an effective skin-resurfacing tool, there are associated complications that physicians and patients need to be made aware of. Abnormal scarring, including the formation of hypertrophic scars and keloids, can potentially occur if dermabrasion is performed beyond the reticular dermal layer. It is also seen in patients with genetic predisposition, such as collagen disorders, and those taking certain medications.

Hyperpigmentation and hypopigmentation can be avoided with proper patient selection and perioperative care. Patients with Fitzpatrick skin types I and II are less likely to experience pigment changes. Patients are instructed to avoid excessive

sun exposure; however, hydroquinone can be prescribed to treat unwanted hyperpigmentation.

Infectious complications can be treated with antibiotic and antiviral therapy. Patients with a history of a herpes outbreak are treated prophylactically with antivirals. Dermabrasion should be used with caution in patients with active acne and may require antibiotic treatment before undergoing the procedure. The formation of milia, small white keratin-filled cysts, may be seen following dermabrasion and usually resolve spontaneously, but they can be treated with incision and drainage when necessary.

MICRODERMABRASION

Microdermabrasion is a cosmetic technique that has gained considerable popularity as a less invasive, painful, and costly method of skin

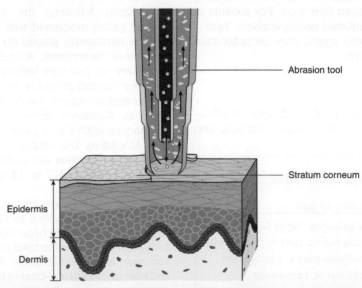

Fig. 4. Microdermabrasion. A fine stream of crystals are used to disrupt the stratum corneum and the dislodged cells are removed by vacuum suction. (*From* AlKhawam BA. Dermabrasion and microdermabrasion. Facial Plast Surg 2009;25(5):307; with permission.)

rejuvenation. The procedure does not need to be performed by a physician, and is, therefore, offered at day spas, aesthetic clinics, and medical offices. Although its effects are not as dramatic as dermabrasion, it offers a more conservative choice in the management of photoaged skin.

The procedure consists of the operator using a device that mobilizes a fine stream of ablative aluminum oxide crystals at the skin with the intent of disrupting the stratum corneum. The cells at the most superficial layer are dislodged and simultaneously removed by vacuum suction (**Fig. 4**). The level of exfoliation achieved is dependent on many factors, including the skin contact time of the microdermabrader as well as the suction strength of the vacuum. Side effects are usually mild and include erythema and tenderness at the procedure site. These complications are treated with nonsteroidal anti-inflammatory drugs.[6]

Microdermabrasion has uses in the treatment of acne scarring and photoaged, damaged skin. However, its noninvasive nature makes it of limited use in the treatment of skin beyond the most superficial layer of the epidermis. Multiple procedures are usually required to achieve a noticeable effect.

SUMMARY

Dermabrasion is an effective skin-resurfacing tool whose results have withstood the test of time. When performed properly, it can achieve dramatic results with a low risk of complications. Although its use has decreased because of the introduction of laser therapy and chemical peels, dermabrasion still retains some benefits over the other modalities in certain circumstances. Dermabrasion can be more effective than chemical peels in dealing with deeper wrinkles and may also be more advantageous in patients with darker complexions. Nonetheless, all 3 techniques may be used alone or in combination to achieve the desired effect.

REFERENCES

1. 2010 Report of the 2009 Statistics. National clearinghouse of plastic surgery statistics. Arlington Heights (IL): American Society of Plastic Surgeons; 2010. Available at: http://www.plasticsurgery.org/Documents/news-resources/statistics/2010-statisticss/Member-Surgeon-Data/2010-ASPS-member-surgeon-cosmetic-trends-statistics.pdf. Accessed May 21, 2011.
2. Kromeyer E. Cosmetic treatment of skin complaints. New York: Oxford University Press; 1930.
3. Iverson P. Surgical removal of traumatic tattoos on the face. Plast Reconstr Surg 1947;2(5):427–32.
4. Gartner LP, Hiatt JL. Color textbook of histology. 2nd edition. Baltimore (MD): Saunders; 2001.
5. Gold M. Dermabrasion in dermatology. Am J Clin Dermatol 2003;4(7):467–71.
6. Shim EK, Barnette D, Hughes K, et al. Microdermabrasion: a clinical and histopathologic Study. Dermatol Surg 2001;27:524–30.

The Art and Science of New Advances in Cosmeceuticals

Zoe Diana Draelos, MD*

KEYWORDS

- Cosmeceuticals • Antiaging preparations • Antioxidants
- Acne • Skin pigmentation

The cosmeceutical category is an undefined, unclassified, and unregulated area of skin treatment that is yet in its infancy. Traditional cosmeceuticals involve the topical application of biologically active ingredients, which affect the skin barrier and overall skin health. The ability of these ingredients to enhance skin functioning depends on how they are formulated into creams, lotions, and so forth, which can maintain the integrity of the active ingredients, deliver these ingredients in a biologically active form to the skin, reach the target site in sufficient quantity to exert an effect, and properly release the ingredients from the carrier vehicle.

In the United States and Europe, cosmeceuticals are sold as cosmetics, making marketing, packaging, and aesthetic appeal important considerations.[1] However, in Japan, a novel category of quasi-drugs exists that encompasses these biologically active formulations sold directly to consumers. Because cosmeceuticals intend to deliver on a higher level than cosmetics that simply color and scent the skin, cosmeceuticals should be clinically tested for efficacy not only to insure a proven skin benefit but also to substantiate marketing claims.[2]

Cosmeceuticals are viewed as cosmetics in the United States and must be careful to make only appearance claims. For example, they can claim to improve the appearance of wrinkles, but not get rid of wrinkles. Improving appearance is a cosmetic claim, whereas getting rid of wrinkles is a functional drug claim. Cosmeceuticals can also brighten skin and improve radiance, but they cannot treat abnormal pigmentation. Treating abnormal pigmentation is a drug claim. The recognition that there are governmental limitations on efficacy claims restricts cosmeceutical development because products can only be assessed in terms of their ability to improve skin appearance but not function. Improving function would remove the cosmeceutical from the cosmetic category and place it in the drug category.

COSMECEUTICAL DEVELOPMENT

Basically, cosmeceuticals are functional cosmetics, which means that the ingredients that are included in formulations must come from a list of raw materials that are generally recognized as safe, else the cosmeceutical would be classified as a drug. The easiest source of new cosmeceutical ingredients is the plant kingdom. Plants are rich in endogenous antioxidants because they must survive in an environment rich in UV radiation insults. Plant extracts are also thought to be safe and meet the Food and Drug Administration criteria for substances that can be put in over-the-counter (OTC) formulations. It is generally thought that substances that are safe for oral consumption can be assumed safe when applied topically. This thinking has led to a renewed interest in herbal preparations, which form the basis for functionality in many cosmeceuticals.

The search for novel herbs has led to the gathering of flowers, seeds, roots, leaves, twigs, and berries from plants all over the world. This gathering can be a complex process because the

No conflicts of interest to disclose.
Department of Dermatology, Duke University School of Medicine, Durham, NC, USA
* 2444 North Main Street, High Point, NC 27262.
E-mail address: zdraelos@northstate.net

Clin Plastic Surg 38 (2011) 397–407
doi:10.1016/j.cps.2011.02.002

constituents of a plant extract are influenced by the season in which the plant material was picked, the growing conditions, and the processing of the botanic. Once a possible functional cosmeceutical active ingredient has been identified and synthesized, it is typically applied to a fibroblast cell culture and the supernatant is placed on a gene chip to look for upregulation or downregulation of key skin mediators. For example, the ingredient may downregulate matrix metalloproteinases (MMPs), leading to a decrease in collagen degradation, providing the data for an antiaging claim. Sometimes the ingredient is further tested in a rodent model for confirmation of the desired skin benefits. The active ingredient is then placed in a vehicle suitable for human application, and clinical studies are undertaken. Successful human clinical studies pave the way for successful introduction into the marketplace via ingredient licensing arrangements.

COSMECEUTICAL CONCERNS

Although cosmeceuticals represent the future of skin care, there are also some concerns that should be considered. Not all plant extracts are beneficial to the skin. Many plants contain toxic metabolites, irritants, or allergens in addition to beneficial antiinflammatory agents. For example, feverfew, botanically known as *Tanacetum parthenium*, is a perennial flowering plant that contains antiinflammatory ingredients in its leaves. The leaves contain oils, such as terpinenes and linalool; flavonoid antioxidants; and parthenolides that are sesquiterpene lactones.[3] Parthenolide is a skin irritant that must be removed before feverfew extra can be incorporated into cosmetic preparations. Parthenolide is a distant relative of poison ivy, which is also a natural botanic extract inappropriate for skin application.

Other considerations include the growing habits of the plant. Some plants can only be seasonally harvested, unable to provide raw materials for year-round product manufacture. Other plants grow so slowly that overharvesting of the plant is possible, creating endangered plants. Many plants that grow in the Brazilian rain forest are being overharvested for cosmetic use, giving rise to a new concern in skin care manufacture known as sustainability. Sustainability is focused on ensuring the safe and continuing propagation of all plant materials. Even though many consumers want "natural" plant-derived ingredients because they are concerned about heath issues, the use of highly specific synthetic plant isolates may be more environmentally friendly and may lower the incidence of allergic or irritant contact dermatitis.

Another solution is to develop plant cell cultures known as bioreactors.[4] Care must be taken to protect plant materials from extinction.

COSMECEUTICAL CLASSIFICATION

The number of ingredients that can be formulated into cosmeceuticals is limited only by the imagination of the cosmetic chemist. Because cosmeceuticals are unregulated, the potential uses of cosmeceuticals are also unlimited. Cosmeceuticals could be developed to improve skin radiance, minimize acne, create the appearance of plump lips, optimize skin texture, shine hair, decrease nail brittleness, shrink facial pore appearance, create skin luminosity, improve the appearance of stretch marks, encourage pigmentation evenness, and so forth. If it would sell, it would be created. This article focuses on the more traditional use of cosmeceuticals relevant to skin care, including acne and antiaging uses.

COSMECEUTICALS FOR ACNE

A variety of preparations have been introduced for skin care that fall outside the prescription and the OTC drug realm. Oral and topical antibiotics and engineered retinoids form the basis for prescription-only therapies. Benzoyl peroxide, salicylic acid, and sulfur are the major ingredients from the acne monograph that are found as sole active ingredients in the concentration specified in most OTC acne drugs. The unregulated cosmeceutical acne category is based on natural acne-inhibiting substances of salicylic acid from willow bark, elemental sulfur, and tea tree oil.

Willow Bark (Salicin)

The white willow, known as Salix, contains a chemical known as salicin in its bark, which is a rich source of tannins and flavonoids. Salicin is the precursor of salicylic acid, comprising about 1% of the white willow bark extract, whereas other glycosides comprise about 12%. Salicylic acid is a colorless crystalline oil-soluble phenolic compound incorrectly classified as a β-hydroxy acid in which the OH group is adjacent to the carboxyl group. Synthesis of salicylic acid involves the treating of sodium phenolate, the sodium salt of phenol, with carbon dioxide at 100 atm pressure and 390 K temperature followed by acidification with sulfuric acid.

Salicylic acid, also known as 2-hydroxybenzoic acid, has a rich history in medicine. Salicylic acid is used as an antiinflammatory inhibiting arachidonic acid (because it is chemically related to aspirin), a flavoring agent with the characteristic wintergreen taste, a liniment for sore muscles, and an acne treatment. Hippocrates in the fifth century BC wrote about a bitter powder extracted from the willow back that would ease pain and reduce fever. The active extract of the willow back, called salicin, was isolated in crystalline form by Henri Leroux, a French pharmacist, in 1828.

Salicylic acid is used as a comedolytic in concentrations up to 2% in monographed products because it can penetrate into the follicle and dislodge the comedonal plug from the follicular lining.[5] However, salicylic acid does not kill *Propionibacterium acnes* and does not prevent the development of antibiotic resistance. Thus, salicylic acid may be less effective than benzoyl peroxide in acne treatment, but it is also less irritating and less allergenic. Some proprietary salicylic acid preparations have shown parity to 5% benzoyl peroxide.[6] Salicylic acid is sometimes used in hypoallergenic acne treatments and acne treatments for mature individuals.

Some individuals experience allergic reactions when salicylic acid is ingested; however, salicylic acid is generally accepted as a safe ingredient. An overdose of salicylic acid can lead to salicylate intoxication, presenting as a state of metabolic acidosis with a compensatory respiratory alkalosis. This intoxication has not been reported with topical applications, and salicylic acid acne preparations are considered safe and effective even during pregnancy.

Sulfur

The oldest treatment of acne predating benzoyl peroxide and salicylic acid is sulfur. Sulfur is a known bacteriostatic and antifungal.[7] Sulfur is a yellow nonmetallic element that has been used for centuries to treat various dermatologic conditions. A Roman physician first described the use of a sulfur mineral bath for the treatment of acne in an early medical text named *De Medicina*. The mechanism of action of sulfur is not totally understood, but it is thought to interact with cysteine in the stratum corneum, causing reduction of sulfur to hydrogen sulfide. Hydrogen sulfide in turn degrades keratin producing the keratolytic effect of sulfur.[8] Sulfur has been labeled as a comedogenic agent, but this is controversial.[9] Sulfur is available in concentrations of 3% to 8% in OTC acne formulations.

Tea Tree Oil

Tea tree oil is the most common herbal essential oil used for acne treatment. Tea tree oil, obtained from the Australian tree *Melaleuca alternifolia*, contains several antimicrobial substances, including terpinen-4-ol, alpha-terpineol, and alpha-pinene.[10] It appears as a pale golden oil with a fresh camphoraceous odor. Tea tree oil is used for medicinal purposes, such as antiseptic, antifungal, and antibacterial.[11]

The antibacterial activity of 10% tea tree oil has been shown against *Staphylococcus aureus*, including methicillin-resistant *S aureus*, without resistance.[12] Lower concentrations, however, have demonstrated bacterial resistance. Tea tree oil has been found to be as effective in the treatment of acne as 5% benzoyl peroxide based on a reduction in comedones and inflammatory acne lesions; however, the onset of action was slower for tea tree oil.[13] The tea oil group experienced fewer side effects than the benzoyl peroxide group. Another randomized placebo-controlled study in 60 subjects with mild to moderate acne vulgaris found that 5% topical tea tree oil produced a statistically significant reduction in total lesion count and acne severity index as compared with placebo.[14] Tea tree oil may also reduce the amount of inflammation present around acne lesions, thereby reducing redness.[15]

Tea tree oil is toxic when swallowed. It also has produced toxicity when applied topically in high concentrations to cats and other animals.[16] When used in low concentration topically for the treatment of acne, tea tree oil has not produced toxicity problems. However, tea tree oil is a known cause of allergic contact dermatitis. An Italian study of 725 subjects patch tested with undiluted, 1%, and 0.1% tea tree oil found that 6% of subjects experienced a positive reaction to undiluted tea tree oil, 1 subject experienced an allergic reaction to 1% tea tree oil, and no subjects experienced a reaction to the 0.1% dilution.[17] Thus, the incidence of allergic reactions to tea tree oil is concentration dependent.

COSMECEUTICALS FOR ANTIAGING

By far, the biggest use of cosmeceuticals is for improving the appearance of aged skin, which is perhaps because of the lack of prescription and OTC drugs for this purpose because there is really nothing else that has been introduced, besides tazarotene and tretinoin that have been proven to improve aging skin. This lack of OTC drugs for improving aging skin leaves a void in the market between colored cosmetics that temporarily improve skin appearance and prescription retinoids that have poor aesthetics, causing peeling and possibly burning sensation during the first 2 weeks of use. Cosmeceuticals may be the modern name for "hope in a jar"; however, this article examines the science behind the ingredients that are currently used to achieve a desired skin benefit.

COSMECEUTICAL PROTEINS

Cosmeceutical proteins have a rich history. One of the first modern cosmeceutical additives introduced was hydrolyzed animal protein. Hydrolyzed protein was obtained by cooking and denaturing cowhide. The hydrolyzed protein was combined with the occlusives petrolatum and mineral oil to serve as a humectant, attracting water to the epidermis and stratum corneum, which was trapped by the occlusives. As the sophistication of cosmeceuticals advanced, other sources of protein were used such as avian protein, beer protein, egg protein, and caviar protein. The source of the protein was not as important as the size of the protein because smaller molecules are preferred for better skin penetration and aesthetics.

As the concept of skin penetration grew, new engineered proteins were developed to influence skin functioning at a more fundamental level. These proteins were formed from amino acids selected to achieve a specific functional goal and to obtain more accurately labeled peptides.[18] The first peptides introduced were carrier peptides, which were adapted to the antiaging skin care market from wound healing. From the carrier peptides, the next development was signal peptides designed to mimic a natural body structure and turn on or off production of an endogenous protein. Neurotransmitter peptides were then developed that interrupted acetylcholine release. Enzyme-modulating peptides directly or indirectly inhibiting enzyme functioning were produced. Each of these peptide families is discussed.[19]

Carrier Peptides

The first commercialized peptides were carrier peptides. These peptides were designed to hook to another ingredient and facilitate transportation of the agent to the active site. The first carrier peptide was designed to deliver copper, a trace element necessary for wound healing. From a wound healing application, a peptide known as GHK-Cu was commercialized into a line of skin care products to minimize the appearance of fine lines and wrinkles. GHK-Cu is composed of glycine and histidyl and lysine hooked to copper and was found to induce dermal keratinocytes

proliferation. GHK was originally isolated from human plasma and then synthetically engineered.

Signal Peptides

The largest peptide family currently used in marketed cosmeceuticals is the signal peptides. Signal peptides stimulate collagen, elastin, fibronectin, proteoglycan, and glycosaminoglycan production, creating the appearance of younger-looking skin. The most popular signal peptide is palmitoyl pentapeptide (Pal-KTTKS), commercially known as Matrixyl (Sederma, Paris, France). Pal-KTTKS, is composed of the amino acids lysine, threonine, and serine. The peptide is a procollagen I fragment that stimulates the production of collagen I, III, and IV in vitro. Pal-KTTKS is used in a low concentration of 4 parts per million because it theoretically acts as a signal, whereby one molecule has a cascading effect. The idea is to present the body with procollagen fragments that downregulate the production of collagenase, thereby increasing dermal collagen and minimizing the appearance of aging.

Neurotransmitter Peptides

Neurotransmitter peptides function by inhibiting the release of acetylcholine at the neuromuscular junction. These peptides are similar to botulinum toxin in that both selectively modulate synaptosome-associated proteins of 25,000 Da, more commonly known as SNAP-25. Botulinum toxin A proteolytically degrades SNAP-25, whereas acetyl hexapeptide-3, a neurotransmitter peptide, mimics the N-terminal end of the SNAP-25 protein that inhibits the soluble N-ethyl-maleimide-sensitive factor attachment protein receptor (SNARE) complex formation. Acetyl hexapeptide-3 is commercially known as Argireline (Centerchem, Norwalk, CT, USA). Acetyl hexapeptide-3 supposedly functions topically to relax muscles, much like a weak short-lived botulinum toxin, by inhibiting vesicle docking through prevention of the SNARE complex formation. This muscle relaxation reduces the appearance of facial wrinkles.

A second commercialized neurotransmitter peptide is pentapeptide-3, commercially known as VIALOX (Centerchem, Norwalk, CT, USA). Pentapeptide-3 is a competitive antagonist at the acetylcholine receptor. This peptide also reduces muscle contraction and theoretically the depth of wrinkles on the face.

Enzyme-Modulating Peptides

Enzyme-modulating peptides directly or indirectly inhibit the function of a key enzyme in some metabolic process. Many of these enzyme-modulating peptides are extracted from botanic sources rather than engineered through protein chemistry. Soy proteins, already used in cosmeceuticals for the reduction of pigmentation and the inhibition of hair growth, possess another peptide that inhibits the formation of proteases. Rice proteins possess a peptide that inhibits MMP activity. These naturally occurring peptides are used in cosmeceutical facial moisturizers in combination with the previously discussed synthesized peptides.

COSMECEUTICALS FOR PIGMENTATION

Another popular market for cosmeceuticals is pigmentation improvement. With the removal of hydroquinone from the OTC markets in Europe and Asia, cosmetic chemists have focused on developing a hydroquinone alternative that would improve even skin tone. Hydroquinone has remained the gold standard as the most effective pigment-lightening ingredient, but health concerns have arisen because it seems that oxidized hydroquinone is toxic to melanocytes rather than simply a tyrosinase inhibitor.[20] A variety of vitamins and botanics have also been evaluated for their beneficial effects on melanization.

Ascorbic Acid

Ascorbic acid, also known as vitamin C, is used in cosmeceuticals for the treatment and prevention of hyperpigmentation because it interrupts melanogenesis by interacting with copper ions to reduce dopaquinone and blocks dihydrochinindol-2-carboxyl acid oxidation.[21] Ascorbic acid, an antioxidant, is rapidly oxidized when exposed to air with limited stability. For this reason, many cosmeceuticals are using the more stable magnesium ascorbyl phosphate, which is metabolized to ascorbic acid in the skin.[22] However, high concentrations of ascorbic acid must be used with caution because the low pH can be irritating to the skin. Pigment-lightening cosmeceuticals may contain ascorbic acid as a pH adjustor or to function as an antioxidant preservative. It is important to recognize that ascorbic acid is a multifunctional ingredient with minimal pigment-lightening capabilities.

Licorice Extract

Licorice extracts are found in cosmeceuticals to decrease facial redness and reduce pigmentation. The extract contains liquiritin and isoliquertin, which are glycosides containing flavonoids, that induce skin lightening by dispersing melanin.[23] To observe clinical results, 1 gm/d of liquiritin must be applied for 4 weeks. Irritation is not a side effect because it is so frequently observed with hydroquinone and ascorbic acid, but efficacy is minimal.

α-Lipoic Acid

α-Lipoic acid is found in a variety of antiaging cosmeceuticals to function as an antioxidant, but it may also have very limited pigment-lightening properties.[24] α-Lipoic acid is a disulfide derivative of octanoic acid that is able to inhibit tyrosinase. However, α-lipoic acid is a large molecule, and cutaneous penetration to the level of the melanocyte is challenging, significantly reducing its efficacy.

Kojic Acid

Kojic acid, chemically known as 5-hydroxymethyl-4H-pyrane-4-one, is one of the most popular cosmeceutical skin-lightening agents found in cosmetic-counter skin-lightening creams distributed worldwide. Kojic acid is a hydrophilic fungal derivative obtained from *Aspergillus* and *Penicillium* species. Kojic acid is the most popular agent used in the Orient for the treatment of melasma; however, it is highly unstable.[25] Newer formulations have incorporated kojic dipalmitate, but the efficacy of this derivative has not been well studied. Some research indicates that kojic acid is equivalent to hydroquinone in pigment-lightening ability.[26] The activity of kojic acid is attributed to its ability to prevent tyrosinase activity by binding to copper.

A new skin-lightening preparation combines kojic acid with emblica fruit extract and glycolic acid. It is necessary to combine preparations because no single pigment-lightening agent seems to work as well as hydroquinone alone. The emblica fruit contains tannins to inhibit melanization, while the glycolic acid causes exfoliation of the unevenly pigmented skin and enhances penetration of the kojic acid and emblica fruit extract. Careful combinations such as this optimize cosmeceutical lightening.

Aleosin

Aleosin is a low–molecular weight glycoprotein obtained from the aloe vera plant. Aleosin is a natural hydroxymethylchromone functioning to inhibit tyrosinase by competitive inhibition at the dopa oxidation site.[27,28] In contrast to hydroquinone, aleosin shows no cell cytotoxicity; however, it has a limited ability to penetrate the skin because of its hydrophilic nature. The effects of aleosin have been largely demonstrated in pigmented skin equivalents but not in human use studies.[29]

Aleosin is sometimes mixed with arbutin to enhance its skin-lightening abilities.

Arbutin

Arbutin, chemically known as 4-hydroxyphenyl-beta-glucopyranoside, is obtained from the leaves of *Vaccinicum vitis-idaea* and other related plants. Arbutin is a naturally occurring glucopyranoside derivative of hydroquinone that causes decreased tyrosinase activity without affecting messenger RNA expression.[30] Arbutin also inhibits melanosome maturation. Arbutin is not toxic to melanocytes and is used in a variety of pigment-lightening preparations in Japan at concentrations of 3%. Higher concentrations are more efficacious than lower concentrations, but a paradoxic pigment darkening may occur. Arbutin-beta-glycosides have been produced that are less cytotoxic than arbutin.[31]

N-acetylglucosamine

N-acetylglucosamine (NAG) is a monosaccharide composed of glucose and chitin. Chitin, chemically known as poly-NAG, is a common polymer found in nature that is structurally related to cellulose. NAG inhibits the conversion of protyrosinase to tyrosinase, thus decreasing pigmentation. The appearance of pigmentation was reduced when 2% NAG was applied with 4% niacinamide in an 8-week split-face study.[32] The niacinamide functions to inhibit the transfer of melanosomes to keratinocytes.

COSMECEUTICAL ANTIOXIDANTS

Antioxidants form one of the most popular categories of cosmeceutical ingredients because the major cause of cutaneous aging is oxidation of skin structures from highly reactive oxygen molecules in the environment. It is amazing to think that the life-giving oxygen required to survive is also the same oxygen responsible for aging in the human body. The primary source of cosmeceutical antioxidant ingredients is botanic extracts because all plants must protect themselves from oxidation as a result of UV exposure.

Antioxidant botanics function by quenching singlet oxygen and reactive oxygen species, such as superoxide anions, hydroxyl radicals, fatty peroxy radicals, and hydroperoxides. There are many botanic antioxidants available from raw material suppliers to the cosmeceutical industry, which can be classified into 1 of the 3 categories: carotenoids, flavonoids, and polyphenols. Carotenoids are chemically related to retinoids, whereas flavonoids possess a polyphenolic structure that accounts for their antioxidant, UV protectant, and metal chelation abilities. Polyphenols represent a chemical subset of flavonoids. These antioxidants can be used singly or in combination in cosmeceutical formulations.

Carotenoids

Carotenoids are derivatives of vitamin A and have found widespread use in cosmeceuticals because of the established topical antiaging benefits associated with the prescription retinoid tretinoin. The carotenoids are a large family of orange-, red-, and yellow-appearing substances that perform vital antioxidant roles when ingested and are less well established as topical antioxidants.[33]

Of all the topical carotenoids, retinol is the best understood because it is necessary for vision and possesses a well-characterized skin receptor.[34] Prescription retinoids, such as tazarotene and tretinoin, are well studied for their ability to induce the skin changes; however, OTC retinoids may show some of the same effects, to a lesser degree.[35,36]

It is theoretically possible to interconvert the retinoids from one form to another. For example, retinyl palmitate and retinyl propionate, chemically known as retinyl esters, can become biologically active after cutaneous enzymatic cleavage of the ester bond and subsequent conversion to retinol. Retinol is the naturally occurring vitamin A form found in red, yellow, and orange fruits and vegetables. Retinol is the pigment responsible for vision but is highly unstable. Retinol can be oxidized to retinaldehyde and then oxidized to retinoic acid, also known as prescription tretinoin. It is this cutaneous conversion of retinol to retinoic acid that is responsible for the biologic activity of some of the new stabilized OTC vitamin A preparations designed to improve the appearance of benign photodamaged skin.[37] However, only small amounts of retinyl palmitate and retinol can be converted by the skin, accounting for the increased efficacy seen with prescription preparations containing retinoic acid.

The main problem with prescription retinoids is their irritancy. As the biologic efficacy of the retinoid increases, so does the irritancy. This is also the case with the OTC retinoids.[38] Retinol is more irritating than the retinyl esters and also more unstable. It is for this reason that cosmeceutical formulations not manufactured under strict oxygen-free conditions prefer to add retinyl palmitate to moisturizing creams. However, the retinyl palmitate may present to act as an antioxidant for the lipids present in the moisturizer.

The topical benefit of retinol has been documented by well-controlled studies.[39] It is commonly thought among dermatologists that retinol is of benefit,[40] but it is difficult in moisturizer studies that do not include vehicle control to separate the retinol benefit from the moisturizer benefit. Nevertheless, of all the carotenoids available for formulation, retinol has the most evidence to support topical application.[41]

Flavonoids

Flavonoids are aromatic compounds, frequently with a yellow color, that occur in higher plants. About 5000 flavonoids have been identified with a similar chemical structure possessing 15 carbon atoms and possessing a variety of biologic activities.[42] Flavonoids can be divided into flavones, flavonols, isoflavones, and flavanones, each with a slightly different chemical structure. At present, the most common isoflavones incorporated into cosmeceuticals are daidzein and genistein derived from soybeans. Other sources of flavonoids include curcumin, silymarin, pycnogenol, and gingko.

Soy

The soybean-derived isoflavones genistein and daidzein function as phytoestrogens when orally consumed and have been credited with the decrease in cardiovascular disease and breast cancer seen in Asian women.[43] These isoflavones are present when the soy is fermented.[44] Some of the cutaneous effects of soy have been linked to its estrogenic effect in postmenopausal women. Topical estrogens have been shown to increase skin thickness and promote collagen synthesis.[45] Genistein increases collagen gene expression in cell culture; however, there are no published reports of this collagen-stimulating effect in topical human trials. Genistein has also been reported to function as a potent antioxidant, scavenging peroxyl radicals and protecting against lipid peroxidation in vivo.[46] The only studies that document the ability of soy to protect against UV-B–induced skin damage are in mice in which a topical application of nondenatured soy extracts reduced UV-B–induced cyclooxygenase-2 expression, prostaglandin-E2 secretion, and inhibited p38 MAP kinase activation.[47]

Curcumin

Curcumin is a popular natural yellow food coloring used in everything from prepackaged snack foods to meats. Curcumin is sometimes used in skin care products as a natural yellow coloring in products that claim to be free of artificial ingredients. Curcumin comes from the rhizome of the turmeric plant and is consumed orally as an Asian spice, frequently found in rice dishes to color the

otherwise white rice yellow. However, this yellow color is undesirable in cosmetic preparations because yellowing of products is typically associated with oxidative spoilage. Tetrahydrocurcumin, a hydrogenated form of curcumin, is off-white in color and can be added to skin care product not only to function as a skin antioxidant but also to prevent the lipids in the moisturizer from becoming rancid. The antioxidant effect of tetrahydrocurcumin is said to be greater than vitamin E by cosmetic chemists. Tetrahydrocurcumin is said to provide antioxidant skin benefits by quenching oxygen radicals and inhibiting nuclear factor $\kappa\beta$.[48,49]

Silymarin

Silymarin is an extract of the milk thistle plant (Silybum marianum), which belongs to the aster family of plants, including daisies, thistles, and artichokes. The plant is named milk thistle because the oldest recorded use of the extract was to enhance human lactation, and the plant produces a white milky sap. The extract consists of 3 flavonoids derived from the fruit, seeds, and leaves of the plant. These flavonoids are silybin, silydianin, and silychristine. Homeopathically, silymarin is used to treat liver disease, but it is a strong antioxidant preventing lipid peroxidation by scavenging free radical species. The antioxidant effects of silymarin have been demonstrated topically in hairline mice by the 92% reduction of skin tumors following UV-B exposure.[50,51] The mechanism for this decrease in tumor production is unknown, but topical silymarin has been shown to decrease the formation of pyrimidine dimers in a mouse model.[52]

Pycnogenol

Pycnogenol is an extract of French marine pine bark (Pinus pinaster), which grows only on the southwest coast of France in Les Landes de Gascogne. The extract is a water-soluble liquid containing several phenolic constituents, including taxifolin, catechin, and procyanidins. Pycnogenol also contains several phenolic acids, including p-hydroxybenzoic acid, protocatechuic acid, gallic acid, vanillic acid, p-couric acid, caffeic acid, and ferulic acid.[53] Pycnogenol is a trademarked ingredient that is a potent free radical scavenger that can reduce the vitamin C radical, returning the vitamin C to its active form.[54] The active vitamin C in turn regenerates vitamin E to its active form, maintaining the natural oxygen scavenging mechanisms of the skin intact.

Pycnogenol is the ideal antiaging additive because it demonstrates no chronic toxicity, no mutagenicity, no teratogenicity, and no allergenicity.[55] In B16 melanoma cells, pycnogenol was shown to inhibit tyrosinase activity and melanin biosynthesis.[56] Many discussions of antioxidant flavonoids include a mention of pycnogenol, but little quality data are presented.[57]

Ginkgo

Ginkgo biloba, also named the maidenhair tree, is the last member of the Ginkgoaceae family, which grew on earth some 200 to 250 million years ago. For this reason, ginkgo contains flavonoids not found in other botanics. *Gingko* possesses bibobalide (a sesquiterpene), ginkgolides (diterpenes with 20 carbon atoms), and other aromatic substances, such as ginkgol, bilobdol, and ginkgolic acid. *Ginkgo* is a plant with numerous purported benefits that is a common part of homeopathic medicine in the Orient for 4000 years. The plant leaves are said to contain unique polyphenols such as terpenoids (ginkgolides, bilobalides), flavonoids, and flavonol glycosides that have antiinflammatory effects. These antiinflammatory effects have been linked to antiradical and antilipoperoxidant effects in experimental fibroblast models.[58] Ginkgo flavonoid fractions containing quercetin, kaempferol, sciadopitysin, ginkgetin, and isoginkgetin have been demonstrated to induce human skin fibroblast proliferation in vitro. Increased collagen and extracellular fibronectin were also demonstrated by radioisotope assay.[59] Thus, ginkgo extracts are added to many cosmeceuticals to function as antioxidants and promoters of collagen synthesis after resurfacing based on nonhuman models of oxidative damage.

Polyphenols

Polyphenols are a subset of flavonoids used in many cosmeceuticals. The 3 main sources of polyphenols are teas, fruits, and seeds. Green tea, pomegranate fruit, and grape seeds are used as examples.

Green tea

Tea, also known as Camellia sinensis, is a botanic popular in the Orient for 5000 years used both topically and orally. There are several different types of teas: green, black, oolong, and white. The different teas come from the same plant, but different processing imparts different properties. Green tea is made from unfermented tea leaves and contains the highest concentration of polyphenol antioxidants.[60] Black tea leaves are fermented days before heating. Oolong tea originates in the Fujian province of China, and the leaves are treated much like black tea, except that the withering and fermentation times are minimized. White tea comes from young tea leaves that are harvested for a few days each spring when the plant emerges

from the ground. These leaves are said to be very high in antioxidants. The highest quality white tea is obtained from buds that are just ready to open known as needles or tips.

Green tea is manufactured from both the leaf and bud of the plant. Orally, green tea is said to contain beneficial polyphenols, such as epicatechin, epicatechin-3-gallate, epigllocatechin, and eigallocatechin-3-gallate (EGCG), which function as potent antioxidants.[61] EGCG is the most potent of the polyphenols sold as a white caffeine-free powder.[62] Oral studies with EGCG have demonstrated the increased fat oxidation and improvements in heart rate and serum glucose levels with 300 mg. Other alkaloids present in green tea include caffeine, theobromine, and theophylline.

Green tea can be easily added to topical creams and lotions designed to combat the signs of photoaging, but it must be stabilized itself with an antioxidant, such as butylated hydroxytoluene. The Mayo Clinic Drugs and Supplements rate the evidence to support green tea as a photoprotectant as a C.[63]

A study by Katiyar and colleagues[64] demonstrated the antiinflammatory effects of topical green tea application on C3H mice. A topically applied green tea extract containing GTP ([−]-epigallocatechin-3-gallate) was found to reduce UV-B–induced inflammation as measured by double skinfold swelling. The investigators also found protection against UV-induced edema, erythema, and antioxidant depletion in the epidermis. This work was further investigated by applying GTP to the back of humans 30 minutes before UV irradiation, which resulted in decreased myeloperoxidase activity and decreased infiltration of leukocytes as compared with untreated skin.[65]

The application of topical green tea polyphenols before UV exposure has also been shown to decrease the formation of cyclobutane pyrimidine dimers.[66] These dimers are critical in initiating UV-induced mutagenesis and carcinogenesis, which represent the end stage of the aging process. Thus, green tea polyphenols can function topically as antioxidants, antiinflammatories, and anticarcinogens, making them a popular cosmeceutical additive.[67,68]

Pomegranate fruit

Pomegranate, botanically known as Punica granatum, is a deciduous tree bearing a red fruit native to Afghanistan, Pakistan, Iran, and northern India.[69] It was brought to California by the Spanish settlers in 1769 and is commercially cultivated for its juice. Pomegranate juice, commonly consumed in the Middle East, provides about 16% of the adult requirement of vitamin C per 100 mg serving.

It also contains pantothenic acid, also known as vitamin B5, potassium, and antioxidant polyphenols. These substances have been demonstrated to protect against UV-A– and UV-B–induced cell damage in SKU-1064 human skin fibroblasts.[70] Pomegranate juice has also been purported to reduce oxidative stress and affect low-density lipoprotein level and platelet aggregation in humans and apolipoprotein E–deficient mice.[71,72]

Grape seed

Grape seed extract, botanically known as Vitis vinifera seed extract, contains a combination of polyphenols, including flavonoids, tannins, and stilbenes.[73] The most interesting of the stilbenes is resveratrol. Resveratrol has been shown to modulate sirtuins that regulate DNA transcription. Ingestion of resveratrol in rodent models has demonstrated effects similar to caloric restriction in prolonging life and is therefore of great interest as an oral supplement. Resveratrol is found in the skins of red grapes and is incorporated into red wine. Japanese knotweed is another source.

In addition, grape seed extract contains unique procyanidin antioxidants. These dimers and oligomers of catechin, epicatechin, and their gallic acid esters are known as oligomeric proanthocyanidins, which comprise 65% of grape polyphenols. These polyphenols have been shown to decrease glycol oxidation of proteins, thus inhibiting aging. The oral benefits of grape seed have been better investigated than the value of topical application.

SUMMARY

Some of the key messages in this article are as follows:

1. Cosmeceuticals use OTC ingredients to serve as functional cosmetics.
2. Acne cosmeceuticals are based on botanic ingredients such as tea tree oil, willow bark extract, and sulfur designed to function as keratolytics, antiinfectives, and antiinflammatories.
3. Antiaging cosmeceuticals are based on botanic extracts and peptides, which are protein fragments designed to mimic structural aspects of the skin.
4. Pigment lightening cosmeceuticals contain botanic extracts intended to interrupt pigment production at key steps in the melanin synthetic pathway.

From the prior discussions, it is obvious that most of the data supporting cosmeceuticals come from oral ingestion of the botanic materials in rodents. Oral consumption is not the same as topical application, and rodents are not the same

as humans. It is not practical or wise to extrapolate too far. If this article was written based on double-blind placebo-controlled human studies of topical cosmeceutical application, it would be about 2 paragraphs. Clearly, much more validation is needed for cosmeceuticals before they can become part of mainstream medical practice. But then, there are so little data, probably because no one really wants to know what botanic extracts actually affect. If a botanic was found that increased dermal collagen, it would be a drug and not a cosmetic, and OTC sale would be forbidden. Indeed, cosmeceutical manufacturers walk a fine line.

In addition, research studies are very difficult to conduct. The ideal topical trial would be to isolate an ingredient and compare the ingredient plus the moisturizing vehicle with the moisturizing vehicle alone. The problem with this study design is that the moisturizing vehicle is also an active. If current cosmeceutical claims are analyzed, most claims are moisturizing claims. For example, a cream may claim to improve skin firmness by 38% after 48 hours of use. This claim is a moisturizer claim not solely related to the special cosmeceutical ingredient. Both arms of the vehicle-controlled study might be expected to show similar results. There really is no true placebo for comparison.

The need for cosmeceutical research is ever present. This article has tried to highlight the chemistry of botanic extracts in the current marketplace and review the best research available. In some ways, more questions have been raised than answered; yet, ideas for intellectual discourse have been provided. Herein lies the physician cosmeceutical challenge.

REFERENCES

1. Griffiths TW. Cosmeceuticals: coming of age. Br J Dermatol 2010;162(3):169–70.
2. Armer M, Maged M. Cosmeceuticals versus pharmaceuticals. Clin Dermatol 2009;27(5):428–30.
3. Fowler JF, Woolery-Lloyd H, Waldorf H, et al. Innovations in natural skin care ingredients and their use in skin care. J Drugs Dermatol 2010;9(6 Suppl):s72–9.
4. Schurch C, Blum P, Zulli F. Potential of plant cells in culture for cosmetic purposes. Phytochem Rev 2007;7(3):599–605.
5. Eady EA, Burke BM, Pulling K, et al. The benefit of 2% salicylic acid lotion in acne. J Dermatol Ther 1996;7:93–6.
6. Bissonnette R, Bolduc C, Seite S, et al. Randomized study comparing the efficacy and tolerance of a lipophilic hydroxy acid derivative of salicylic acid and 5% benzoyl peroxide in the treatment of facial acne vulgaris. J Cosmet Dermatol 2009;8(1):19–23.

7. Gupta AK, Nicol K, Gupta AK, et al. The use of sulfur in dermatology. J Drugs Dermatol 2004;3(4):427–31.

8. Lin AN, Reimer RJ, Carter DM. Sulfur revisited. J Am Acad Dermatol 1988;18(3):553–8.

9. Mills OH Jr, Kligman AM. Is sulphur helpful or harmful in acne vulgaris? Br J Dermatol 1972; 86(6):620–7.

10. Raman A. Antimicrobial effects of tea-tree oil and its major components on Staphylococcus aureus, Staph. epidermidis and Propionibacterium acnes. Lett Appl Microbiol 1995;21(4):242–5.

11. Hammer KA, Carson CF, Riley TV. Susceptibility of transient and commensal skin flora to the essential oil of Melaleuca alternifolia. Am J Infect Control 1996;24(3):186–9.

12. Shemesh A, Mayo WL. Australian tea tree oil: a natural antiseptic and fungicidal agent. Aust J Pharm 1991;72:802–3.

13. Bassett IB, Pannowitz DL, Barnetson RS. A comparative study of tea-tree oil versus benzoyl peroxide in the treatment of acne. Med J Aust 1990;153(8):455–8.

14. Enshaieh S, Jooya A, Siadat AH, et al. The efficacy of 5% topical tea tree oil gel in mild to moderate acne vulgaris: a randomized, double-blind placebo-controlled study. Indian J Dermatol Venereol Leprol 2007;73(1):22–5.

15. Koh KJ, Pearce AL, Marshman G, et al. Tea tree oil reduces histamine-induced skin inflammation. Br J Dermatol 2002;147(6):1212–7.

16. Bischoff K, Guale F. Australian tea tree oil poisoning in three purebred cats. J Vet Diagn Invest 1998;10:208.

17. Lisi P, Melingi L, Pigatto P, et al. Prevalenza della sensibilizzazione all'olio exxenziale di Melaleuca. Ann Ital Dermatol Allergol 2000;54:141–4 [in Italian].

18. Zhang L, Falla TJ. Cosmeceuticals and peptides. Clin Dermatol 2009;27(5):485–94.

19. Lintner K, Mas-Chamberlin C, Mondon P, et al. Cosmeceuticals and active ingredients. Clin Dermatol 2009;27(5):461–8.

20. Draelos ZD. Skin lightening preparations and the hydroquinone controversy. Dermatol Ther 2007; 20(5):308–13.

21. Espinal-Perez LE, Moncada B, Castanedo-Cazares JP. A double blind randomized trial of 5% ascorbic acid vs 4% hydroquinone in melasma. Int J Dermatol 2004;43(8):604–7.

22. Kameyama K, Sakai C, Kondoh S, et al. Inhibitory effect of magnesium L-ascorbyl-2-phosphate on melanogenesis in vitro and in vivo. J Am Acad Dermatol 1996;34:29.

23. Amer M, Metwalli M. Topical liquiritin improves melasma. Int J Dermatol 2000;39(4):299–301.

24. Beitner H. Randomized, placebo-controlled, double blind study on the clinical efficacy of a cream containing 5% alpha-lipoic acid related to photoageing of facial skin. Br J Dermatol 2003;149(4):841–9.

25. Lim JT. Treatment of melasma using kojic acid in a gel containing hydroquinone and glycolic acid. Dermatol Surg 1999;25:282–4.

26. Garcia A, Fulton JE Jr. The combination of glycolic acid and hydroquinone or kojic acid for the treatment of melasma and related conditions. Dermatol Surg 1996;22(5):443–7.

27. Choi S, Lee SK, Kim JE, et al. Aloesin inhibits hyperpigmentation induced by UV radiation. Clin Exp Dermatol 2002;27:513–5.

28. Jones K, Hughes J, Hong M, et al. Modulation of melanogenesis by aloesin: a competitive inhibitor of tyrosinase. Pigment Cell Res 2002;15:335–40.

29. Wang Z, Li X, Yang Z, et al. Effects of aloesin on melanogenesis in pigmented skin equivalents. Int J Cosmet Sci 2008;30(2):121–30.

30. Hori I, Nihei K, Kubo I. Structural criteria for depigmenting mechanism of arbutin. Phytother Res 2004;18:475–9.

31. Jun SY, Park KM, Choi KW, et al. Inhibitory effects of arbutin-beta-glycosides synthesized from enzymatic transglycosylation for melanogenesis. Biotechnol Lett 2008;30(4):743–8.

32. Bissett DL, Robinson LR, Raleigh PS, et al. Reduction in the appearance of facial hyperpigmentation by topical N-acetylglucosamine. J Cosmet Dermatol 2007;6(1):20–6.

33. Manela-Azulay M, Bagatin E. Cosmeceuticals vitamins. Clin Dermatol 2009;27(5):469–74.

34. Kligman LH, Do CH, Kligman AM. Topical retinoic acid enhances the repair of ultraviolet damaged dermal connective tissue. Connect Tissue Res 1984;12:139–50.

35. Goodman DS. Vitamin A and retinoids in health and disease. N Engl J Med 1984;310(16):1023–31.

36. Noy N. Interactions of retinoids with lipid bilayers and with membranes. In: Livrea MA, Packer L, editors. Retinoids. New York: Marcel Dekker; 1993. p. 17–27.

37. Duell EA, Derguini F, Kang S, et al. Extraction of human epidermis treated with retinol yields retro-retinoids in addition to free retinol and retinyl esters. J Invest Dermatol 1996;107:178–82.

38. Sorg O, Antille C, Kaya G, et al. Retinoids in cosmeceuticals. Dermatol Ther 2006;19(5):289–96.

39. Kafi R, Swak HS, Schumacher WE, et al. Improvement of naturally aged skin with vitamin A (retinol). Arch Dermatol 2007;143(5):606–12.

40. Hruza GJ. Retinol benefits naturally aged skin [abstract]. J Watch Dermatol 2007.

41. Varani J, Fisher GJ, Kang S, et al. Molecular mechanisms of intrinsic skin aging and retinoid-induced repair and reversal. J Investig Dermatol Symp Proc 1998;3(1):57–60.

42. Arct J, Pytokowska K. Flavonoids as components of biologically active cosmeceuticals. Clin Dermatol 2008;26:347–57.

43. Glazier MG, Bowman MA. A review of the evidence for the use of phytoestrogens as a replacement for traditional estrogen replacement therapy. Arch Intern Med 2001;161:1161–72.

44. Friedman M, Brandon DL. Nutritional and health benefits of soy proteins. J Agric Food Chem 2001; 49(3):1069–86.

45. Maheux R, Naud F, Rioux M, et al. A randomized, double-blind, placebo-controlled study on the effect of conjugated estrogens on skin thickness. Am J Obstet Gynecol 1994;170:642–9.

46. Wiseman H, O'Reilly JD, Adlercreutz H, et al. Isoflavone phytoestrogens consumed in soy decrease F-2-isoprostane concentrations and increase resistance of low-density lipoprotein to oxidation in humans. Am J Clin Nutr 2000;72:395–400.

47. Chen N, Scarpa R, Zhang L, et al. Nondenatured soy extracts reduce UVB-induced skin damage via multiple mechanisms. Photochem Photobiol 2008; 84(6):1551–9.

48. Hatcher H, Planalp R, Cho J, et al. Curcumin: from ancient medicine to current clinical trials. Cell Mol Life Sci 2008;65(11):1631–52.

49. Jagetia GC, Aggarwal BB. "Spicing up" of the immune system by curcumin. J Clin Immunol 2007; 27(1):19–35.

50. Katiyar SK, Korman NJ, Mukhtar H, et al. Protective effects of silymarin against photocarcinogenesis in a mouse skin model. J Natl Cancer Inst 1997;89: 556–66.

51. Katiyar SK. Silymarin and skin cancer prevention: anti-inflammatory, antioxidant and immunomodulatory effects [review]. Int J Oncol 2005;26(1):169–76.

52. Chatterjee L, Agarwal R, Mukhtar H. Ultraviolet B radiation-induced DNA lesions in mouse epidermis: an assessment sing a novel 32P-postlabeling technique. Biochem Biophys Res Commun 1996;229: 590–5.

53. Available at: http://www.drugs.com/npp/pyconogenol. html. Accessed December 7, 2008.

54. Cossins E, Lee R, Packer L. ESR studies of vitamin C regeneration, order of reactivity of natural source phytochemical preparations. Biochem Mol Biol Int 1998;45:583–98.

55. Schonlau F. The cosmetic pycnogenol. J Appl Cosmetol 2002;20:241–6.

56. Kim YJ, Kang KS, Yokozawa T. The anti-melanogenic effect of pycnogenol by its anti-oxidative actions. Food Chem Toxicol 2008;46(7):2466–71.

57. Rona C, Vailati F, Berardesca D. The cosmetic treatment of wrinkles. J Cosmet Dermatol 2004;3(1): 26–34.

58. Joyeux M, Lobstein A, Anton R, et al. Comparative antilipoperoxidant, antinecrotic and scavenging properties of terpenes and biflavones from Ginkgo and some flavonoids. Planta Med 1995;61:126–9.

59. Kim SJ, Lim MH, Chun IK, et al. Effects of flavonoids of Ginkgo biloba on proliferation of human skin fibroblast. Skin Pharmacol 1997;10:200–5.

60. Hsu S. Green tea and the skin. J Am Acad Dermatol 2005;52:1049–59.

61. Katiyar SK, Elmets CA. Green tea and skin. Arch Dermatol 2000;136:989–94.

62. Geria NM. Green, black or white, it fits beauty to a "t". HAPPI 2006;46–50.

63. Chui AD, Chan JL, Kern DG, et al. Double-blinded, placebo-controlled trial of green tea extracts in the clinical and histologic appearance of photoaging skin. Dermatol Surg 2005;31(7pt2):855–60.

64. Katiyar SK, Elmets CA, Agarwal R, et al. Protection against ultraviolet-B radiation-induced local and systemic suppression of contact hypersensitivity and edema responses in C3H/HeN mice by green tea polyphenols. Photochem Photobiol 1995;62:855–61.

65. Elmets CA, Singh D, Tubesing K, et al. Green tea polyphenols as chemopreventive agents against cutaneous photodamage. J Am Acad Dermatol 2001;44:425–32.

66. Katiyar SK, Afaq F, Perez A, et al. Green tea polyphenol treatment to human skin prevents formation of ultraviolet light B-induced pyrimidine dimers in DNA. Clin Cancer Res 2000;6:3864–9.

67. Ahmad N, Mukhtar H. Cutaneous photochemoprotection by green tea. A brief review. Skin Pharmacol Appl Skin Physiol 2001;14:69–76.

68. Mukhtar H, Katiyar SK, Agarwal R. Green tea and skin—anticarcinogenic effects. J Invest Dermatol 1994;102:3–7.

69. Jurenka JS. Therapeutic applications of pomegranate (Punica granatum L.): a review. Altern Med Rev 2008;13(2):128–44.

70. Pacheco-Palencia LA, Noratto G, Hingorani L, et al. Protective effects of standardized pomegranate (Punica granatum L.) polyphenolic extract in ultraviolet-irradiated human skin fibroblasts. J Agric Food Chem 2008;56(18):8434–41.

71. Aviram M, Rosenblat M, Gaitini D, et al. Pomegranate juice consumption for 3 years by patients with carotid artery stenosis reduces common carotid intima-media thickness, blood pressure and LDL oxidation. Clin Nutr 2004;23(3):423–33.

72. Aviram M, Dornfeld L, Rosenblat M, et al. Pomegranate juice consumption reduces oxidative stress, atherogenic modifications to LDL, and platelet aggregation: studies in humans and in atherosclerotic apolipoprotein e-deficient mice. Am J Clin Nutr 2000;71:1062–76.

73. Sharma SD, Katiyar SK. Dietary grape seed proanthocyanidins inhibit UVB-induced cyclooxygenase-2 expression and other inflammatory mediators in UVB-exposed skin and skin tumors of SKH-1 hairless mice. Pharm Res 2010;27(6):1092–102.

An Overview of Botulinum Toxins: Past, Present, and Future

Todd V. Cartee, MD*, Gary D. Monheit, MD

KEYWORDS

- Botulinum • Neurotoxin • Dysport • Botox • Cosmetic

Botulinum toxin (BTX) has revolutionized the field of cosmetic medicine. With more than 11 million injections since 2002,[1] its administration is by far the most common cosmetic procedure being performed in the United States. This achievement is truly impressive for what may be the most toxic chemical on earth. Based on the estimated inhalational lethal dose, a single gram of BTX is capable of killing 1 million people.[2] Fortunately, a vial of BTX for cosmetic use contains about a 200 million-fold smaller quantity of active neurotoxin. The rapid ascent in popularity of BTX with both clinicians and patients can be attributed to its remarkable efficacy; predictable and reproducible results; excellent safety record; and the relative ease, comfort, and speed of administration. Over the past 9 years since its Food and Drug Administration (FDA) approval for the treatment of glabellar lines, physicians have explored myriad applications for BTX not only for the treatment of the aging face and neck but also for a long list of neuromuscular and glandular disorders, muscle contouring, and various pain syndromes. In keeping with the theme of this issue, this review focuses predominantly on aesthetic uses of BTX. The pharmacodynamics, clinical properties, and safety profiles of the 2 BTX products FDA approved for cosmetic use, onabotulinumtoxinA (Botox) and abobotulinumtoxinA (Dysport), are also explored in detail.

STRUCTURE AND MECHANISM OF ACTION

Botulinum toxin is produced by various species of gram-positive, spore-forming bacilli of the genus, Clostridium, but chiefly from strains of C botulinum. Seven serotypes of BTX have been identified to date, which are labeled alphabetically, A to G. Many of these possess additional subtypes; for example, there are 4 described distinct subtypes of serotype A toxins.[3] All of the serotypes have a similar chemical structure and, except subtype C_2, are neurotoxins. Each botulinum toxin is initially synthesized as a continuous 150-kDa gene product. Biologic activity requires posttranslational proteolysis, or nicking, which clips the BTX polypeptide into 2 separate moieties of 100 kDa and 50 kDa in size. This process results in a heavy chain and light chain that remain covalently bound by a single disulfide bridge.[4] In human tissue, the heavy chain is recognized by receptors on presynaptic nerve terminals and the active di-chain neurotoxin is endocytosed. Upon acidification of the endosome, the heavy chain forms a channel in the endosomal membrane and the disulfide bond

Dr Cartee has no relevant conflicts of interest. Dr Monheit receives funding from Allergan Corporation, consultant and clinical investigator, Juvederm; Dermik Laboratories, clinical investigator, Sculptra; Genzyme Corporation, consultant and clinical investigator, Captique, Prevelle; J & J, consultant; Contura, clinical investigator, Aquamid; Ipsen/Medicis, consultant and clinical investigator, Dysport; Electro-Optical Sciences, Inc, consultant and clinical investigator, Melafind; Revance, consultant and clinical investigator; Kythera, clinical investigator; Galderma, consultant and clinical investigator; Mentor, consultant and clinical investigator; Merz, consultant and clinical investigator.
Total Skin and Beauty Dermatology Center, 2100 16th Avenue South, Suite 202, Birmingham, AL 35205, USA
* Corresponding author.
E-mail address: tvcartee@yahoo.com

between the chains is reduced.[5] The liberated light chain translocates to the cytosol where its zinc-dependent protease domain cleaves a member of the soluble NSF attachment protein receptor (SNARE) complex. The loss of any of these proteins abrogates exocytosis of presynaptic acetylcholine-rich vesicles, thereby eliminating signal conduction in afflicted cholinergic neurons. The various serotypes have specific molecular targets: SNAP-25 for toxins A and E; VAMP/synaptobrevin for B, D, F, G; and both SNAP-25 and syntaxin for C.[6]

Botulinum toxin serotype A (BTX-A), the serotype in both onabotulinumtoxinA (Botox/Vistabel; Allergan, Inc) and abobotulinumtoxinA (Dysport), naturally exists as a complex with a surrounding coat of catalytically inactive, protective proteins, known collectively as neurotoxin- associated proteins (NAPs). NAPs, including 4 distinct hemagglutinin proteins and a nontoxic nonhemagglutinin protein, are synthesized by the clostridial bacterium and shield the neurotoxin from potential destruction by gastric acidity. Clostridial cultures yield 3 sizes of progenitor complexes: 300 kDa, 500 kDa, and 900 kDa.[7] Allergan asserts their proprietary purification method for onabotulinumtoxinA (OnaA) isolates the 900-kDa complex exclusively.[8] It has been suggested that the column chromatography purification method used to isolate abobotulinumtoxinA (AboA) results in a heterogeneous mixture of the 3 progenitor complexes, with the smaller complexes conferring more rapid diffusion in tissues.[9] These claims have been disputed by Ipsen[10] and admittedly the authors were unable to identify any convincing studies that establish a direct correlation between tissue diffusion properties and complex size.

Pharmacologic activity of BTX-A requires dissociation of the progenitor complex and release of the active BTX-A 150-kDa monomer. This process does occur at physiologic pH but the kinetics of the dissociation are not fully clarified. Some have suggested that dissociation is nearly immediate.[11] A recent study conducted by Merz Pharmaceuticals (manufacturers of one of the new naked neurotoxin agents discussed later) reported that the 150-kDa toxin was released from both OnaA and AboA in less than 1 minute at neutral pH.[12] The investigators suggested that dissociation may occur in the vial even before injection. The relative kinetics of dissociation versus diffusion have implications for the safety profiles of the various formulations of BTX-A in current or future clinical use and, therefore, these remain contentious issues for their respective manufacturers.

In addition to the well-characterized effects previously detailed, a growing body of evidence indicates that BTX-A targets some noncholinergic

neurons. Inhibition of neurotransmitters, such as substance P, glutamate, and calcitonin gene-related peptide, has been demonstrated, supplying the mechanistic underpinning for the use of BTX-A in the treatment of chronic pain,[13] one of its most exciting new nonaesthetic applications. It is hoped that future research in this area will establish novel therapeutic indications for BTX-A.

HISTORY

Botulism, derived from the Latin *botulus* meaning sausage, was first described in the 1820s when several cases occurred in Germany associated with the ingestion of improperly preserved smoked sausage. The bacterial etiology was discovered in 1895 and the toxin itself was isolated in the 1940s. In the 1970s, Dr Alan Scott pioneered research on the clinical utility of BTX, treating strabismus in a primate model. He eventually graduated to humans and published the first sizable therapeutic trial in 20 patients with strabismus in 1981.[14] Over the ensuing decade, Dr Scott established or inspired numerous ophthalmologic applications, including blepharospasm, nystagmus, entropion, and hemifacial spasm. In 1989, BTX received its first FDA approval for blepharospasm and nystagmus.

In 1987, a serendipitous observation by a patient of Jean Carruthers, MD, an ophthalmologist, spawned the cosmetic use of BTX. The patient, who was receiving BTX-A for blepharospasm, noted a softening of her frown lines. Dr Carruthers happened to be married to a dermatologist, Alistair Carruthers, MD, so the couple was uniquely positioned to initiate clinical research on the use of BTX in rhytid reduction. They published their first clinical study of BTX for glabellar lines in 1992.[15] Sixteen of 17 patients who completed follow-up had a clear benefit with no major adverse events. It would take another decade to achieve FDA approval for this limited indication. In 2004, approval for treatment of primary axillary hyperhidrosis was granted. All other dermatologic usage of BTX remains off-label despite the general comfort most injectors have enjoyed for many years in using BTX for dynamic wrinkling in multiple areas of the face.

BOTULINUM TOXINS IN CLINICAL USE

Currently, 4 botulinum toxin products have FDA approval in the United States. Three contain serotype A complexes: OnaA (Botox), AboA (Dysport), and incobotulinumtoxinA (Xeomin). There is also 1 serotype B injectable: rimabotulinumtoxinB (Myobloc). RimabotulinumtoxinB (RimB) is only approved for treatment of cervical dystonia. It has been employed for other conditions of muscular spasticity but has been rarely used for cosmetic purposes. A recent randomized, placebo-controlled trial demonstrated that RimB is effective for the treatment of glabellar lines with patient satisfaction and adverse event profiles comparable to BTX-A products.[16] However, in this study, the benefit persisted for only 8 weeks with the highest doses tested, and, at 12 weeks, muscular activity in almost all patients had returned to baseline. Furthermore, because of the mild acidity of reconstituted RimB (pH = 5.6), injections may not be tolerated as well as BTX-A. The speed of onset, though, may be shorter (2–3 days) than with BTX-A (3–7 days).[17,18] Because of its shorter duration of action, its role in cosmetics will remain limited to unusual and specific situations where rapid onset is critical or when tachyphylaxis to a BTX-A product has developed. In the latter scenario, RimB has proven effective.[19]

AboA (Dysport) was first licensed for medical usage in Europe in 1990. Clinical studies for aesthetic indications were first performed in Europe in 2002 and 2003, followed by US FDA studies in 2009. FDA approval for treatment of glabellar frown lines occurred in May 2009. **Table 1** summarizes the differences between the

two formulations of BTX-A. Although variations in progenitor complex size as previously described may exist and the excipients differ, it must be stressed that the *active ingredient is thought to be identical and as such the clinical properties* of the two agents are largely similar. Purported variations in clinical behavior are likely to be subtle when controlled for volume, toxin concentration, and injection technique.

The most important difference between OnaA and AboA is in the activity units employed by their respective manufacturers: Botox units (bU) for OnaA and Speywood units (sU) for AboA. Both define 1 unit as the quantity necessary to kill 50% of mice (LD_{50}) with an intraperitoneal injection. Because of differences in the experimental design of their murine assays, however, the units are not equivalent. The Dysport assay is undeniably more sensitive (ie, less toxin is required to kill a mouse when toxin of any formulation is tested in this assay vs the Botox assay).[20] Indeed, in a small study it was shown that, when tested in the Dysport assay, the LD_{50} of Botox is achieved with 0.32 bU (68% less product than that required for LD_{50} in the Botox assay).[20] Therefore, a Speywood unit corresponds to a smaller quantity of active toxin than does a Botox unit. The exact potency ratio between a Speywood unit and

Table 1
Overview of product composition for the FDA-approved Botulinum toxin serotype A agents

Product	OnaA (Botox)	AboA (Dysport)	IncA (Xeomin)
Manufacturer	Ipsen (Europe) Medicis (USA)	Allergan	Merz Pharmaceuticals
Units per vial	100 bU	300 sU (for cosmetic use)	50 or 100 units
Active ingredient (molecular weight)	Botulinum toxin serotype A complex (900 kDa)	Botulinum toxin serotype A complex (500–900 kDa)[a]	Uncomplexed Botulinum toxin serotype A (150 kDa)
Total toxin protein per vial (active toxin + NAPs[b])	5 ng	2.61 ng	0.6 ng (in 100 units)
Excipients	Human serum Albumin 500 µg NaCl 0.9 mg	Human serum Albumin 125 µg Lactose 2.5 mg	Human serum Albumin 1 mg Sucrose 4.7 mg
Bacterial source	*Clostridium botulinum*, Hall strain[c]	*Clostridium botulinum*, Hall strain[c]	*Clostridium botulinum*, Hall strain[c]
Storage conditions	2–8°C	2–8°C	Up to 25°C
Purification process	Dialysis and acid precipitation then vacuum dried	Column chromatography then freeze dried (lyophilized)	Column chromatography then freeze dried (lyophilized)

IncobotulinumtoxinA is only approved for therapeutic use.
[a] Molecular weight of AboA is not firmly established –See discussion in text.
[b] Neurotoxin-associated proteins.
[c] There are numerous Hall strains and the manufacturers do not necessarily use identical bacteria.
Data from Refs.[54,57–61]

a Botox unit remains an open question. Because, in any competitive marketplace, product interchangeability is not a desirable attribute, the BTX-A manufacturers have predictably emphasized the uniqueness of their formulations and have discouraged the use of any unit conversion factors. Nevertheless, practitioners have sought to define a conversion factor to guide the novice injector when transitioning from one toxin to the other for a given application.

Numerous in vivo and in vitro studies have attempted to define this conversion factor with conflicting results. For a comprehensive review of this literature, please refer to the recently published review by Karsai and Raulin.[21] Only a brief summary of the pertinent human studies follows. A 2004 meta-analysis, using Cochrane Review methodology, identified 4 high-quality comparative clinical studies all examining neurologic indications, 2 employed a 1:4 (OnaA/AboA) dose ratio, 1employed a 1:3 ratio, and the last used 1:3 and 1:4 in separate arms.[22] This analysis concluded that a 1:4 ratio was too high and a 1:3 ratio approached bioequivalence, although the included studies suggested that an even lower ratio might be more appropriate. An independently funded, double-blind study of Dysport versus Botox for the treatment of glabellar lines found a longer duration of action as assessed by electromyographic studies with Dysport used at a 1:3 ratio. This finding led the investigators to conclude the bioequivalent ratio was less than 1:3.[23] Lowe and colleagues[24] examined the relative effects of a 1:2.5 dose ratio on glabellar lines assessed by blinded investigator rating and found greater longevity with Botox. Therefore, although the preponderance of current evidence supports a dose ratio of no more than 1:3, a more precise definition awaits additional controlled, head-to-head comparisons with ideally objective measurements of muscle activity. The investigators recommend a conversion factor of 1:2.5, which has become the most commonly quoted unit dose ratio among experienced injectors. The multiple studies that underpinned the FDA-approved dosages for glabellar lines (50 sU of Dysport and 20 bU of Botox) demonstrated comparable efficacy with the two BTX-A products, further supporting the 1:2.5 ratio as a starting point for cosmetic applications.

The perception that an increased capacity for a toxin to diffuse from the site of injection translates into increased side effects has encouraged a lively debate among the manufacturers of the BTX-A products. The question of diffusion has mostly been investigated in humans by measuring anhidrotic haloes after injecting equal volumes of each agent into the forehead. Some comparative studies of Botox and Dysport have demonstrated that anhidrotic haloes are significantly larger for Dysport.[9,25] The only double-blind randomized study used a Botox/Dysport unit ratio of 1:3, and one could argue that the increased anhidrotic haloes observed in this study with Dysport is a consequence of not using equipotent dosages. In other words, diffusion is primarily driven by concentration gradients, and it would be expected that a higher injected concentration of neurotoxin would result in greater diffusion. In an unblinded study, Trindade De Almeida and colleagues[25] examined 3 different dose ratios: 1:2.5, 1:3, and 1:4. They found significantly increased anhidrotic haloes with all dose ratios (the mean absolute increase in area of the anhidrotic halo was 1.2 cm^2 with the lowest Dysport dose). These results were challenged by a similarly designed comparative trial conducted by Hexsel and colleagues,[26] which found no significant difference in the field of anhidrosis using only the more widely accepted equipotent dose ratio of 1:2.5. Hexsel and colleagues[26] reported taking great care to standardize injection technique, which would certainly influence results. Of note, the first two studies described were sponsored by Allergan and the third by Ipsen. A definitive answer to this question will await an impartial, double-blind study comparing truly equipotent injections of neurotoxins.

In conclusion, it must be emphasized that subtle differences in the properties of the BTX-A formulations may exist. Extant data on product composition, diffusion properties, and relative clinical potencies remains inconclusive. Indeed, the number and types of NAPs probably differ between BTX-A products. NAPs have known biologic relevance in the pathogenesis of food-borne botulism.[27] One recent study demonstrated that a hemagglutinin protein binds E-cadherin to facilitate passage of toxin through epithelial tight junctions within the alimentary canal.[28] This finding raises the unexplored and previously discounted possibility that NAPs could have other specific biologic functions, some that might impinge on the neuromuscular activity of injected BTX-A. Until we possess a better understanding of these various issues, the injector is advised to think and treat independently with each BTX-A product, as one learns a foreign language, and avoid converting for usage.

Botulinum Toxins on the Horizon

Other BTX-A preparations now under consideration for aesthetic usage include 2 additional injectables (incobotulinumtoxinA [IncA; Xeomin] and PurTox) and a topical BTX-A (RT001). PurTox and IncA are both naked neurotoxins (ie, pure formulations of the 150-kDa active-di-chain). They are in phase III trials. Recently published results from a phase III comparative trial of 24 units of either IncA or OnaA in the treatment of glabellar lines exhibited nearly identical response rates and a similar incidence of adverse effects.[29] IncA is already approved in Germany for cosmetic use and was approved in the United States for therapeutic use (blepharospasm and cervical dystonia) on July 30, 2010. Both IncA and PurTox will likely be approved for cosmetic use in the United States within 5 years. The absence of NAPs might theoretically decrease the immunogenicity of the agent (see later discussion of neutralizing antibodies). Of course, the smaller molecular weight has also raised the specter of an increased capacity for tissue diffusion.

RT001 is a particularly exciting new product as it affords an entirely different method of administration. RT001 is a topical gel formulated with the 150-kDa toxin and a proprietary peptide that facilitates transcutaneous delivery. In a recently published placebo-controlled trial, investigators applied RT001 under occlusion to the lateral canthal rhytids for 30 minutes and repeated this at 4 weeks. At 8 weeks, 94.7% exhibited at least a 1-point improvement on a 5-point lateral canthal rhytid scale and 50% experienced a 2-point improvement (vs 0% of placebo).[30] Depth of penetration likely limits its utility to superficial muscles, such as the lateral orbicularis oculi. Because of its potential for frequent painless administration and usage in areas in which injectables pose significant risks (eg, lower eyelids and lateral lips), RT001 may occupy a unique cosmetic niche in the future.

RECONSTITUTION, SUPPLIES, AND STORAGE

The package inserts of Botox and Dysport both advise reconstitution in 2.5 mL of unpreserved saline (1.5 mL is also a listed alternative for Dysport). A randomized, double-blind study has shown that there is less pain and equal efficacy with preserved saline, which is possibly secondary to the anesthetic properties of the benzyl alcohol that is added as a bacteriostatic agent.[31] A 2004 consensus conference of opinion leaders on the cosmetic use of Botox reported that most injectors use a preserved diluent. This consensus conference also reported that a wide range of dilution volumes is in common usage.[32] The field of effect of an injected toxin is dependent both on diffusion (as previously discussed) and spread, a physical parameter that describes the forced dispersion of the toxin as a consequence of injection pressure and volume. Thus, the field of effect increases

proportionately with the volume injected assuming other variables are held constant. This consideration is important when precise localization of effect is desired, such as at the inferior orbital rim, and has led many injectors to favor a more concentrated toxin solution. Certainly, smaller volumes are prudent for inexperienced injectors. Also, in theory, larger volumes could decrease efficacy. The albumin that is included in the BTX-A vials (present at 25,000-fold excess relative to the toxin; see **Table 1**) coat potential nonspecific protein binding sites on glassware and plastics used for storage and injection. As the albumin becomes more dilute, the extent of blocking decreases, which creates the potential for loss of toxin caused by adherence to the vial or syringe. The diluent volume at which this phenomenon might become germane is undefined but may be substantial. A recent study demonstrated that dilutions of 10 units/mL to 100 units/mL produced indistinguishable results in the treatment of glabellar rhytids.[33]

The authors reconstitute OnaA in 1 mL of preserved saline and AboA in 3 mL, which yields a concentration of 1 unit per 0.01 mL for both agents (**Table 2**). Thus, each gradation on an insulin syringe corresponds to 1 unit. This approach affords an added safety measure and reduces the potential for error when support staff are instructed to draw up a specified quantity of BTX.

The manufacturers of both BTX-A products recommend usage within 4 hours of reconstitution. However, there is no loss of efficacy after up to 6 weeks of storage of reconstituted OnaA at 4°C.[34] Although it is advised to slowly and carefully add diluent to the vial to avoid bubbles, a comparison of an agitated, foamy solution of BTX-A to an unagitated solution failed to reveal significant differences in response or duration of effect.[35]

Table 2
Dilution table for OnaA (100-unit vial) and AboA (300-unit vial)

Diluent Volume (mL)	OnaA Units (bU) per 0.1 mL	AboA Units (sU) per 0.1 mL
1.0	**10.0**	30.0
1.5	6.7	20.0
2.0	5.0	15.0
2.5	4.0	12.0
3.0	3.3	**10.0**
4.0	2.5	7.5
5.0	2.0	6.0

Authors' preferred concentrations are in bold.

The authors prefer to inject using an insulin syringe with a 31-gauge needle. These syringes have no dead space between the syringe barrel and needle, minimizing waste. They have easily visualized gradations, which correspond 1:1 with units of BTX-A when reconstituted as previously described. Finally, the ultrafine needle is well tolerated by patients.

ONSET AND DURATION OF ACTION

Clinically detectable rhytid reduction occurs 3 to 7 days after injection, although the onset of action of OnaA has not been formally studied. In contrast, the self-reported onset of action of AboA was specifically investigated in its 4 phase III FDA trials. Patients were asked to maintain diaries during the initial 7 days following injection. The patients' self-reported median onset of action ranged from 2 to 4 days with 13.4% to 32.5% responding in the first 24 hours. (Schlessinger J, Kane M, Monheit GD. Time-to-onset of response of abobotulinumtoxinA in the treatment of glabellar lines: a subset analysis of phase 3 clinical trials of a new botulinum toxin type A. Submitted for publication.) Some have proposed, therefore, that AboA has a more rapid clinical efficacy than OnaA but head-to-head comparative analyses of this endpoint do not exist. Furthermore, the mechanistic rationale for speedier onset is unclear. With both agents, maximum benefit may not occur for 2 weeks after injection.

The longevity of the BTX-A response is variable and depends on dose (which determines the extent of denervation) and patient characteristics, such as age and baseline muscle strength. The duration of effect usually falls within a range of 3 to 5 months. There is some evidence that patients experience longer responses with repeated injections. This finding may be caused by slower neural regeneration but may also be a consequence of a conditioned behavioral change in facial expressiveness (ie, the prolonged inability to frown leads to diminished frowning even when muscle strength returns).

PRESENT USES
General Principles

1. Dose must be tailored to the individual patient, taking into account idiosyncratic anatomy, individual muscle size, tone and strength, baseline asymmetries, and perhaps most importantly, desired outcome.
2. A thorough knowledge of the anatomy in an area of injection is required to optimize efficacy and safety.

3. Neurotoxin monotherapy is most gratifying for patients with predominantly dynamic wrinkling or small facial asymmetries or ptoses. Patients with enhanced resting muscle tone that report looking angry or sad all of the time are also good candidates. Permanently etched lines, which usually represent wrinkling from photodamage or volume loss, generally require combined approaches with other modalities for satisfactory results.

TREATMENT OF THE UPPER FACE
Glabellar Lines

Injection of the glabella is the original and by far most common cosmetic usage of BTX-A. Numerous randomized, placebo-controlled trials have demonstrated the efficacy of both AboA and OnaA for this indication.

Anatomy

The glabellar complex depresses the medial brow and consists of the paired corrugator supercilii, which flank the central procerus muscle. Each corrugator originates medially on the frontal bone at the glabella just lateral to its junction with the nasal bone (this bony juncture is referred to as the nasion and underlies the anatomic concavity at the nasal root). The muscle fibers travel superolaterally to insert on the skin of the forehead just superior to the midpupillary eyebrow. As such, the corrugators adduct and depress the medial brow and produce the *vertical glabellar lines*. Laterally, the corrugators decussate with the medial portion of the orbicularis oculi, which also contributes to the glabellar complex.

The procerus originates from the fascia overlying the nasal bones and fans out superiorly to insert broadly in the skin of the lower central forehead. Contraction produces the *horizontal frown lines* at the nasal root.

Injection

Patients are requested to frown maximally. Muscle size and strength can be qualitatively categorized as a mild, moderate, or severe frown (**Fig. 1**) and the dose adjusted accordingly. Also, it is important to compensate for asymmetry in corrugator strength, which is common, with differential BTX dosing. Occasionally, patients present with a broad procerus or even 2 apparent procerus bellies, a bifid procerus. In these patients, we typically divide the procerus dose into 2 injections into each belly.

The standard 5-injection point approach is appropriate for most patients with 2 injections in each corrugator and 1 injection in the procerus as diagrammed in **Fig. 2**. The procerus and medial corrugators are injected deeply and directly into

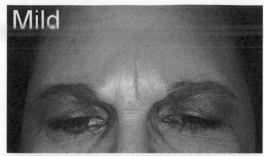

Mild

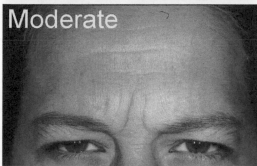

Moderate

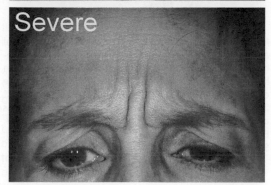

Severe

Fig. 1. Frown severity.

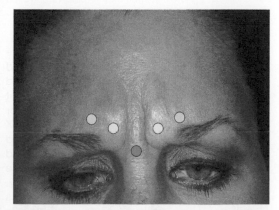

Fig. 2. Injection sites for glabellar line treatment: Blue dots indicate the corrugator insertion/orbicularis oculi fibers, yellow dots indicate the corrugator bodies, and the green dot indicates the procerus.

the bodies of the muscles, which are easily identified at maximal frown in most patients. The lateral corrugator is injected slightly more superficially where it inserts into the dermis and medial to the midpupillary line. These lateral injections also target fibers of the orbicularis oculi. All injections should be 1.0 cm (approximately 1 fingerbreadth) above the orbital rim to limit the risk of eyelid ptosis from the spread of toxin to the levator palpebrae muscle.

The total dose of OnaA should be 20 bU and the total dose of AboA should be 50 sU in women with moderate frown, divided evenly among the 5 injections. As always, doses must be adjusted for the strength of individual muscles and the patients' desired outcome. A dose-ranging study exhibited improved results with men who received 40 bU in the glabella versus 20 bU. Higher doses did not result in more adverse events and no cases of ptosis were reported in this small study.[36] The authors do use a higher dose of toxin in men and may add 2 additional injection points at the midpupillary line in those with bulky corrugators. However, the authors almost never exceed a total dose of 40 bU in any patients.

In the initial clinical trials with AboA, men did not have as robust a response to the 50 sU dose as did women, presumably because of increased muscle mass. This finding inspired a further study that varied the AboA dose with corrugator/procerus volume. Men with mild frown (small muscle mass) received 60 sU, moderate 70 sU, and severe 80 sU. Correlating the dose with muscle mass raised the response rate of men to that of women and increased the longevity of response in all patients.[37]

Forehead Lines

Although an off-label usage, BTX-A provides excellent smoothing of forehead rhytids and is generally a gratifying procedure for patients when performed properly. However, the more severe forms of forehead wrinkles cannot be corrected by BTX-A denervation alone and may need soft-tissue augmentation. This need can be determined by the degree of wrinkling and the affect of BTX in reducing the wrinkle. Moderate to severe dynamic wrinkles at rest and at maximal frown usually indicate filling material or even surgical intervention may be needed for full forehead and brow correction. Perhaps more so than any other region of the face, the placement and dosage of toxin can be highly customized, and optimal results are achieved when factors, such as forehead height and width, muscular strength, symmetry, and baseline brow position, are all incorporated into a treatment plan.

Anatomy

Contraction of the frontalis muscle produces horizontal forehead lines. This muscle is a paired muscle that originates in the galea aponeurotica inferior to the coronal suture essentially at the frontal hairline. Its fibers run vertically and insert in the subcutis and deep dermis of the eyebrow at the superciliary arch (the bony projection of the frontal bone superior to the orbital rim). The frontalis is frequently absent at the midline, although this is variable. The frontalis is the only significant brow elevator. Its inferiormost portion is critical for opposing brow depression by the orbicularis oculi at rest.

Injection

The goal for the treatment of forehead wrinkles is to soften the undesirable lines without causing brow ptosis or eliminating all expressiveness on the upper face. A conservative approach is preferred, informing patients preoperatively that more than 1 treatment may be needed to reach the desired level of wrinkle reduction while avoiding undesirable side effects. Patients are asked to forcefully raise their eyebrows and the strength of the frontalis is assessed. Any discrepancy in brow position at baseline and at maximal contraction is noted and brought to the attention of the patients. A compensatory downward dose adjustment should be made on the side with the lower eyebrow. In the average brow, 2 to 4 bU or 5 to 10 sU are injected in 4 to 6 sites at least 2.5 to 3.0 cm above the orbital rim. Administration more inferiorly greatly increases the risk of brow ptosis. In toxin naïve patients, the authors almost always begin at the lower end of that dosage range. A common strategy is to place the line of injection parallel and inferior to a deep furrow crossing the middle to upper third of the forehead (**Fig. 3**). For high foreheads (typically men) or those with many fine wrinkles, the same total dose may be divided into 2 lines of injection across the forehead separated by 1 cm. A lateral arch to the eyebrow is characteristic of the female brow pattern. This arch can be accentuated in female patients by placing less toxin lateral to the midpupillary line or raising this injection point 1 cm relative to the midforehead and central forehead injections. The authors commonly use a V-shaped configuration for injections in women (**Fig. 4**). Although often desirable in women, this should be avoided in male patients. This approach can also produce an excessively arched brow (the mephisto sign or Dr Spock look) that will require

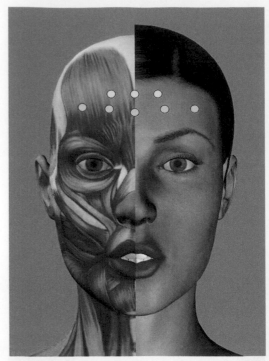

Fig. 3. Standard forehead line treatment: a typical approach is 4 to 6 injection points across middle of forehead (yellow dots indicate optional injection points in high foreheads). Lateral injection points determine degree of eyebrow movement. Keep injections at least 2.5 to 3.0 cm above brow to avoid brow ptosis and loss of expressivity. (*Adapted from* de Maio M, Rzany B. Botulinum toxin in aesthetic medicine. Berlin: Springer-Verlag; 2007; with permission.)

correction with a small dose of additional toxin 1 to 2 cm superior to the apex of the arch.

Unless no significant glabellar lines are present, the authors commonly inject the glabella

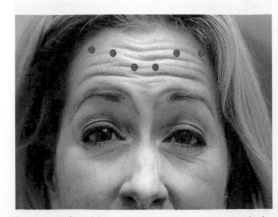

Fig. 4. Forehead line treatment in women. Variation favored by authors to accentuate the lateral arching of the feminine brow pattern.

simultaneously whenever treating forehead wrinkles. This practice generally produces better overall aesthetic results and the concomitant paralysis of the brow depressors reduces the incidence of brow ptosis.

Lateral Eyebrow Lift

The paresis of muscles of facial expression not only smoothes dynamic wrinkles but can also influence the resting position of various facial elements. This property has been successfully exploited to lift the eyebrow, correcting mild brow ptosis, restoring a youthful brow arch, and giving the eye a more open appearance. The eyebrow position is determined by the balance of the resting tone of the brow elevator (the frontalis) and depressors (glabellar complex and orbicularis oculi). Unilateral injection into the medial brow depressors, as occurs with treatment of glabellar lines, elevates the medial and central brow modestly (<1 mm). Glabellar complex treatment alone has also been shown to lift the lateral brow by as much or more than the medial brow.[38] This unexpected result was postulated to stem from inadvertent paralysis of the inferomedial portions of the frontalis with a consequent increased tone in the lateral frontalis.

The vertical fibers of the lateral orbicularis oculi function to depress the lateral brow. BTX-A injected into these fibers can produce a significant lateral brow elevation, as much as 4.88 mm in one study, although a 2-mm elevation is more likely.[39] For this chemical brow lift, the authors typically inject 5 units of OnaA or 10 units of AboA intradermally at the lateral tail of the eyebrow 5 to 7 mm superolateral to the orbital rim (**Fig. 5**A). If performed in isolation, an additional injection into each corrugator body is typically added to complete the chemical brow lift. More commonly, the lateral brow lift injection is done in tandem with other upper face treatments, especially injection of the glabellar complex and forehead. In combination with medial and central frontalis denervation, which tends to lower the medial brow, a pleasingly arched female pattern eyebrow can be shaped (**Fig. 5**B).

Crow's Feet

Lateral periorbital wrinkling is one of the earliest signs of aging. Hyperkinetic lateral canthal lines are effectively treated with neurotoxin. In older patients, static wrinkling caused by photodamage becomes more prominent and is less responsive to BTX alone. It is important to manage expectations in these patients as they may need a resurfacing procedure in addition to toxin to achieve the desired wrinkle reduction.

Anatomy

The orbicularis oculi is the sphincter of the eye. It is divided into 3 parts: orbital, palpebral, and lacrimal. All 3 work in concert during forced closure of the eye. The orbital portion runs circumferentially around the orbital rim and is the primary portion targeted by BTX-A in the treatment of crow's feet (CF).

Injection

CF are typically treated with 3 equal injections of 2 to 4 bU or 5 to 10 sU evenly spaced along an arc lying at least 1 cm external to the orbital rim to avoid diffusion to the palpebral portion of the orbicularis oculi or to the levator palpebrae muscle (**Fig. 6**A, B). The middle injection is placed in line with the lateral canthus. Injections flanking this point at 8 to 10 mm are then placed, but their exact

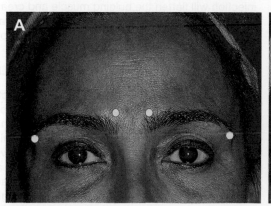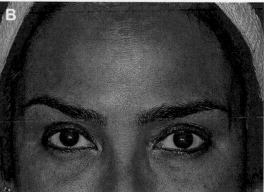

Fig. 5. The chemical brow lift. (*A*) Injection sites for a chemical brow lift if performed alone are shown (5–10 sU or 3–5 bU per injection site). This patient had a male pattern eyebrow without perceptible arching. She received AboA treatment to the lateral tail of each eyebrow (10 sU per side), into the corrugators bodies (total 20 sU), and to the frontalis (20 sU). (*B*) Posttreatment at 33 days reveals an elevated and laterally arched feminine brow.

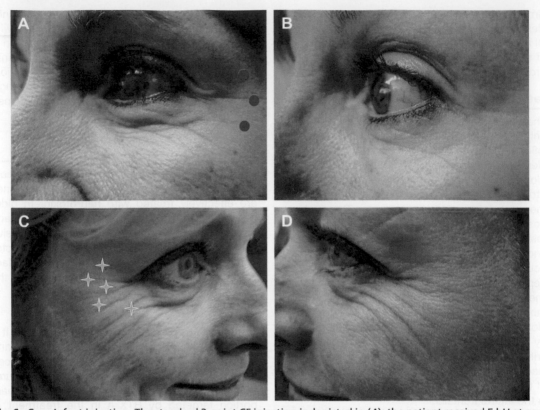

Fig. 6. Crow's feet injection. The standard 3-point CF injection is depicted in (*A*); the patient received 5 bU at each point and had an excellent response (*B*). (*C*) A variation that employs the same total dose (20–30 sU or 10–15 bU per side) but divided into 5 smaller injections for broad and wide canthal lines. (*D*) It is common for CF to have a significant inferior extension as in the pictured patient. It is imperative not to chase CF beyond the zygoma or one risks denervation of the zygomaticus muscles.

positioning depends on the width of the individual's canthal lines (**Fig. 6**C). The highest CF injection is inferior to the lateral eyebrow tail injection previously described for a chemical brow lift. The authors commonly lower this superior CF injection slightly when a CF treatment and a chemical brow lift are performed concomitantly. The skin of the temple is thin with little subcutis and the orbicularis oculi is located more superficially then most facial muscles. Injections, therefore, should be intradermal, producing a visible bleb.

The authors also commonly treat lower eyelid wrinkles with a series of 3 to 4 evenly spaced low dose, infraorbital injections of 0.5 to 1.0 bU or 1 to 2 sU (**Fig. 7**), usually injected in conjunction with and in the same manner as the CF injections. These multiple, low-dose intradermal injections can produce a notable smoothing of wrinkles with an excellent safety profile. The zygoma is a critical landmark for CF treatment. BTX should never be placed inferior to the zygoma (**Fig. 6**D), and any injections medial to the zygoma must be placed at or above the orbital rim. Violation of this rule can lead to unintended paresis of the

zygomaticus major or minor muscles resulting in an ipsilateral mouth droop and a dissatisfied patient.

An additional injection of 1 bU or 2 sU can be judiciously placed in the lower lid at the midpupillary line 2 mm below the tarsal plate (**Fig. 8**). This injection will flatten the bulging muscle and create an image of an open eye. Overaggressive treatment may, though, create an unwanted ectropion.

TREATMENT OF THE MID AND LOWER FACE

As experience with BTX-A increases, many practitioners have ventured beyond the traditional applications of BTX-A in the upper face. Although not as extensively chronicled, BTX-A has definite utility in the rejuvenation of the mid and lower face but, in most patients, is best employed as adjuvant therapy with soft-tissue fillers or resurfacing procedures. The latter point has been highlighted in a recent prospective study. Ninety patients were randomized to receive (1) OnaA to the lips, depressor anguli oris (DAO), and mentalis muscles; (2) hyaluronic acid filler (Juvederm Ultra

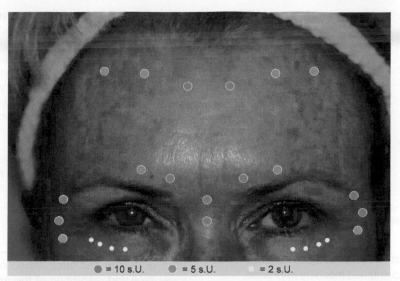

= 10 s.U.   = 5 s.U.   = 2 s.U.

Fig. 7. Treatment of infraorbital wrinkles. A series of 3 to 4 *low dose, superficial* injections can effectively and safely smooth infraorbital rhytids (*yellow dots*). Injection must be at or superior to the orbital rim to avoid inadvertent paresis of mouth elevators and at or lateral to the midpupillary line to prevent epiphora (watering eye). The patient pictured had a complete upper face treatment: chemical brow lift, forehead, glabella, and CF. The picture illustrates the kind of tailored dosing strategy that produces optimal results with neurotoxins. The CF injections were reduced to 2 because of her narrow lateral canthal lines and orbit. A total standard dose of 50 sU was injected into the glabella but the dose was concentrated in her broad, well-developed procerus with less toxin administered laterally.

or Ultra Plus) to the lips, oral commissures, marionette lines, and chin; or (3) combined treatment with both. Multiple objective outcome measures were assessed, as was patient satisfaction. The group receiving both OnaA and dermal filler performed significantly better in all endpoints. Notably, the toxin-only group demonstrated the least efficacy.[40]

Bunny Lines

Multiple dynamic wrinkles on the upper nasal dorsum are common and can even be

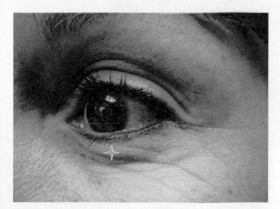

Fig. 8. Location of lower palpebral injection: a tiny dose of toxin into the lower eyelid can create a more youthful, open eye (2 sU or 0.5–1.0 bU).

accentuated in BTX recipients as frowning patients compensate for glabellar paralysis.

Anatomy
The nasalis muscle has 2 portions. The alar portion dilates the nares and possesses minimal functional or cosmetic relevance. Nasoglabellar lines are a consequence of contraction of the transverse portion of the nasalis. The nasalis covers the nasal sidewalls, originating on the maxillary bones bilaterally and travelling medially to insert on a thin aponeurosis overlying the nasal bridge.

Injection
A single injection can be aimed at the point of maximal nasalis contraction (ie, the center of an imaginary circle encompassing the bunny lines). This point is usually one-third the way up the nasal sidewall and about 1 cm superior to the alar groove (**Fig. 9**). A dose of 2 to 4 bU or 5 to 10 sU per side is adequate for most patients.

Lips

Vertical perioral rhytids are a consummate feature of the aging face and can be bothersome, especially to female patients. Frequent puckering and pursing of the lips and activities, such as cigarette smoking, can contribute to the development of dynamic wrinkling in this area. However, perioral lines commonly possess a multifactorial etiology, including

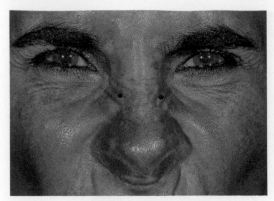

Fig. 9. Bunny line injection points: 10 sU or 5 bU units per point intradermally into nasal sidewall.

photoaging and chronologic aging, and, as such, benefit from a combined modality approach.

Anatomy
The elegant choreography of musculature that enables the diverse functionality of the human mouth (speech, music, mastication, and expression) is complex and a full discussion is beyond the scope of this review. Perioral BTX targets the central portion of the orbicularis oris, a wide, thin muscular band encircling the lips. The orbicularis oris controls closure and protrusion of the mouth.

Injection
For the upper cutaneous lip, 1 or 2 injections of 0.5 bU or 1.0 sU are placed on each side of the philtrum

along the vermilion border (**Fig. 10**). BTX should never be placed where unintended paresis of the lateral lip elevators could occur. Therefore, the injections should be medial to a vertical line dropped from the lateral edge of the ala to the vermilion. The lower lip is treated similarly with 1 injection (0.5 bU or 1.0 sU) along the lower vermilion border either in line with the upper vermilion injection (if 1 injection) or bisecting the upper vermilion injections (if 2 injections).

The authors rarely, if ever, employ BTX alone to address perioral rhytids but do find it a useful complement to hyaluronic acid fillers in patients with a significant component of dynamic wrinkling.

Drooping Oral Commissures

Loss of dermal and subcutaneous volume in the lower face and resorption of the mandibular body occur inexorably with age. These processes frequently culminate in the formation of prominent melomental folds or marionette lines and an accompanying inferior displacement and downturn of the corners of the mouth. Adequate correction of this problem requires volume replacement, but a small, precise dose of BTX to the DAO muscles can provide a modest lift to the oral commissures, remedying an inverted smile.

Anatomy
The DAO is a triangular muscle with a broad base along the mandibular body beginning anterior to the masseter and extending to and a little beyond

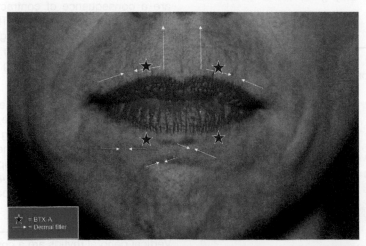

Fig. 10. Treatment of perioral rhytids: superficial perioral rhytids can be ameliorated with 1 to 2 microdoses of toxin per side (0.5 bU or 1.0 sU) placed near the upper vermilion border between the philtral crest and an imaginary vertical line dropped from the lateral edge of the ala (*blue stars*). These microdoses are coupled with a single injection per side at the lower vermilion border, if indicated. In approaching perioral rhytids, the authors usually combine toxin with dermal fillers. The pictured patient received hyaluronic acid filler along both philtral crests along the entire upper vermilion border (excluding the philtrum) and focally for depressions in the lower cutaneous lip (*white arrows*).

the oral commissure. It inserts at the oral commissure where its fibers interdigitate with the orbicularis oris and risorius muscles and contribute to the modiolus complex. As its name implies, DAO contraction generates an inferolateral pull on the corner of the mouth.

Injection
The DAO can be identified by instructing patients to clench their teeth, which facilitates palpation of the anterior border of the masseter. The DAO is then injected with 5 bU or 10 sU at a point 1 cm anterior to the masseter a few millimeters above the inferior border of the body of the mandible (**Fig. 11A**). Contraction of the DAO can usually be palpated at this location by directing patients to forcefully downturn the corners of their mouth. When treating DAOs, precise localization of toxin is critical. If BTX is injected at a point too high or too medial, then weakening of the orbicularis oris or depressor labii inferioris (**Fig. 11B**), respectively, could ensue with accompanying asymmetric smile, lip protrusion, and oral sphincteric incompetence. To avoid these untoward effects, BTX must never be placed close to the oral commissure.

Dimpled Chin and Mental Crease
Occasionally individuals will present with puckering and dimpling of their chin when they voluntarily or involuntarily contract their mentalis muscle. In others, a hyperkinetic mentalis produces a deep mental crease that is a source

of self-consciousness. Although not common, these complaints can be ameliorated with partial denervation of the mentalis.

Anatomy
The mentalis is a paired muscle that originates low in the incisive fossa on the midline anterior surface of the mandible and inserts in the integument on either side of the frenulum of the lower lip. Contraction protrudes the lower lip but can also create a corrugated appearance to the chin.

Injection
Bilateral, symmetric 5 bU or 10 sU injections are made 2 mm above the inferior border of the body of the mandible about 5 mm lateral to midline (**Fig. 12**). Some injectors prefer a single midline injection (**Fig. 12**). Instructing patients to raise their lower lip to their nose will accentuate the mentalis and aid in localization of toxin. The depth of injection does not appear to be critical.

Platysmal Bands
Although the progress in nonsurgical rejuvenation of the face over the past decade has been nothing short of sensational, the same, unfortunately, cannot be said of the aging neck, which still poses a conundrum to the cosmetic surgeon. Attempts to eliminate horizontal neck creases with BTX have been discouraging. Despite overall frustration, neurotoxins have a clear role in the treatment of one bothersome component of the senescent neck, platysmal bands. As we age, there is an invariable loss of elasticity and soft-tissue support

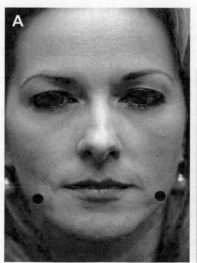
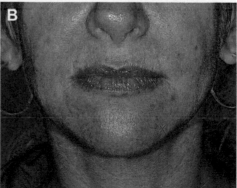

Fig. 11. Depressor anguli oris injection points: (*A*) The DAO is injected approximately 1 cm medial to the lateral edge of the masseter. Although the DAO is actually centered somewhat medial to this point, the injection targets its lateral fibers and is adequate to lift the oral commissure. (*B*) Injection too far medially (*red Xs*) risks paresis of the depressor labii inferioris and an asymmetric smile.

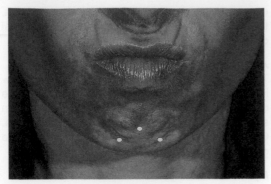

Fig. 12. Dimpled chin injection points: the mentalis is treated with 2 symmetric injections as shown (*blue dots*). A variation is single midline injection at a higher point (*yellow dot*) nearer the center of the body of the mentalis.

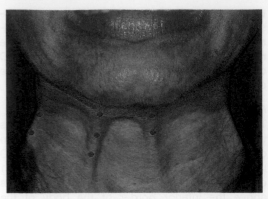

Fig. 13. Platysmal bands injection points: platysmal bands are treated with a series of 2 to 5 injections (2–4 bU or 5–10 sU each) spaced 2 cm apart along the length of the band. The total dose per band should be kept less than 50 sU or 25 bU. Pinching the band before injection can be helpful. Avoid deep injections in the neck.

of the neck. The resultant thinning and flaccidity of the neck skin makes platysmal contraction more prominent. This factor combined with an age-related separation and clumping of anterior fibers of the platysma generates readily apparent, tense, muscular cords vertically in the neck known as platysmal bands.

Anatomy

The platysma is a broad sheet of muscle that originates from the superficial fascia of the upper chest, clavicular, and parasternal regions. It envelops the anterior and lateral neck except for a thin strip devoid of fibers at the midline. The platysma crosses the mandible and then blends into the superficial muscular aponeurotic system encasing the muscles of facial expression of the lower face.

Injection

Two to 4 bU or 5 to 10 sU are injected into each platysmal band superficially beginning near the jawline and progressing caudally at 2-cm intervals (**Fig. 13**). Typically 2 to 5 injections and a total of 12 to 25 bU per band are required. To limit the total dose, no more than 3 or 4 bands are treated in one session. Excessive doses of BTX in the neck can produce hoarseness and dysphagia from denervation of laryngeal musculature.

COMPLICATIONS

The overall safety record of BTX is exceptional. A recent meta-analysis of placebo-controlled trials with OnaA for either lateral canthal or glabellar rhytids found only 3 adverse events (AEs) were more common than placebo among 1170 subjects: eyelid sensory disorder (2.4%), which includes subjective symptoms of tightness and heaviness; eyelid edema (1.1%), and eyelid ptosis (1.8%).[41]

Adverse sequelae of BTX administration can be divided into 2 major categories: product-related complications and technical complications. Importantly, all AEs to date have been ephemeral in nature and, to the authors' knowledge, no credible long-term complications have even been proposed, much less established.

Product-Related Complications

Considering the protracted list of side effects with most modern pharmaceuticals and the prodigious number of patients exposed to BTX, the number and frequency of true drug reactions to BTX is remarkably low. The injection of a foreign protein might be expected to trigger immunologic phenomena, but these are exceedingly rare. Type I immediate hypersensitivity reactions characterized by urticaria or anaphylaxis are listed as possible AEs on the package insert for OnaA. However, a literature search for these and other allergic complications revealed only one reported case of anaphylaxis.[42] This case was a fatal AE occurring in response to an unapproved BTX-lidocaine amalgam.[43] No cases of urticaria were found. There were only a handful of reports of cutaneous eruptions or potential hypersensitivity reactions that could be reasonably attributed to BTX-A or an associated excipient.[44–48] A 2005 comprehensive review of FDA AE reporting revealed 47 cases of unspecified "nonserious rash" and 13 "serious" cases of "allergic reactions/rash" out of millions of exposures, with 85% of the latter serious reactions following noncosmetic usage.[49]

Similarly, BTX does not appear to provoke significant cell-mediated immunity with few, if any, well-established reactions consistent with a delayed type hypersensitivity. There has been one report of postinjection nodules diagnosed as sarcoidosis[50] and one report of a fixed drug eruption elicited by the lactose included with AboA.[48] Three of the documented BTX-related eruptions previously mentioned had a morbilliform character comparable to a classic drug exanthem[45,47] (although 2 of these did not recur on rechallenge). BTX, in sufficient doses and durations, will, however, engender significant humoral immunity, including neutralizing antibodies. These antibodies have been reported in patients treated for cervical dystonia who receive repetitive treatments, each typically well in excess of 100 bU.[51,52] Despite intensive investigations by the manufacturers and others, neutralizing antibodies have not been discovered in patients treated for cosmetic purposes except for one patient after receiving 240 bU (4 injections of 60 bU) for masseter hypertrophy.[53,54]

Complications Related to Technique

Untoward sequelae that can occur at any site from BTX includes bruising, edema, erythema, pain, and transient numbness. These complaints are common to all percutaneous injections. Headache (usually mild) can develop, especially with treatments of the upper face, but in the aforementioned meta-analysis the incidence of headache in the BTX and placebo arms was not statistically different (10.6% vs 9.5%).[41] Alam and colleagues[55] described a rare, idiosyncratic severe headache reaction that can last up to 1 month, and patients should be counseled of this improbable outcome.

The second major group of technical complications is dose-dependent direct pharmacologic effects and involves either overtreatment of a targeted muscle (eg, brow ptosis from forehead paralysis) or unintentional paresis of adjacent musculature (eg, blepharoptosis following glabellar complex treatment). Most of these potential sequelae have been discussed in the relevant sections previously mentioned and are all avoidable with appropriate consideration of placement and dose. Much has been made of the different diffusion characteristics of current and future BTX-A products and how this may impinge on the relative safety of the agents. It is important, however, to temper this theoretical debate with the reality of published clinical experience. Per

Table 3
BTX-A dosages for common cosmetic applications

Indications	Total Usual Dose	Number of Injections	Dose Range
Glabella	50 sU 20 bU	5 (7 in some men)	40–80 sU 15–40 bU
Forehead	40–50 sU[a] 15–20 bU[a]	4–6	20–70 sU 10–30 bU
Crow's feet	60 sU 30 bU	3 per side	30–60 sU 18–30 bU
Lateral eyebrow lift	20 sU 10 bU	1 per side	10–20 sU 6–10 bU
Lower eyelid wrinkles	8–12 sU[b] 4–6 bU[b]	3–4 per side[b]	6–14 sU[b] 3–8 bU[b]
Bunny lines	20 sU 10 bU	2	10–20 sU 6–10 bU
Perioral wrinkles	4–6 sU 2–3 bU	4–6	4–6 sU 2–3 bU
Drooping oral commissure (DAOs)	20 sU 10 bU	2	10–20 sU 6–10 bU
Dimpled chin (mentalis)	20 sU 10 bU	2	10–20 sU 6–10 bU
Platysmal bands	20–35 sU 10–15 bU (per band)	2–5 per band (maximum 4 bands per treatment)	15–50 sU 12–25 bU (per band)

Total dose and dose range assume bilateral treatment, unless otherwise indicated.
[a] The authors almost always begin with a lower dose in new patients (20–30 sU or 10–12 bU).
[b] Does not include the optional extra injection 1 to 2 mm inferior to eyelid margin described in the text.

their respective package inserts, the incidence of lid ptosis accompanying the treatment of glabellar lines with 20 bU of OnaA was 3% compared with 2% with 50 sU of AboA. A review of the overall experience at one center administering AboA to 500 patients for facial rhytids in multiple anatomic locations was recently published. Dr Hevia used a consistent 1:2.67 unit dose ratio (OnaA/AboA) and a concentration of 133 sU/mL. There was a 0.6% overall incidence of ptosis (2 cases of lid ptosis and 1 case of brow ptosis) and no other significant AEs.[56] To the authors' knowledge, at recommended dosages and volumes, evidence of detectable differences attributable to less precise localization of one agent versus another in actual clinical practice does not yet exist. This fact should offer reassurance to the injector when administering either of the currently FDA-approved agents. See **Table 3** for a summary of Botox dose ranges for the most typical cosmetic applications.

SUMMARY

The advent of BTX-A in the 1990s effectively launched the modern era of nonsurgical aesthetic medicine. Many of the components of the senescent face, which previously required surgical intervention, are now readily addressed with neurotoxin. Its wide acceptance paved the way for the adoption of numerous other injectables, which are now commonplace in the cosmetic surgeon's office.

The two BTX-A products currently approved in the United States for cosmetic use share the same active ingredient and largely similar clinical properties. Because of the absence of unit equivalency and unbiased comparative trials, injectors should not consider the agents interchangeable. OnaA and AboA are best conceptualized as unique pharmaceuticals until more data is available.

BTX-A in monotherapy can be used to correct dynamic wrinkling of the upper face with an outstanding safety profile. BTX-A in the lower face is best thought of as a complement to soft-tissue fillers and resurfacing procedures but still plays an important role. In all areas, administration of BTX-A must be individualized based on patients' gender, muscle mass, and baseline symmetry. The patients' desired outcome is also an essential component in designing a treatment plan. Most patients and physicians target a natural look that softens wrinkles while maintaining some facial expressivity. The frozen look, so common when practitioners were first acclimating to BTX, should be a relic of the past. Similarly, in all

applications optimal results and patient satisfaction may necessitate combining multiple aesthetic modalities.

The upcoming approval of two additional BTX-A injectables alongside a topical formulation will offer the aesthetic surgeon a diverse armamentarium to denervate facial musculature. Insight into how these new products behave differently from those currently available must await further investigations and more clinical experience. If nothing else, the infusion of healthy price competition among these agents should only serve to make neurotoxins accessible to more of our patients.

REFERENCES

1. Data on file, Allergan, Inc. Safety analysis; from Allergan website. Available at: http://www.botoxcosmetic.com/botox_physician_info/clinical_information.aspx. Accessed on October 1, 2010.
2. Arnon SS, Schechter R, Inglesby TV, et al. Botulinum toxin as a biological weapon: medical and public health management. JAMA 2001;285(8):1059–70.
3. Henkel JS, Jacobson M, Tepp W, et al. Catalytic properties of botulinum neurotoxin subtypes A3 and A4. Biochemistry 2009;48(11):2522–8.
4. Lacy DB, Tepp W, Cohen AC, et al. Crystal structure of botulinum neurotoxin type A and implications for toxicity. Nat Struct Biol 1998;5(10):898–902.
5. Koriazova LK, Montal M. Translocation of botulinum neurotoxin light chain protease through the heavy chain channel. Nat Struct Biol 2003;10(1):13–8.
6. Schiavo G, Matteoli M, Montecucco C. Neurotoxins affecting neuroexocytosis. Physiol Rev 2000;80(2): 717–66.
7. Inoue K, Fujinaga Y, Watanabe T, et al. Molecular composition of Clostridium botulinum type A progenitor toxins. Infect Immun 1996;64(5):1589–94.
8. Lietzow MA, Gielow ET, Le D, et al. Subunit stoichiometry of the Clostridium botulinum type A neurotoxin complex determined using denaturing capillary electrophoresis. Protein J 2008;27(7–8): 420–5.
9. Cliff SH, Judodihardjo H, Eltringham E. Different formulations of botulinum toxin type A have different migration characteristics: a double-blind, randomized study. J Cosmet Dermatol 2008;7(1):50–4.
10. Pickett A. Dysport®: pharmacological properties and factors that influence toxin action. Toxicon 2009;54(5):683–9.
11. Karl-Heinz E, Taylor HV. Dissociation of the 900 kDa neurotoxin complex from C. botulinum under physiological conditions. Toxicon 2008;51(Suppl 1):10.
12. Eisele K-H, Fink K, Vey M, et al. Studies on the dissociation of botulinum neurotoxin type A complexes. Toxicon 2011;57:555–65.

13. Benedetto AV, editor. Botulinum toxin in clinical dermatology. Boca Raton (FL): Taylor & Francis; 2006.

14. Scott AB. Botulinum toxin injection of eye muscles to correct strabismus. Trans Am Ophthalmol Soc 1981; 79:734–70.

15. Carruthers JD, Carruthers JA. Treatment of glabellar frown lines with C. botulinum-A exotoxin. J Dermatol Surg Oncol 1992;18(1):17–21.

16. Carruthers A, Carruthers J, Flynn TC, et al. Dose-finding, safety, and tolerability study of Botulinum toxin type B for the treatment of hyperfunctional glabellar lines. Dermatol Surg 2007;33:S60–8.

17. Lowe NJ, Yamauchi PS, Lask GP, et al. Botulinum toxins types A and B for brow furrows: preliminary experiences with type B toxin dosing. J Cosmet Laser Ther 2002;4(1):15–8.

18. Flynn TC, Clark RE. Botulinum toxin type B (MYO-BLOC) versus Botulinum toxin type A (BOTOX) Frontalis Study: rate of onset and radius of diffusion. Dermatol Surg 2003;29(5):519–22.

19. Alster TS, Lupton JR. Botulinum toxin type B for dynamic glabellar rhytides refractory to Botulinum toxin type A. Dermatol Surg 2003;29(5):516–8.

20. Hambleton P, Pickett AM. Potency equivalence of botulinum toxin preparations. J R Soc Med 1994; 87(11):719.

21. Karsai S, Raulin C. Current evidence on the unit equivalence of different Botulinum Neurotoxin A formulations and recommendations for clinical practice in dermatology. Dermatol Surg 2009;35(1):1–8.

22. Sampaio C, Costa J, Ferreira JJ. Clinical comparability of marketed formulations of botulinum toxin. Mov Disord 2004;19(Suppl 8):S129–36.

23. Karsai S, Adrian R, Hammes S, et al. A randomized double-blind study of the effect of Botox and Dysport/Reloxin on forehead wrinkles and electromyographic activity. Arch Dermatol 2007;143(11): 1447–9.

24. Lowe P, Patnaik R, Lowe N. Comparison of two formulations of botulinum toxin type A for the treatment of glabellar lines: a double-blind, randomized study. J Am Acad Dermatol 2006;55(6):975–80.

25. Trindade De Almeida AR, Marques E, De Almeida J, et al. Pilot study comparing the diffusion of two formulations of Botulinum Toxin Type A in patients with forehead hyperhidrosis. Dermatol Surg 2007; 33:S37–43.

26. Hexsel D, Dal'Forno I, Hexsel C, et al. A randomized pilot study comparing the action halos of two commercial preparations of Botulinum toxin type A. Dermatol Surg 2008;34(1):52–9.

27. Sugawara Y, Fujinaga Y. The botulinum toxin complex meets E-cadherin on the way to its destination. Cell Adh Migr 2011;5(1):34–6.

28. Sugawara Y, Matsumura T, Takegahara Y, et al. Botulinum hemagglutinin disrupts the intercellular epithelial barrier by directly binding E-cadherin. J Cell Biol 2010;189(4):691–700.

29. Sattler G, Callander MJ, Grablowitz D, et al. Noninferiority of IncobotulinumtoxinA, free from complexing proteins, compared with another Botulinum toxin type A in the treatment of Glabellar Frown Lines. Dermatol Surg 2010;36:2146–54.

30. Brandt F, O'Connell C, Cazzaniga A, et al. Efficacy and safety evaluation of a novel botulinum toxin topical gel for the treatment of moderate to severe lateral canthal lines. Dermatol Surg 2010;36:2111–8.

31. Alam M, Dover JS, Arndt KA. Pain associated with injection of Botulinum A Exotoxin reconstituted using isotonic sodium chloride with and without preservative: a double-blind, randomized controlled trial. Arch Dermatol 2002;138(4):510–4.

32. Carruthers J, Fagien S, Matarasso SL, et al. Consensus recommendations on the use of botulinum toxin type a in facial aesthetics. Plast Reconstr Surg 2004;114(6):1S–22S.

33. Carruthers A, Carruthers J, Cohen J. Dilution volume of botulinum toxin type A for the treatment of glabellar rhytides: does it matter? Dermatol Surg 2007;33(1 Spec No.):S97–104.

34. Hexsel DM, De Almeida AT, Rutowitsch M, et al. Multicenter, double-blind study of the efficacy of injections with botulinum toxin type A reconstituted up to six consecutive weeks before application. Dermatol Surg 2003;29(5):523–9 [discussion: 529].

35. Trindade De Almeida AR, Kadunc BV, Di Chiacchio N, et al. Foam during reconstitution does not affect the potency of botulinum toxin type A. Dermatol Surg 2003;29(5):530–1 [discussion: 532].

36. Carruthers A, Carruthers J. Prospective, double-blind, randomized, parallel-group, dose-ranging study of botulinum toxin type A in men with glabellar rhytids. Dermatol Surg 2005;31(10):1297–303.

37. Kane MA, Brandt F, Rohrich RJ, et al. Evaluation of variable-dose treatment with a new U.S. Botulinum Toxin Type A (Dysport) for correction of moderate to severe glabellar lines: results from a phase III, randomized, double-blind, placebo-controlled study. Plast Reconstr Surg 2009;124(5):1619–29.

38. Carruthers A, Carruthers J. Eyebrow height after botulinum toxin type a to the glabella. Dermatol Surg 2007;33:S26–31.

39. Maas CS, Kim EJ. Temporal brow lift using botulinum toxin a: an update. Plast Reconstr Surg 2003;112(5): 109S–12S.

40. Carruthers A, Carruthers J, Monheit GD, et al. Multicenter, randomized, parallel-group study of the safety and effectiveness of OnabotulinumtoxinA and Hyaluronic acid dermal fillers (24-mg/mL Smooth, Cohesive Gel) alone and in combination for lower facial rejuvenation. Dermatol Surg 2010;36:2121–34.

41. Brin MF, Boodhoo TI, Pogoda JM, et al. Safety and tolerability of onabotulinumtoxinA in the treatment

of facial lines: a meta-analysis of individual patient data from global clinical registration studies in 1678 participants. J Am Acad Dermatol 2009; 61(6):961–70. e1–11.

42. PubMed search string: (botulinum or Botox) AND (rash OR urticaria OR anaphylaxis OR allergy OR allergic).

43. Li M, Goldberger BA, Hopkins C. Fatal case of BO-TOX-related anaphylaxis? J Forensic Sc 2005;50(1): 169–72.

44. Bowden JB, Rapini RP. Psoriasiform eruption from intra-muscular botulinum A toxin. Cutis 1992;50(6):415–6.

45. Brueggemann N, Doegnitz L, Harms L, et al. Skin reactions after intramuscular injection of Botulinum toxin A: a rare side effect. J Neurol Neurosurg Psy-chiatr 2008;79(2):231–2.

46. LeWitt PA, Trosch RM. Idiosyncratic adverse reac-tions to intramuscular botulinum toxin type A injec-tion. Mov Disord 1997;12(6):1064–7.

47. Mezaki T, Sakai R. Botulinum toxin and skin rash reaction. Mov Disord 2005;20(6):770.

48. Cox NH, Duffey P, Royle J. Fixed drug eruption caused by lactose in an injected botulinum toxin preparation. J Am Acad Dermatol 1999;40(2):263–4.

49. Coté TR, Mohan AK, Polder JA, et al. Botulinum toxin type A injections: adverse events reported to the US Food and Drug Administration in therapeutic and cosmetic cases. J Am Acad Dermatol 2005;53(3): 407–15.

50. Ahbib S, Lachapelle JM, Marot L. Sarcoidal granu-lomas following injections of botulic toxin A (Botox)

for corrections of wrinkles. Ann Dermatol Venereol 2006;133(1):43–5 [in French].

51. Mejia NI, Vuong KD, Jankovic J. Long-term botu-linum toxin efficacy, safety, and immunogenicity. Mov Disord 2005;20(5):592–7.

52. Kessler KR, Skutta M, Benecke R. Long-term treat-ment of cervical dystonia with botulinum toxin A: effi-cacy, safety, and antibody frequency. German Dystonia Study Group. J Neurol 1999;246(4):265–74.

53. Lee S-K. Antibody-induced failure of botulinum toxin type a therapy in a patient with masseteric hyper-trophy. Dermatol Surg 2007;33:S105–10.

54. Dysport [package insert].

55. Alam M, Arndt KA, Dover JS. Severe, intractable head-ache after injection with botulinum a exotoxin: report of 5 cases. J Am Acad Dermatol 2002;46(1):62–5.

56. Hevia O. Retrospective review of 500 patients treated with abobotulinumtoxinA. J Drugs Dermatol 2010;9(9):1081–4.

57. Wortzman MS, Pickett A. The science and manufacturing behind botulinum neurotoxin type A-ABO in clinical use. Aesthetic Surg J 2009; 29(Suppl 6):S34–42.

58. Pickett A, Perrow K. Formulation composition of botulinum toxins in clinical use. J Drugs Dermatol 2010;9(9):1085–91.

59. BOTOX cosmetic [package insert].

60. Xeomin cosmetic [package insert].

61. Carruthers A, Carruthers J. Botulinum toxin products overview. Skin Therapy Lett 2008;13(6):1–4.

Principles and Practice of Cutaneous Laser and Light Therapy

Andrew A. Nelson, MD[a,b,]*, Gary P. Lask, MD[c]

KEYWORDS

- Laser • Review • Selective photothermolysis
- Vascular lesions • Laser hair removal
- Skin resurfacing/rejuvenation

KEY MESSAGES

- Many different lasers (light amplification by stimulated emission of radiation) can be used to treat patients. The concept of selective photothermolysis guides the proper selection of laser wavelength, fluence, and pulse duration to selectively treat a target while minimizing damage to the surrounding tissue.
- Vascular lesions (vascular malformations, telangiectasias, rosacea) can be effectively treated with pulsed dye lasers (PDLs) (585–595 nm). Alternatively, diode (810 nm) and long-pulsed alexandrite lasers (755 nm) can also be used.
- Laser hair removal can be safely and effectively performed in nearly all patients. Options for laser hair removal include long-pulsed alexandrite (755 nm), diode (810 nm), and long-pulsed Nd:YAG (1064 nm) lasers.
- Pigmented lesions and tattoos can be effectively treated with Q-switched lasers. The ideal wavelength to be used depends on the color and depth of the pigment.
- Laser skin rejuvenation and resurfacing can be accomplished with many different devices. The newest technologies are fractional technologies, which treat only a portion of the skin surface, thereby potentially minimizing the downtime and side effects.

Lasers and light sources have offered unparalleled advances in dermatologic therapy in the last decades. Laser therapy has evolved rapidly from the first ruby laser in 1960[1] to the numerous different technologies that are available today. As the number of lasers available has increased, so has the need for a full understanding of the technology underlying these devices. In order to offer patients the best and safest treatment options, it is necessary to understand the technologies and theories behind the lasers. With this knowledge, it is then possible to select not only the proper laser but also the ideal settings such as energy fluence, pulse duration, and cooling. This article discusses the basic concepts of lasers and light sources as well as the indications for their usage.

BASIC CONCEPTS OF LASER LIGHT

Laser light describes a specific type of light produced by these devices. The medium of the laser determines the wavelength of light produced. Laser light has several characteristics that make it unique: (1) it is monochromatic, meaning that it is of 1 specific wavelength; (2) it is collimated, meaning that the rays of light are parallel; (3) it is coherent,

The authors have nothing to disclose.
[a] Department of Dermatology, Tufts University School of Medicine, Boston, MA, USA
[b] South End Dermatology & Skin Care, 321 Columbus Avenue, Suite 2R, Boston, MA 02116, USA
[c] Division of Dermatology, Dermatologic Surgery Service and Laser Center, David Geffen School of Medicine at the University of California-Los Angeles, 200 UCLA Medical Plaza, Suite 450, Los Angeles, CA 90095, USA
* Corresponding author. South End Dermatology & Skin Care, 321 Columbus Avenue, Suite 2R, Boston, MA 02116.
E-mail address: andrew.nelson.md@gmail.com

Clin Plastic Surg 38 (2011) 427–436
doi:10.1016/j.cps.2011.02.007

meaning that the rays of light are in phase with each other; and (4) it is of high intensity.[2] These properties allow lasers to produce a single wavelength of high intensity, which can be focused and targeted accurately, and to specifically target tissue while sparing surrounding structures, producing a predictable clinical end point.

It is important to differentiate lasers from light sources. Lasers, as described earlier, produce a high-intensity beam of a single specific wavelength. By contrast, light sources such as intense pulsed light (IPL), produce a broader spectrum of light. Most IPL sources use flashlamps that emit multiple wavelengths, including visible and near-infrared lights, ranging from approximately 500 to 1200 nm.[3] Filters can be placed on the IPL handpieces to restrict the wavelengths of light produced. However, despite these filters, it is not possible for IPL machines to produce true monochromatic light.

CHROMOPHORES, LASER PARAMETERS, AND SELECTIVE PHOTOTHERMOLYSIS

There are 3 main parameters to consider when using lasers: wavelength, fluence, and pulse duration. In general, the wavelength of a laser is fixed and depends on the specific laser selected. Fluence and pulse duration, on the other hand, can be adjusted by the treating physician. It is important to have a basic understanding of how these 3 parameters can be used to accurately and selectively target tissue while sparing the surrounding structures.

Lasers and light sources cause their clinical effects when the light is absorbed by molecules known as chromophores. In the skin, there are 3 main chromophores: melanin, hemoglobin, and water.[4] These chromophores absorb certain wavelengths of light (**Fig. 1**), which results in heat produced in the targeted tissue through transfer

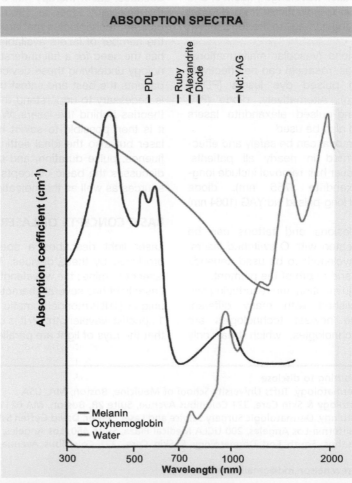

Fig. 1. Absorption spectra for the 3 main chromophores in the skin.

of energy. It is possible to target a specific chromophore by selecting a wavelength that is absorbed by that chromophore, with minimal absorption by other competing chromophores.[5] For example, hemoglobin has a relative absorption peak at approximately 595 nm, which is the wavelength of PDLs. Thus, PDLs are used to specifically target hemoglobin and vascular structures, while attempting to spare competing chromophores such as melanin and water. Depending on which chromophore the treating physician is attempting to target, a laser producing the corresponding wavelength should be selected.

As the chromophores absorb light, heat is produced in the tissue. This heat is responsible for the clinical outcome. A certain amount of heat is necessary to denature the targeted tissue.[6] If this amount of heat is not achieved, no clinical effect occurs. However, if too much heat is produced, thermal injury such as scarring can result.[4] The fluence of a laser represents the amount of energy produced by the laser; this value is an adjustable parameter selected by the treating physician when using the device. Physicians should select a sufficiently high fluence to damage the intended target tissue, but not so high as to cause surrounding tissue damage and scarring. Darker skin types, with more melanin and thus a greater concentration of that chromophore, can be more likely to develop collateral tissue damage and scarring. Thus, the ideal fluence to achieve a clinical end point, while preventing unwanted adverse effects, depends on the skin type of the patient. Many laser companies produce suggested treatment parameters for their device, classified according to the skin type of the patient.

Finally, the proper pulse duration for the device should be selected. The pulse duration determines how long the tissue is exposed to the laser energy. Once the targeted tissue is heated by the laser, this heat begins to spread into surrounding tissue. The thermal relaxation time is defined as the time necessary for the heated, targeted tissue to lose half of its heat to the surrounding tissues.[7] In general, in order to have selective treatment, physicians want to heat the targeted tissue faster than the rate at which the heat is lost to surrounding tissue.[4] The rate at which a chromophore absorbs and releases heat is related to its size and shape. Larger targets, such as hair follicles, have longer thermal relaxation and heating times than smaller targets, such as tattoo pigments. The ideal pulse duration for a laser is approximately equal to or less than the thermal relaxation time. Thus, lasers that target small tattoo pigments use pulse durations of nanoseconds or even picoseconds, whereas lasers that target hair follicles may use pulse durations of several milliseconds.[8]

Laser therapeutics was revolutionized by the concept of selective photothermolysis, first described by Anderson and Parrish[5] in 1983. The basic concept is that by using a laser with a preferentially absorbed wavelength, sufficient fluence, and pulse duration approximately equal to or less than the thermal relaxation time, it is possible to selectively target tissue while sparing surrounding structures. This concept still guides clinical decision making in laser treatment. By understanding the importance of the 3 main parameters, it is possible to use selective photothermolysis to target specific tissue components while avoiding damage to surrounding, unintended targets.

COOLING DEVICES

Although selective photothermolysis allows for the specific targeting of a chromophore, there remains some level of absorption of energy by competing chromophores and heat transfer to unintended tissues. Epidermal damage from the unwanted absorption of energy by epidermal melanin represents one of the most common difficulties in laser treatments. If the epidermal melanin absorbs too much energy, such as in darker skin types with larger melanosomes, blistering and scarring of the epidermis can occur. Skin cooling devices were developed to protect the epidermis from unintended damage. Typically, these devices spray a cool agent across the skin, provide cool contact with a chilled solid surrounding the aperture of the laser, or place a cool gel between the laser and the skin. These devices allow for precooling of the skin before the laser energy is delivered to the skin, as well as parallel cooling of the skin during the laser energy delivery.[9] Depending on the type of laser, as well as its pulse duration, the ideal cooling device varies. Manufacturers typically include a guideline for the cooling device settings incorporated into their lasers.

With an understanding of these basic concepts in laser technology, it is possible to apply these principles to clinical practice. The following sections focus on laser technologies as they apply to clinical situations. Thus, rather than discussing each laser individually, the authors discuss the most common clinical indications encountered by laser surgeons and then discuss the typical lasers used. A complete discussion of the specific details, treatment parameters, and end points is beyond the scope of this article. Rather, the goal of this article is to provide a solid foundation of knowledge, which can be expanded as the proceduralist gains more knowledge and experience with laser technologies.

VASCULAR LESIONS

Facial erythema and telangiectasias remain some of the most common complaints of cosmetic patients. These lesions often develop in patients with rosacea, or in those with a long history of photodamage, and can be a common sign of the aging process. These lesions can be easily treated with laser technologies. In order to effectively treat these lesions, it is necessary to target the oxyhemoglobin within the vessels.

PDL (585–595 nm)

Multiple lasers can be used to target the chromophore oxyhemoglobin; however, the most commonly used laser for treatment of these lesions remains the PDL. PDL was initially developed to treat capillary malformations, port-wine stains, in children.[10] After PDL treatments, blood vessels were observed to contain agglutinated erythrocytes, fibrin, and thrombi. One month after treatment, these damaged vessels were replaced by normal-appearing vessels.[11] Since its initial development, the use of PDL has been expanded to include facial telangiectasias, erythrotelangiectatic rosacea, facial rejuvenation, and infantile hemangiomas.[12] PDL has also been used to successfully treat many other skin conditions with increased vascularity, including psoriasis, scars, verruca, and skin malignancies such as basal cell carcinoma.[13]

The original PDL devices used short pulse durations (0.45–1.5 milliseconds), which are shorter than the thermal relaxation times of facial vessels. As a result, red blood cells in the targeted vessels coagulated with a clinical result of purpura.[14] This purpura can require up to 2 weeks to fully resolve. While these purpuric treatments are effective, many patients do not wish to have obvious purpura. Newer PDL technologies, including variable and longer-pulsed PDLs, use adjustable pulse durations from 0.45 to 40 milliseconds. As the pulse duration is increased, the risk of purpura is decreased by a more uniform, slow heating of the blood vessels. Longer-pulse durations with lower-energy fluences, commonly referred to as nonpurpuric settings, have been shown to be similarly effective in the treatment of erythema and telangiectasia.[15] When treating larger-diameter blood vessels, it is important to bear in mind that these larger-caliber vessels have longer thermal relaxation times; it is therefore useful to treat these larger vessels with longer pulse durations in order to achieve clinical efficacy.

Manufacturers of PDLs produce tables of suggested treatment parameters for their specific device. The exact energy fluence and pulse duration depends on the clinical indication, as well as whether the proceduralist is using purpuric or nonpurpuric settings.

Alternative Vascular Lasers and Light Sources

Although the PDL remains the gold standard for the treatment of vascular lesions, other technologies have roles as well. Another commonly used technology is IPL. As mentioned previously, IPL is actually a light source producing a broad spectrum of light, which is then restricted with filters. Although IPL does not target hemoglobin as specifically as PDL, it is efficacious in treating erythema and telangiectasia.[16] IPL is particularly beneficial in treating diffuse background erythema on the face or upper part of chest because it has a much larger treatment size (approximately 8 × 35 mm) compared with PDL and other laser devices. IPL also has the advantage of treating multiple chromophores at the same time, because of its broad spectrum of light, which can be useful when treating patients with erythema and lentigines or conditions such as poikiloderma.[17]

Because hemoglobin has several relative absorption peaks, multiple other lasers have been used to treat vascular lesions. These lasers include the alexandrite laser (755 nm), the diode laser (810 nm), and the long-pulsed Nd:YAG laser (1064 nm).[12] These lasers have longer wavelengths, which in turn penetrate further into the dermis, potentially allowing for the treatment of deeper vascular targets. In addition, they have longer pulse durations compared with PDL, which can allow for the treatment of larger-diameter veins. Unfortunately, these wavelengths are not absorbed as efficiently by hemoglobin and they often have less clinical efficacy compared with PDL. These lasers should typically be used only in cases refractory to PDL treatment, and should be used by experienced proceduralists in these cases.

LASER HAIR REMOVAL

Laser hair removal remains one of the most common cosmetic procedures performed in the United States. Similar to other clinical applications, laser hair removal is also guided by the principle of selective photothermolysis. The target chromophore in laser hair removal is melanin, which is located at the base of the hair follicle. Unfortunately, the stem cells responsible for the growth and regrowth of hair are more superficial, located in the bulge region of the hair shaft.[8] Laser hair removal works by targeting the melanin at the base of the hair shaft, thereby generating heat; this heat then diffuses to the bulge region of the hair shaft, which damages and ultimately destroys the stem cells. Because the diameter of the hair follicles is relatively large, the thermal relaxation time is long. This long thermal relaxation time requires the use of lasers with longer pulse durations, in the order of milliseconds, to effectively heat and destroy the follicular stem cells.[18] Thus, long-pulsed lasers with wavelengths absorbed by melanin are the treatment of choice for laser hair removal.

The ideal candidate for laser hair removal is a patient with light skin and dark terminal hairs. These patients have significant melanin in the hair follicle to absorb the laser energy and little epidermal melanin to serve as a competing chromophore; these patients can be effectively treated with a variety of laser devices.[19] Blond hair and vellous hairs, which do not contain significant amounts of melanin, do not respond well to laser hair removal. Darker skin type patients, with significant epidermal melanin, are more challenging to treat; in early clinical trials, there were reports of some patients developing blistering, hypopigmentation, and scarring after laser hair removal.[20] Several advances have been developed to allow for safe laser hair removal in these darker skin type patients. Ideally, epidermal melanin would be spared and only the hair follicle melanin would absorb energy to reduce the likelihood of these adverse effects. Longer wavelengths are absorbed less effectively by epidermal melanin and penetrate further into the dermis; these properties help to protect epidermal melanin in darker skin types. Epidermal cooling devices and long pulse durations further help to protect the epidermal melanin from being targeted. With these advances, it is possible for patients of all skin types to undergo safe and effective laser hair removal.

Specific Lasers for Laser Hair Removal

Most proceduralists use 1 of 3 lasers to perform laser hair removal: the long-pulsed alexandrite laser (755 nm), the diode laser (810 nm), or the long-pulsed Nd:YAG laser (1064 nm). Alexandrite and diode lasers can be safely used in patients with lighter skin types, up to an approximately skin type III or IV. For darker skin types, IV to VI, the long-pulsed Nd:YAG laser is the treatment of choice. Whereas the Nd:YAG laser is safer for those with darker skin types than the alexandrite or diode laser, its efficacy is decreased compared with these devices; thus, for lighter skin type

patients, use of the diode or alexandrite device is the treatment of choice.[21] It is important to determine the proper skin type of the patient before determining the treatment parameters for laser hair removal. The ideal fluences and pulse durations for each laser depend on the exact device, as well as the skin type of the patient. Laser manufacturers typically provide tables of suggested treatment parameters for their device based on patient skin types.

Proceduralists should set reasonable expectations for their patients before beginning laser hair removal treatments. First, patients must be aware that several treatment sessions will be necessary to effectively perform laser hair removal. These sessions should be sufficiently far apart such that the hair has reentered its anagen (growth) phase when it produces melanin; if the sessions are too close together, the treatment will be ineffective. Typically, sessions are scheduled approximately every 6 weeks. Second, blonde and gray hairs are not likely to respond to the treatment; vellous and fine hairs are similarly refractory to laser hair removal. There are some reports of laser hair removal actually leading to increased hair growth; treatments should be discontinued if the patient reports increased hair growth. Finally, patients should not be tan at the time of their treatments. Tanning causes redistribution of melanin in the epidermis, increasing the size and concentration of melanin granules. These changes effectively increases the risk of adverse effects such as burning, hypopigmentation, hyperpigmentation, and possibly even scarring. If patients present for their laser hair removal session tan, they should not be treated at that time. Unfortunately, despite the best efforts and treatments, there are some patients who do not respond well to hair removal treatments or who do not achieve permanent hair reduction.

LASER PIGMENT AND TATTOO REMOVAL

Pigmented lesions, including lentigines, nevus of Ota, as well as tattoos can now be safely and effectively treated with Q-switched lasers. Q-switched lasers deliver high-intensity energy in extremely short pulse durations. These short pulse durations allow the laser to selectively target small molecules, such as individual melanocytes or tattoo particles.[22] Recently, lasers with even shorter pulse durations, picosecond pulse duration lasers, have been developed to more effectively treat tattoos.[23] Immediately after treatment, the targeted pigment turns white, likely corresponding to dispersion and destruction of the pigment particle.[24] This whitening is a transient phenomenon, and the color of the pigment returns minutes to hours after the treatment. This destroyed and dispersed pigment is then absorbed and eliminated by phagocytes in the skin, gradually reducing the color and intensity of the pigment over the next several weeks. Q-switched lasers can be used to safely and effectively treat epidermal and dermal pigmentation. Despite the increased safety of modern Q-switched lasers, adverse effects including scarring can occur. In general, use of Q-switched lasers with high energy in short pulse durations can be painful for patients. Patients generally require either a topical or an intralesional anesthetic to be treated comfortably. There is an additional risk of scarring or dyspigmentation associated with these devices, particularly in darker skin type patients. Finally, patients often require multiple treatments for clinical efficacy; patients presenting for tattoo removal should be counseled that many treatment sessions (approximately 6–10) may be necessary to significantly improve their appearance and that the tattoo may never be removed completely.

Specific Q-Switched Lasers

There are 4 main wavelengths used in Q-switched lasers: the frequency-doubled Nd:YAG (532 nm), ruby (694 nm), alexandrite (755 nm), and Nd:YAG (1064 nm) lasers. Similar to other clinical situations, selecting which laser and corresponding wavelength to use for treatments is based on selective photothermolysis. Shorter wavelengths, such as that produced by the frequency-doubled Nd:YAG laser (532 nm), tend to be absorbed more superficially, preferentially treating lesions such as freckles and lentigines. Longer-wavelength lasers penetrate more deeply into the dermis, specifically treating tattoos or dermal pigment. Superficial lesions such as solar lentigines respond well to treatment with a 532-nm laser. Deeper dermal lesions, such as tattoos or dermal melanocytosis, tend to respond, better to 694-nm or 755-nm lasers; in patients with darker skin types, the 1064-nm laser is the device of choice to reduce the likelihood of hypopigmentation and scarring. Thus, selecting the appropriate laser is based on the depth of the pigment; the deeper the pigment is located, the longer the wavelength necessary to effectively target the pigment. Furthermore, the color of the pigment being targeted also influences the choice of wavelength. Blue-black tattoo ink can be effectively treated with any of these wavelengths. Red and yellow colors, on the other hand, tend to be best treated with the frequency-doubled Nd:YAG (532 nm) wavelength regardless of their depth in the dermis. Green colors are best treated with either the ruby (694 nm) or alexandrite (755 nm) wavelengths.[25] When selecting the device to use, the proceduralist should first consider the color of the pigment to be targeted. Then, the physician should attempt to estimate the depth of the pigment in the skin. With these 2 considerations in mind, the proceduralist can select the best laser option for the patient. Once the proper laser and corresponding wavelength are determined, the physician must determine the energy fluence. The energy fluence necessary depends on the skin type of the patient, as well as the color and density of the pigment particle. The pulse duration of these Q-switched devices is fixed, so the physician does not need to determine this parameter. If there are questions regarding the exact nature or composition of the pigment, or if the patient has a darker skin type, performing a test spot laser treatment before a full treatment can be beneficial. The test spot should be performed on a noncritical, less-visible lesion or portion of the tattoo or pigmented lesion; the patient should then return to have the area examined in 2 to 4 weeks. If the patient has developed any signs of hypopigmentation or scarring, the patient should be either tested again at significantly lower-energy fluences or should not be treated at all. While the test spot can help the proceduralist to determine if the full treatment will be efficacious, the greatest utility is in reducing the risk of adverse effects. This practice will greatly reduce the risk and incidence of potentially serious adverse effects from Q-switched laser treatments. Despite these precautions, even performing a test spot cannot always predict which patients will have adverse effects after a full treatment.

LASER SKIN REJUVENATION

For years, laser devices have been noted to cause thermal damage to collagen, ultimately resulting in collagen stimulation, remodeling, and new collagen formation. Stimulating new dermal collagen formation may ultimately help to reduce the appearance of photoaging, solar elastosis, and loss of collagen that is present in the aging face. Most of these technologies attempt to target water in the dermis as the target chromophore. Heat is generated by the absorption of energy, and this heat stimulates the existing collagen to remodel and undergo neocollagenosis. Many different technologies, using a variety of different wavelengths and treatment parameters, have been reported to stimulate collagen through this mechanism.

PDL

Although PDL technology was developed to target hemoglobin in vascular lesions, it has also been reported to improve scars, particularly acne scars and hypertrophic scars. Initial reports also indicated promising results with significant improvement in facial rhytides and skin tightening after PDL treatments.[26] However, in practice, most proceduralists have found the results to be modest.[27] PDL can be useful in skin rejuvenation, although most think that the observed improvements are related to the device's ability to improve facial redness and reduce facial telangiectasias, rather than directly affecting collagen, facial rhytides, or skin tightening.[28]

Infrared Devices

Multiple different near-infrared devices have been developed and marketed for skin rejuvenation.[29] These devices typically use wavelengths in the range of 1300 to 1600 nm. The relatively longer wavelengths of these devices allow for deeper penetration into the dermis. Mild fibrosis and thickening of the dermis has been noted histologically after treatment with these devices. Given these histologic changes, it is reasonable to infer that the devices would be effective in improving the appearance of damaged collagen and improving photoaging. However, in clinical practice, these devices have been associated with minimal to moderate improvement in the appearance of facial rhytides and skin tightening.[30] Specific devices include the CoolTouch CT3 Plus (Nd:YAG, 1320 nm; CoolTouch Inc, Roseville, CA, USA), Smoothbeam (diode, 1450 nm; Candela Corporation, Wayland, MA, USA), and Titan (1100 to 1800 nm; Cutera Inc, Brisbane, CA, USA), among others. A complete discussion of each of these devices is beyond the scope of this article.

Radiofrequency Devices

Radiofrequency is electromagnetic wave frequency between audio and infrared wave lengths that ranges from approximately 1.0×10^5 nm to 3.0×10^{13} nm. When the device is used to treat tissue, ionic flow is generated in the tissue, which causes molecular frictional heating. Thus, the heat is actually generated from the tissue, rather than from the device itself. This heat is relatively low level, so that it is confined to the tissue, without generating excess radiation or destruction of nearby unintended tissue.[31] Radiofrequency devices, such as Thermage (Solta Medical Inc, Hayward, CA, USA), have been reported to result in skin tightening and collagen remodeling, thereby helping with skin rejuvenation.[32] In practice, these results are often modest. A full discussion of these devices is outside of the scope of this article because they are not true laser devices.

LASER SKIN RESURFACING

The first modalities for skin resurfacing were fully ablative carbon-dioxide (CO_2) and erbium lasers. These lasers target water in the epidermis and do not penetrate deeply into the dermis. As a result, they are effective in removing (ablating) the epidermis of patients, thereby causing their clinical effects. These devices were effective in treating facial discoloration and rhytides. However, they were also associated with significant downtime and healing phases of several weeks to months after treatment. Because the epidermis is fully ablated, the barrier function of the skin is reduced; as a result, serious bacterial and viral infections can occur. Furthermore, these ablative resurfacing devices had significant risks of posttreatment transient hyperpigmentation and hypopigmentation, permanent hypopigmentation, and scarring.[33] As a result, newer fractional technologies with potentially less risk of these adverse events have become more popular. This following section focuses on these fractional technologies and their clinical applications.

Fractional Technology

Fractional photothermolysis was a concept developed by Manstein and colleagues in 2004.[34] The basic concept is simple: rather than uniformly treating the entire epidermis, only a portion of the skin is treated with columns of energy. These columns of energy treat both the epidermis and the underlying dermis, creating targeted areas of thermal damage known as microthermal treatment zones (MTZs). The area of skin between these MTZs is unaffected, which stimulates collagen remodeling and serves as a reservoir for tissue regrowth. By treating only a portion of the skin surface, it is theoretically possible to treat with greater energy and have deeper penetration, while reducing the risk of adverse events such as scarring. Furthermore, the downtime associated with healing from these devices should be decreased because only a portion of the skin surface is treated. Fractional devices, in general, have 2 main parameters controlled by the proceduralist. The first is the pattern density, which refers to how many MTZs are placed within the treatment area; a greater density implies that more of the skin surface is being treated with each pass of the device. The second treatment parameter is the energy; the energy per MTZ dictates how far the MTZ penetrates into the dermis. By varying these 2 parameters, it is possible to control the depth and confluence of the treatment, resulting in the safest and most efficacious treatment. Fractional technology has been at the forefront of the development of minimally invasive rejuvenation. The authors' colleagues, Petelin, Saedi, and Zachary discuss fractionation and its effect on the laser field elsewhere in this issue, a testament to the significance of this discovery. Interested readers can thoroughly read further about this technology from multiple sources and experts.

Nonablative Fractional Devices

The first fractional device was actually a nonablative erbium-doped laser at 1550 nm (Fraxel, Reliant Technology, Atlanta, GA, USA). This device was shown in clinical studies to cause significant improvement in facial texture and rhytides. Since its initial development, Fraxel has also been used to treat other conditions including acne, striae, scarring, and even disorders of pigmentation, such as melasma.[35] While treatments with Fraxel are generally well tolerated by patients, topical anesthesia is necessary; the authors pretreat patients with topical anesthetics (combination preparations of lidocaine and prilocaine [EMLA] or lidocaine [LMX]) for 1 hour before performing the Fraxel treatment for patient comfort. Immediately after the treatment, the patient's skin is red and may be slightly swollen. These changes resolve in 1 to 2 days, but the collagen remodeling continues for 4 to 6 weeks after the treatment. Patients should be reminded that the full effects of a nonablative fractional rejuvenation treatment may not be visible for up to 2 months after the treatment. In addition, in order to see the full effects, a series of 4 to 6 treatments will likely be necessary.

Since the initial development of Fraxel, other manufacturers have produced similar nonablative fractional rejuvenation devices. The specific treatment parameters for each device vary; the ideal treatment parameters depend on the condition being treated, the patient's skin type, and the specific device being used.

For the most part, Fraxel has been well tolerated by patients. In 2005, the first study of side effects associated with nonablative fractional photothermolysis was reported; transient posttreatment erythema was noted by all patients. Other common side effects included facial edema, dry skin, flaking, superficial scratches, pruritus, pigmentary changes, and an acneiform eruption.[36] A more recent retrospective study documented other potentially serious side effects including scarring, pinpoint bleeding, and blistering; these adverse effects were thought to be related to higher energy fluences and bulk heating associated with nonablative fractional photothermolysis treatments.[37] There is also a risk of herpes simplex virus and varicella zoster virus reactivation after nonablative fractional photothermolysis.[2]

Ablative Fractional Devices

While traditional fully ablative technologies were effective in treating photodamaged skin, the downtime associated with the procedure and increased risk of serious adverse events associated with these devices render them less desirable for patients. Extending the concept of fractional treatment to ablative skin resurfacing allows for potentially some of the benefits of fully ablative treatments while decreasing the associated risks and downtime. Recently, several manufacturers have developed devices incorporating fractional ablative CO_2 or erbium lasers. In clinical studies, these devices have been shown to reduce the appearance of fine lines, periocular rhytides, dyspigmentation, and improve skin tone and tightness.[38] In order for patients to comfortably undergo these treatments, a topical anesthetic is absolutely necessary and nerve blocks of facial sensory nerves may be beneficial.

In clinical studies, fractional ablative devices seem to offer substantial improvements in a patient's appearance. In addition, the downtime associated with fractional ablative devices is significantly shorter than that associated with traditional fully ablative devices.[30] However, there are still potential adverse effects associated with these fractional ablative technologies.[39] First, there is still healing and downtime associated with the devices. Immediately after treatment, the skin is significantly erythematous and there may be areas of pinpoint bleeding. The patient's skin peels following the treatment, typically for 3 to 7 days, depending on how aggressively the treatment was performed; during this time, the patient needs to apply protective petrolatum several times daily and clean the skin meticulously to prevent infection. The patient's skin is likely to remain erythematous for 2 to 4 weeks, again depending on the aggressiveness of the treatment. This duration is a substantial improvement in the length of the downtime compared with traditional fully ablative resurfacing, but is still a significant time commitment for the patient. Despite the use of fractional technologies, there remains a risk of hypopigmentation and scarring, although this seems to be less likely than with fully ablative technologies. It is important that patient's understand this procedure, the expected healing process, and the potential clinical outcomes. The proceduralist must set reasonable expectations because this is not a no-downtime procedure. Despite these potential adverse effects, fractional ablative resurfacing can be an effective treatment to help rejuvenate and resurface photoaged skin.

SUMMARY

Laser therapeutics has evolved rapidly in the last 2 decades. Seemingly every year or two, there is a new device being developed or a new application of an existing device being promoted. It is important to have a strong background in the concepts and technologies underlying lasers. With this background, and an understanding of selective photothermolysis, it is possible to select the proper laser, energy fluence, and pulse duration to safely, reliably, and effectively treat patients.

REFERENCES

1. Maiman TH. Stimulated optical radiation in ruby. Nature 1960;187:493–4.
2. Carroll L, Humphreys TR. LASER-tissue interactions. Clin Dermatol 2006;24:2–7.
3. Babilas P, Schreml S, Szeimies RM, et al. Intense pulsed light (IPL): a review. Lasers Surg Med 2010;42:93–104.
4. Hirsch RJ, Wall TL, Avram MM, et al. Principles of laser-skin interactions. In: Bolognia JL, Jorizzo JL, Rapini RP, editors. Dermatology. New York: Mosby Elsevier; 2008. p. 2089–97.
5. Anderson RR, Parrish JA. Selective photothermolysis: precise microsurgery by selective absorption of pulse radiation. Science 1983;220:524–7.
6. Polla BS, Anderson RR. Thermal injury by laser pulse: protection by heat shock despite failure to induce heat shock response. Lasers Surg Med 1987;7:398–404.
7. Hruza GJ, Geronemus RG, Dover JS, et al. Lasers in dermatology. Arch Dermatol 1993;129:1026–33.
8. Anderson RR. Lasers in dermatology – a critical update. J Dermatol 2000;27:700–5.
9. Zenzie HH, Altchuler GB, Smirnov MZ, et al. Evaluation of cooling methods or laser dermatology. Lasers Surg Med 2000;26:130–44.
10. Glassberg E, Lask GP, Tan EM, et al. The flashlamp-pumped 577-nm pulsed tunable dye laser: clinical efficacy and in vitro studies. J Dermatol Surg Oncol 1988;14:1200–8.
11. Tan OT, Carney M, Margolis R, et al. Histologic responses of port wine stains treated by argon, carbon dioxide, and tunable dye lasers. Arch Dermatol 1986;122:1016–22.
12. Hare McCoppin HH, Goldberg DJ. Laser treatment of facial telangiectases: an update. Dermatol Surg 2010;36:1221–30.
13. Karsai S, Roos S, Hammes S, et al. Pulsed dye laser: what's new in non-vascular lesions? J Eur Acad Dermatol Venereol 2007;21:877–90.
14. Garden JM, Tan OT, Kershcmann R, et al. Effect of dye laser pulse duration on selective cutaneous vascular injury. J Invest Dermatol 1986;87:653–7.
15. Bernstein EF, Kligman A. Rosacea treatment using the new-generation, high-energy, 595 nm, long pulse-duration pulsed-dye laser. Lasers Surg Med 2008;40:233–9.
16. Angermeier MC. Treatment of facial vascular lesions with intense pulsed light. J Cutan Laser Ther 1999;1: 95–100.
17. Rusciani A, Motta A, Fino P, et al. Treatment of poikiloderma of Civatte using intense pulsed light source: 7 years of experience. Dermatol Surg 2008;34:314–9.
18. Altshuler GB, Anderson RR, Manstein D, et al. Extended theory of selective photothermolysis. Lasers Surg Med 2001;29:416–32.
19. Casey AS, Goldberg D. Guidelines for laser hair removal. J Cosmet Laser Ther 2008;10:24–33.
20. Breadon JY, Barnes CA. Comparison of adverse events of laser and light-assisted hair removal systems in skin types IV–VI. J Drugs Dermatol 2007; 6:40–6.
21. Sadighha A, Mohaghegh Zahed G. Meta-analysis of hair removal laser trials. Lasers Med Sci 2009;24: 21–5.
22. Polla LL, Margolis RJ, Dover JS, et al. Melanosomes are a primary target of Q-switched ruby laser irradiation in guinea pig skin. J Invest Dermatol 1987;89: 281–6.
23. Izikson L, Farinelli W, Sakamoto F, et al. Safety and effectiveness of black tattoo clearance in a pig model after a single treatment with a novel 758 nm 500 picosecond laser: a pilot study. Lasers Surg Med 2010;42:640–6.
24. Dover JS, Margolis RJ, Polla LL. Pigmented guinea pig skin irradiated with Q-switched ruby lasers. Arch Dermatol 1989;25:43–9.
25. Alexiades-Armenakas MR, Dover JS, Arndt KA. Laser therapy. In: Bolognia JL, Jorizzo JL, Rapini RP, editors. Dermatology. New York: Mosby Elsevier; 2008. p. 2099–120.
26. Rostan E, Bowes LE, Iyer S, et al. A double-blind, side-by-side comparison study of low fluence long pulse dye laser to coolant treatment for wrinkling of the cheeks. J Cosmet Laser Ther 2001;3: 129–36.
27. Hsu TS, Zelickson B, Dover JS, et al. Multicenter study of the safety and efficacy of a 585 nm pulsed-dye laser for the nonablative treatment of facial rhytides. Dermatol Surg 2005;31:1–9.

28. Jørgensen GF, Hedelund L, Haedersdal M. Long-pulsed dye laser versus intense pulsed light for photodamaged skin: a randomized split-face trial with blinded response evaluation. Lasers Surg Med 2008;40:293–9.

29. Nelson JS, Majaron B, Kelly KM. What is nonablative photorejuvenation of human skin? Semin Cutan Med Surg 2002;21:238–50.

30. Sadick NS. Update on non-ablative light therapy for rejuvenation: a review. Lasers Surg Med 2003;32:120–8.

31. Elsaie ML. Cutaneous remodeling and photorejuvenation using radiofrequency devices. Indian J Dermatol 2009;54:201–5.

32. Alster TS, Tanzi E. Improvement of neck and cheek laxity with a nonablative radiofrequency device: a lifting experience. Dermatol Surg 2004;30:503–7.

33. Bernstein LJ, Kauvar ANB, Grossman MC, et al. The short and long term side effects of carbon dioxide laser resurfacing. Dermatol Surg 1997;23:519–25.

34. Manstein D, Herron GS, Sink RK, et al. Fractional photothermolysis: a new concept for cutaneous remodeling using microscopic patterns of thermal injury. Lasers Surg Med 2004;34:426–38.

35. Sherling M, Friedman PM, Adrian R, et al. Consensus recommendations on the use of an erbium-doped 1,550-nm fractionated laser and its applications in dermatologic laser surgery. Dermatol Surg 2010;36:461–9.

36. Fisher G, Geronemus R. Short-term side effects of fractional photothermolysis. Dermatol Surg 2005;31:1245–9.

37. Graber EM, Tanzi EL, Alster TA. Side effects and complications of fractional laser photothermolysis: experience with 961 treatments. Dermatol Surg 2008;34:301–7.

38. Hunzeker CM, Weiss ET, Geronemus RG. Fractionated CO2 laser resurfacing: our experience with more than 2000 treatments. Aesthet Surg J 2009;29:317–22.

39. Fife DJ, Fitzpatrick RE, Zachary CB. Complications of fractional CO2 laser resurfacing: four cases. Lasers Surg Med 2009;41:179–84.

Radio Frequency Energy for Non-invasive and Minimally Invasive Skin Tightening

R. Stephen Mulholland, MD, FRCS(C)

KEYWORDS

- Radiofrequency • Nonablative • Fractional radiofrequency
- Invasix • RFAL • Skin tightening • Skin contraction
- Tissue tightening

Much of the surgical effort in plastic surgery is devoted to the enhancement of patients with skin laxity. The gold standard of skin laxity therapy has always been, and remains, skin excision. Whether face-lift, breast-lift, abdominoplasty, or brachioplasty, removal of excess skin through well-placed incisions most often results in excellent clinical results and a happy patient. However, the scars, stigmata, morbidity, and fear of excisional procedures keep most patients looking for less-invasive skin-tightening procedures and, in many cases, away from the plastic surgeon's office.

As this timely issue in *The Clinics in Plastic Surgery* is devoted to noninvasive and minimally invasive plastic surgery, this article focuses on the rapidly growing area of "nonexcisional" skin tightening. The aging baby boomers are a formidable demographic force. There is a person turning 60 years old every 10 seconds, and it is estimated that more than one-fourth of the total US population in 2006 was between 42 and 60 years old.[1] This represents more than 100 million potential patients with skin laxity of the head, neck, and body. As there are approximately

150,000 face-lifts, breast-lifts, arm-lifts, and tummy-tucks per year in the United States, only 1% to 2% of patients with skin laxity ever present for a skin excisional procedure.[2] Over the past 10 years, there have been tremendous technological developments and marked growth in skin-tightening devices that can be performed noninvasively or minimally invasively. In fact, skin tightening is one of the fastest growing market segments, accounting for $56.9 million in device sales and 668,100 patient treatments.[2] With a sales growth of 10.3% annually, it is anticipated that this market will grow to 2 million treatments in 2013.[2]

Clearly, many aging patients will accept less significant results with noninvasive and minimally invasive skin tightening than the more effective skin-excisional procedures. It is important for plastic surgeons to keep current with patient alternatives and to become familiar with and in some cases, master, the nonsurgical options available to patients with lax skin. Further, many plastic surgeons can and do benefit from offering noninvasive skin tightening to those patients who might not want surgery and offer nonsurgical skin tightening for those patients who undergo skin excision

Disclosures. Dr Mulholland has received consulting fees and complimentary technology and/or technology discounts from Invasix, Thermage Inc., Cynosure, Lumenis, ESC, and Sciton. He has stock as well as stock options in Invasix, Ltd.

Private Practice Plastic Surgery, SpaMedica® Clinics, 66 Avenue Road, Suite 4, Toronto, ON M5R 3N8, Canada
E-mail address: mulhollandmd@spamedica.com

Clin Plastic Surg 38 (2011) 437–448
doi:10.1016/j.cps.2011.05.003

and are looking to "protect their investment." Whether the nonexcisional skin-tightening procedures are part of a postoperative maintenance treatment regimen, or a totally nonsurgical skin-tightening program in the plastic surgeon's office, skin-tightening devices can be a valuable adjunct in treating patients with lax skin.

Practice growth for the plastic surgeon can benefit from using the right noninvasive skin-tightening strategy, as controlling the patients' "upstream" nonsurgical experiences through neurotoxins, soft tissue fillers, skin tightening, color correction and texturizing laser, and light and radiofrequency (RF) technologies can enhance the downstream volume of patients presenting for surgical procedures, as they already have a noninvasive relationship with their surgeon. Excisional surgeons who offer noninvasive, nonexcisional treatments in their practice have the ability to offer patients all options in the skin-laxity market.

This article reviews the noninvasive and minimally invasive options for skin tightening, focusing on peer-reviewed articles and presentations and those technologies with the most proven or promising RF skin-tightening results for surgeons who perform skin excision. RF has been the mainstay of noninvasive skin tightening and has emerged as the "cutting edge" technology in the minimally invasive skin-tightening field. Because these RF skin-tightening technologies are capital equipment purchases with a significant cost associated, this article also discusses some business issues and models that have proven to work in the plastic surgeon's office for noninvasive and minimally invasive skin-tightening technologies.

It is the author's hope that this information provides a good overview of the evolution, growth, and opportunities for nonexcisional RF skin-tightening technologies available to plastic surgeons who treat skin laxity.

CLASSIFICATION OF SKIN-TIGHTENING DEVICES

Over the past 2 decades, there has been an explosion in noninvasive and minimally invasive therapies to enhance skin rejuvenation. Characteristics of the aging face include fine rhytids and dynamic rhytids in early aging followed by fixed, deep rhytids both dynamic and static in the glabella area of the forehead and around the eyes. There is a loss of dermal substrate, including functional collagen, elastin, and ground substances.[3] The epidermis tends to thicken and there is general loss of subcutaneous fibrous connectivity with loss of midface soft tissue volume, periosteal absorption, and ptosis of soft tissues, leading to

a more prominent naso-labial fold, labial mental lines, the elongation of the lid-cheek junction, and jowls. Superficial epidermal-dermal changes include dyschromias, brown discoloration, hyperpigmentation, erythema, telangiectasia, rosacea, and dark melanin dyschromia, especially in photo-damaged skin.[3] For the past 15 years there has been tremendous growth and development of technologies that address these various aging facial changes.

Older chemical ablative techniques and macrodermabrasion gave way to ablative laser resurfacing, including carbon dioxide and erbium YAG lasers.[4-6] Full-face laser ablation, although tremendous at rhytid reduction and significant superficial skin tightening, often led to an unacceptable degree of postoperative recovery and erythema, swelling, and downtime, in addition to long-term complications of demarcation, pigmentation abnormalities, and scarring.[7,8] As the aging population over the past 10 to 15 years has increasingly sought esthetic enhancement procedures, there has also been an increasing desire to seek therapies that have less recovery downtime and morbidity than traditional ablative laser or chemical treatments.[2]

The busy social and professional lives of our patients have necessitated the growth and expansion of a whole minimally invasive or noninvasive area of skin rejuvenation. Enhanced improvements in laser technology design and experiences and procedures around the world have resulted in the evolution of many nonablative technologies that have attempted to simulate the results of ablative carbon dioxide and erbium YAG lasers. Although the downtime and recovery from these nonablative laser and light-based technologies is far more desirable than full ablative lasers, multiple treatments are often required and the long-term results of rhytid reduction, skin tightening, diminishment of pores, and texture irregularities are often subtle at best.[9-11]

These nonablative laser and light devices work by a photon interaction with a dermal chromophore, melanin, deoxygenated or oxygenated hemoglobin, and/or dermal water. The end pathway of these photon-chromophore interactions is the generation of heat, which may lead to a resolution of the chromophore, a subablative, noncoagulative inflammatory response, and, over time, mild to modest enhanced dermal levels of elastin, collagen, and ground substance.[10] This nonablative, selective photothermolytic remodeling process will often result over several months, in very subtle rhytid improvement, some subtle to moderate tightening or texture improvements, and, depending on the device, improvements in melanin and/or vascular discoloration. Examples of these devices include early infrared devices, such as the Cool Touch Infrared Laser (1320 nm) (Roseville, CA, USA), the 1064 Neodymium Lag Laser, the 1440 ND YAG Laser, the Smooth-beam Infrared Laser (1450 nm diode) (Wayland, MA, USA), as well as numerous intense pulse-light technologies (585 to 1100 nm) and pulse-dye laser technology (585 nm and 595 nm). Virtually every wavelength between 500 nm and 2000 nm has been developed and used in conjunction with some aspect of skin rejuvenation: color correction, skin tightening, or rhytid textural diminishment. Although all of these technologies work to a greater or lesser degree, they often fall far short of the type of skin-tightening results that patients are seeking.[9–11] The advantages of these noninvasive, nonablative technologies and probably why they have proliferated, is that many esthetic physicians have a comfort level using them. The technical barrier to entry in using these nonablative devices is minimal. Often, nonablative technologies lend themselves well to delegation to nonmedical health professional staff under a physician direction and can be combined with Botox, soft tissue fillers, microdermabrasion, and other minimally invasive techniques to achieve quite pleasing esthetic results.[12] Color correction has been an important part of nonablative enhancement over the past 10 to 15 years. Intense pulse-light photorejuvenation and pulse-dye technologies have dominated the sector of laser technology revolving around correction of vasculature and melanin-based dyschromia.[12]

The need for a nonablative technology that results in significant tissue tightening without disrupting the epidermal-dermal junction, led to the development of nonablative RF skin-tightening technologies. The RF tightening technologies, led by Thermage™ (Solta Medical, Hayward, CA, USA) and, later, by Syneron Medical Ltd (Yokneam Illit, Israel) and other companies, have created a nonablative, transepidermal skin-tightening array of treatment protocols and techniques that have proven to be quite successful in achieving moderate and potentially pleasing skin tightening for patients.[3,12–18] In deciding on a method of classifying these RF skin-tightening technologies, a more anatomic approach has been adopted that takes into account the very exciting growth areas of minimally invasive RF skin tightening through the delivery of skin-tightening laser or RF energy to the immediate subdermal space and by-passing altogether or combining at a later date classic transepidermal-dermal RF skin heating. The following list sets out the classification system. One can divide skin-tightening devices into 2 broad categories: transepidermal delivery of energy and subdermal delivery of energy.

Classification of RF and energy-based skin-tightening devices

1. Transepidermal Energy Delivery
   a. Transepidermal Laser Energy Devices
      Various wavelengths, pulse durations, and pulse configurations: 585, 595 pulse-dye technology, nm pulse dye, 755 nm, 810 nm, 900, 980 nm diodes, 1064 nm, 1320 nm, 1440 nm, and 1500 nm series lasers
   b. Infrared lamp technology, 700 nm and 2000 nm infrared lamps
      i. Sciton SkinTyte (Palo Alto, CA, USA)
      ii. Cutera Titen (Brisbane, CA, USA)
   c. Monopolar RF energy
      i. Thermage™ (Solta Medical, Hayward, CA, USA)
      ii. Accent (Caesarea, Israel)
   d. Bipolar RF energy in combination with other light sources
      i. Syneron Medical Ltd (Yokneam Illit, Israel) intense pulse light and bi-polar RF
      ii. 810 nm diode and bipolar RF
      iii. 950 nm diode and bipolar RF
      iv. Infrared lamp bipolar
   e. Multipolar Transepidermal Skin-Tightening RF Devices
      i. TriPollar (Pollogen, Tel Aviv, Israel)
      ii. Octopolar, Freeze (Tel Aviv, Israel)
   f. Intense pulsed light
      i. 500 nm to 1200 nm intense pulse-light systems
      ii. Lumenis Lume 1 (Yokneam, Israel), the Palomar Starluxe (Burlington, MA, USA), Syneron Medical Ltd E-Max (Yokneam Illit, Israel), the Sciton BBL (Palo Alto, CA, USA), the Alma laser Harmony (Caesarea, Israel)
2. Transepidermal Fractional Energy Delivery
   a. Transepidermal fractional carbon dioxide resurfacing
      i. Active and DeepFX Lumenis (Yokneam, Israel)
      ii. Fraxel Repair, Solta Medical (Hayward, CA, USA)
      iii. Affrim CO_2 Smart Skin, Cynosure (Westford, MA, USA)
   b. Transepidermal fractional delivery of infrared wavelengths
      i. Fraxel Renew, Solta Medical (Hayward, CA, USA)
      ii. Affirm MPX 1320/1440, Cynosure (Westford, MA, USA)
      iii. Lux 1540, Palomar (Burlington, MA, USA)
      iv. Matrix IR, Syneron Medical Ltd (Yokneam Illit, Israel)
      v. Fractional Pearl, Cutera (Brisbane, CA, USA)

c. Fractional infrared delivery of erbium YAG Er:YSGG (Yttrium Scandium Gallium Garnet)
   i. Profractional, Sciton (Palo Alto, CA, USA)
d. Fractional transepidermal RF energy
   i. E-Matrix and Matrix RF, Syneron Medical Ltd (Yokneam Illit, Israel)
   ii. Fractora, Invasix (Yokneam, Israel)
3. Subdermal Delivery of Energy
   a. Subdermal delivery of fiber-optic laser energy
      i. SmartLipo, Cynosure (Westford, MA, USA)
   b. Subdermal delivery of RF energy
      i. BodyTite, NeckTite, FaceTite, and Cellu-Tite RF
      ii. Liposuction and skin-tightening devices, Invasix (Yokneam, Israel).

This anatomic classification is significant because a clinician can now divide the skin-tightening opportunities using RF energy sources and laser devices into those that deliver their energy across the epidermal-dermal junction, resulting in nonablative treatment of the epidermal-dermal junction, or a complete dermal ablative procedure through traditional ablative carbon dioxide and erbium YAG technology, or a fractional transepidermal nonablative and/or ablative experience. All of these devices will interact with dermal water, resulting in a photothermalytic thermal response and, depending on whether the device is principally ablative, nonablative coagulative, or a combination, an inflammatory stimulus of various magnitudes will affect the tissue. The more ablative devices will require an epidermal-repair process and some remodeling of the ablated or coagulative nonablative injury to the dermal substrate. Generally, the more ablative the laser or photon device, the better the tightening results will be.[3]

Into this transepidermal delivery of laser energy has evolved the transepidermal delivery of RF energy. Through minimal to no epidermal-dermal ablation, one can deliver RF energy into the dermis, where, rather than targeting traditional chromophores, such as hemoglobin, melanin, or water, all molecules in the RF pathways are oscillated 1 million to 6 million times per second.[3,14] It is the resistance to RF traveling through tissue that results in molecular oscillation and thermal energy. RF, either fractional or nonfractional, can be selective and targeted in different depths of the dermis and combined with other energy sources.[3,14]

The subdermal space has recently become the focus of an intense excitement for skin-tightening technologies and esthetic physicians. As reviewed in this article, new evidence and research has shown that if the energy source, either a laser-based or RF-based device, is placed in the immediate subdermal space, significant soft tissue skin contraction and correction of laxity can be induced without an excisional procedure or epidermal-dermal ablation. With this new subdermal delivery of RF, the kind of nonexcisional skin-tightening results that many patients are looking for is approached, without seeking the gold standard excisional rhytidectomy or skin-repositioning procedures. The maturation in the transepidermal delivery of monopolar RF (Thermage™) has given patients and clinicians noninvasive options for skin tightening when even subdermal, nonexcisional delivery techniques remain too aggressive.

BASIC SCIENCE OF RF SKIN TIGHTENING

The basic science of skin tightening is really the basic science of controlled dermal heat generation, which is the common final pathway for laser and RF devices. In standard chemical ablation, the chemical agent results in a nonthermal chemical dissolution and coagulation of the associated dermal proteins and the wound healing that occurs over several weeks results in new collagen, elastin, and skin tightening. As the ablative chemical and dermabrasion techniques gave rise to ablative carbon dioxide and erbium YAG lasers, so does the promise of more selective depth control and precision injury. The photothermolytic process involved the photons (10,600 nm for carbon disoxide and 2940 nm for erbium) being attracted to dermal water, resulting in ablative and nonablative coagulative disruption.[4–6] Immediate disruption of the collagen triple helix accounted for immediate, "on-the-table" skin-tightening effects and then a secondary tightening effect over 6 months from secondary neocollagenesis, elastin, and ground substance production.[3,4] The original ablative laser technologies were associated with excessive patient morbidity, potential complications and patient downtime, and resulted in the growth and development of nonablative technologies that attempted to affect the collagen triple helix the same as the more ablative laser wavelengths.[7–12,15–18] The proliferation of wavelengths and energies from intense pulsed light, pulse dye, the infrared diodes, and infrared heating lamps resulted in a nonablated, intact epidermal-dermal junction, whereas dermal water was the principal chromophore for the infrared devices. Hemoglobin and melanin were the chromophores for very near infrared and invisible skin-tightening light devices. Although there was some superficial papillary dermal collagen and ground substance response to these devices, the clinical results were often difficult to see with standard photography and follow-up results.[9–11] Unless the results were a correction of vascular or melanin dyschromia's discernable tightening and textural improvement, results were difficult to detect.

With the evolution, growth, and refinement of Thermage™ and monopolar transepidermal RF technology, moderate, consistent, and pleasing skin tightening can be achieved very reproducibly and comfortably.[14] Since the inception and release of Thermage™ in 2002, the evolution to what type of monopolar nonablative RF skin tightening was available in 2010 (the time of this writing) is a testament to a company that has been very much committed to basic science research and understanding the evolution of the effect of RF on biologic tissues. Over the past 8 years, advances have been seen in tip geometry and shape.[3,14] Although there are other nonablative transepidermal RF devices available, Thermage™ remains the number 1 monopolar RF delivery system in the world.[2,15–18] Thermage™ also has the most abundant nonablative, RF peer-reviewed science behind it and in this article is the main focus of the transepidermal discussion of RF energy delivery for skin tightening. Thermage™ consists of 3 important components: a generator, a coolant, and an applicator tip. Refined and patented delivery of the monopolar RF energy occurs across a thin membrane.[3,14] Synchronous cryogen-based cooling and a very sophisticated volumetric delivery of RF energy, depending on the tip size and configuration and pulse configuration, heat a specific volumetric amount of papillary superficial reticular dermis.[3,14] Over the past 8 years, refinement in Thermage™ tip sizes has improved treatment time.[14] Elegant studies of preauricular biopsies before rhytidectomy have shown that multiple passes at lower Thermage™ fluences result in better, more significant, and enhanced collagen and elastin ground substance production and tissue tightening than fewer passes and higher fluence.[19]

Over the years, transepidermal, monopolar Thermage™ delivery of RF energy has become a much more patient-acceptable procedure with less pain and recovery.[14] The monopolar energy delivered by the Thermage™ tip is delivered to a specific volumetric amount of the dermis or subcutaneous space. RF energy does not rely on a classic chromophore or chromophore photon interaction, as in the laser-based technologies but rather it is the resistance to RF energy traveling through tissue that results in generation of heat. It is the volumetric generation of heat through the oscillatory vibration of molecules along the resistant pathways of RF that results in energy. The RF energy can be used on all skin types and is chromophore independent. The clinical results of Thermage™ monopolar RF energy is discussed in the next section on clinical outcomes.

The basic science of subdermal thermal energy delivery is a very new area of intense clinical interest. Barry DiBernardo, in his seminal work[20] on subdermal delivery of fiber-optic laser energy, specifically a 1064 nm laser fiber, Smart Lipo, Cynosure, was able to show that subdermal delivery of thermal energy resulted in significant tissue tightening using quantitative and reliable techniques. Studies were able to show that area contraction of the skin of 17% can occur over 3 months following subdermal thermal laser energy delivery.[20] That degree of soft tissue area contraction is a very significant amount of soft tissue tightening given that this skin tightening occurs in a nonexcisional fashion. The subdermal laser heating is indeed minimally invasive, as opposed to noninvasive, as local anesthesia must be used and a stab access port must be created to insert the heating device under the skin and into tissue. Most esthetic surgeons who inject a large volume of fillers, make small excisions and are comfortable with human facial anatomy, and are capable of local anesthesia and subdermal delivery of a laser fiber. There is an increased complication rate and risks to subdermal laser and RF delivery. What Dr DiBernardo[20] was able to show was that by keeping the epidermal temperatures at 40 to 42°C and a subreticular dermal temperature of 50 to 55°C, the result is a nonablative, coagulative disruption of deep reticular collagen fibers and that a neocollagenesis, which was biopsy proven, occurs over the subsequent 3 to 6 months with significant measurable and quantitative skin and tissue tightening.

The basic science behind the delivery of this subdermal thermal laser energy is quite straightforward. The laser emits a wavelength of light, which can be from 900 nm up to 1400 nm, and in the presence of local anesthesia and subdermal tumescent fluid, the infrared laser photon will be attracted to the chromophore's water and to a lesser extent, hemoglobin and adipose tissue. These chromophores interact with the photons, resulting in a selective photothermolytic response and release of heat. When the tissue heats to critical temperatures higher than 50 to 55°C, it will result in a nonablative coagulative disruption of collagen and then new collagen forms and tissue tightening occurs over approximately 3 to 6 months.

Taking this subdermal laser-tightening paradigm further, Invasix (Yokneam, Israel) introduced into the marketplace a bipolar RF hand piece and device, which is a novel and proprietary technology that attempts to simulate both the nonablative, transepidermal delivery effects of Thermage™ and the subdermal laser heating effect achieved with a laser fiber optic. There are various Invasix applicators and configurations of the hand pieces, depending on where the internal electrode will be inserted, which can be a very small bipolar hand piece for the face called FaceTite, or neck device called NeckTite, or a much larger device for the body called BodyTite. Each applicator consists of an internal RF probe. This probe can be a hollow RF-emitting suction cannula, if it is to be used for body fat aspiration, used for corporeal body liposuction, or, in the face and neck, it can be a nonaspirating, very small internal RF probe designed to pass directly under the dermis. The internal electrode-probe is coated with Teflon so only the tip emits RF energy. The RF energy from the internal probe then travels directionally in a confined way up to the external electrode, which travels smoothly, in tandem with the internal electrode along the skin (**Fig. 1**). Unlike a monopolar system, which needs to have a return electrode pad somewhere on the body, this bipolar electrode configuration from Invasix allows intense internal RF energy to create heat in the subcutaneous or subdermal space around the internal electrode-probe, while gentle transepidermal dermal heating occurs from the external electrode, which serves as the return electrode for the internally generated RF current (see **Fig. 1**). This unique device, therefore, allows physicians to deliver transepidermal "monopolar" Thermage™ nonablative-type RF heating to the mid and deep dermis and then a more significant RF thermal experience to the

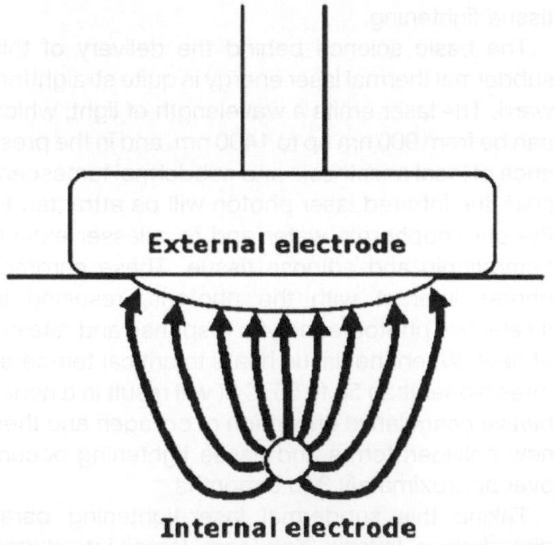

Fig. 1. Radiofrequency energy travels directionally from the internal cannula to the external electrode. The external electrode provides gentle heating of the papillary dermis as well as low and high impedance and temperature cut of control. The internal electrode provides strong coagulative tissue tightening and ablation.

septofascial cutaneous structures in the hypodermis, resulting in matrix-tightening effects in the subdermal and subcutaneous spaces. The various Invasix bipolar applicators, FaceTite, NeckTite, and BodyTite, can be performed under local anesthesia and, like subdermal laser fiber delivery, a physician needs to be skilled in the art of applying anesthesia and know the relevant subcutaneous structures to avoid.

Peer-reviewed results of skin-tightening effects of this novel subdermal and subcutaneous RF delivery, combined with epidermal-transdermal RF delivery from Invasix, have been quite significant.[21–28] Using the BodyTite, RF-assisted liposuction device, the internal cannula can be used to stimulate the septofascial cutaneous fibers in the adipose tissue while the external electrode through transepidermal heat stimulates the dermis. Linear contractions of 15% to more than 30% can be achieved and area contractions averaging 40% to 60% have been reported.[21–23,25] In addition, work with innovative applicators specifically designed for cellulite and treating in the immediate hypodermal space result in an enhanced collagen barrier in the deep hypodermis, which has been shown to improve the appearance of cellulite, both clinically on cell tissue cultures and histologically. Taking the bipolar applicator, called the FaceTite, onto the face, allows the areas of the brow, infraorbital and supraorbital, malar, jowl, and neck to be treated and preliminary results show significant tightening, brow elevation, and jowl and neck tightening. Clinical results for the internal and external delivery of RF energy are discussed in the sections on clinical results and complications.

CLINICAL PROTOCOL AND RESULTS

Over the 8 years that Thermage™ monopolar RF transepidermal delivery has been available, there have been significant advances on both how the RF is delivered and the patient perception of the treatment as well as the clinical outcomes. Recent studies of a very large number of patients show significant improvement over the original Thermage™ treatment algorithm for rhytid reduction in the face and neck skin tightening.[3,14] The original algorithm in Thermage™ systems used very high energy and the patient's discomfort was significant. In the original algorithm, studies were able to demonstrate that approximately 26% of patients exhibited immediate tightening and that 50% to 60% of patients observed evidence of skin tightening that was measurable 6 months after treatment. However, almost one-half of patients found the procedure too painful and only approximately 70% of patients found treatment results met their expectations.[3] With continued evolution in tip size, tip algorithms, and energies delivered, and based on pain as an end point for clinical outcome and biopsy results of different energy thresholds, new Thermage™ multiple-pass algorithms with a larger tip and shorter RF pulse configurations showed that almost 90% of patients observed immediate tightening and that more than 90% of patients had visible and measurable moderate skin tightening 6 months after treatment. Only 5% of patients now find the procedure too painful and more than 94% find the treatment meets their expectations.[14] In addition, studies on the transepidermal delivery of monopolar RF energy or bipolar RF energy, with or without the addition of intense pulse light and infrared energy, showed that the procedure can be done safely in the presence of soft tissue fillers, especially when injected in the supraperiosteal space and even when injected in the deep dermal space[14–17] In addition, these transepidermal RF procedures can be delivered in the presence of neurotoxin and can be combined with intense pulse light sources, either during the same treatment session or at subsequent dates and as well as microdermabrasion to enhance the synergistic esthetic results.

By 2010, the transepidermal delivery of monopolar RF energy or bipolar RF energy with or without the addition of visible light sources had become the standard of nonepidermal dermal ablative skin tightening.[14] When patients are appropriately selected, the outcomes tend to be good.[14] The success of Thermage™ and of the nonablative transepidermal delivery of RF resulted in the evolution of other monopolar RF devices and fractional RF epidermal dermal ablative technologies that would conceivably improve the epidermal-dermal junction superficially, as well as provide some deep RF tightening effect. The market leader in this transepidermal fractional delivery of RF energy has been Syneron Medical Ltd's E-Matrix and Matrix RF.[29] Results from this technology show that consistent and notable skin tightening can occur and that this can be particularly advantageous in patients with acne and that the fractional RF can be combined with other neurotoxins, soft tissue filler, and intense pulse-light color-correction technologies.[12] Other fraction RF devices that have launched and are pending approval by the Food and Drug Administration (FDA) include the Fractora (Invasix) with deep RF transepidermal fractional needle stimulation for additional skin tightening that can be achieved without the insertion of subdermal or subcutaneous devices. New transepidermal RF tightening devices delivering RF energy and therapeutic effect with multiple RF electrodes (TriPollar and octopolar) have been developed.[21–28]

FRACTIONAL LASER RESURFACING

Although not RF in nature, fractional laser resurfacing deserves some special mention because there had been a tremendous resurgence in fractional carbon dioxide and fractional erbium YAG resurfacing. The wonderfully simple advent of fractionating the carbon dioxide or erbium YAG beam leaving intact epidermal dermal tissue between the columns of photons results in very rapid reepithelialization through marginal epithelialization rather than prolonged reepithelialization by a deep dermal adnexa that was an obligatory component in previous carbon dioxide and erbium YAG ablative procedures. By fractionating or treating only a proportion of the epidermal dermal junction in dermis, the areas of laser thermal zones can occupy between 15% and 85% of the dermis. The more surface area covered by the proportion of fractional injury, the longer the recovery and the longer reepithelialization and resolution of erythema takes. There are various fractional carbon dioxide and fractional erbium YAG manufacturers on the market now. Good results have been achieved with all of them, including the Lumenous, Active and Deep FX, the Reliant Repair, the Cynosure Affirm CO_2, and the Sciton Pro Fractional device. The skin-tightening results of these devices, even after multiple treatments, are not quite as impressive as the full ablative nonfractionated carbon dioxide resurfacing of a decade ago, but the rhytid results exceed those of RF nonablative treatment. In addition, if used with appropriate settings, the risks of hypopigmentation and scar formation are much less than their ablative ancestors. The degree of rhytid reduction with fractional transepidermal RF or fractional laser resurfacing can be quite notable.[29]

BIPOLAR TRANSEPIDERMAL AND SUBCUTANEOUS RF ENERGY DELIVERY

The advent and introduction of Invasix's RF-assisted liposuction of BodyTite ushered in a very safe and refined method of RF: subdermal and subcutaneous rejuvenation. The bipolar applicators allow internal RF delivery to the septofascial and fasciocutaneous structures of the hypodermal space during a BodyTite RF-assisted liposuction (RFAL) case, or to the immediate subdermal space when using the NeckTite, FaceTite, or CelluTite applicators. Although the internal electrode can function as an electrode or electrode cannula, depending on the applicator, the external electrode functions both as a return electrode and as a gentle transepidermal nonfractionated RF energy delivery system to the papillary and rhyticular dermis. The electrode is connected to the internal electrode via the hand piece and various depths can be selected, depending on the applicator. The external electrode also constantly measures the all-important epidermal temperature when working superficially, whereas the internal probe can measure the important subdermal or deep subcutaneous temperature. The moving external, Thermage™ like electrode and internal RF electrode have proven to have some very unique uses and clinical results. At the time of this article, the BodyTite is approved by Conformité Européenne, Health Canada, Korean FDA, and Australia, and is sold worldwide and is pending FDA clearance. Studies at 20 US-based institutional review board sites have provided some compelling data. The BodyTite RF-assisted liposuction device has been used to treat all areas of the body.[21–28] Purported advantages include speed; extreme thermal uniformity of tissue heating; safety in thermal monitoring; reduced swelling, pain, and ecchymosis; and synchronous coagulation and aspiration of fat, which can speed up the time required for cutaneous and subcutaneous tightening before, during, or after standard suction-assisted lipoplasty. Perhaps the most important clinically significant effect of internal subdermal and subcutaneous RF is 3-dimensional soft tissue area contraction, which can range from 25% to 60%.[23]

The BodyTite device can be used on its own for small or medium areas, as it aspirates at the same time as the internal electrode emits RF energy and is also a hollow-bore Mercedes tip cannula. The tightening results from BodyTite are impressive, with linear contraction measured between 15% and 40%, the average being 25%.[21–23,25] Area contraction averages, depending on the size of the subcutaneous envelope of the patient can measure between 30% and 60%.[21–23,25] The significant cutaneous skin tightening has allowed the exploration of many new clinical RFAL and RF skin-tightening applications and minimally invasive plastic surgery to evolve. Postpartum individuals or patients who have had massive weight loss with lax abdominal skin and soft tissue may now be acceptable candidates for RF-assisted liposuction contouring and skin tightening rather than full, formal abdominoplasty. RFAL can also be used in combination with a "mini"-abdominoplasty, skin excisions, and diffuse abdominal and flank RF-assisted liposuction.[21–28] Other areas where RFAL appears to be very advantageous in skin tightening and

contour enhancement are the upper arms and inner thighs, back, bra line, and flanks, which traditionally can be very difficult areas for suction-assisted lipoplasty, ultrasound assisted liposuction, or laser assisted liposuction alone.[30,31]

The newest skin-tightening and contour bipolar applicators from Invasix include NeckTite, FaceTite, and RF CelluTite. These RF applicators are smaller and can be used in the submental cervical region where the external electrode of the bipolar configuration continuously moves along the epidermis, providing gentle RF heating to 40°C, as well as epidermal safety temperature and impedance sensing, while the internal electrode heats the subreticular dermal collagen up to 50 to 55°C. The author's experience with long-term contraction results of the cervical mental region with NeckTite applicator have been impressive. Another very small bipolar internal and external electrode applicator, called FaceTite, has been designed for RF tightening of the brow, lids, cheeks, and face. Like NeckTite, FaceTite is performed under local anesthesia and the internal electrode can be passed directly under the reticular dermis of the brow, lower lid, cheeks, upper lip, and jawline, heating the reticular dermis up to 50 to 55°C. The external epidermal electrode provides RF heat to the papillary and reticular dermis, heating it to 40°C and constantly measuring epidermal temperature, cutting off the RF energy when the physician-selected threshold is met. FaceTite RF skin tightening can be applied to the brow, to the under eye, to the cheek, and to the nasal labial fold, upper lip, and perioral region. Because of the thermal containment between the 2 electrodes, it is unlikely for the facial nerve to suffer a thermal injury, which can occur by passing non-confined laser energy beams in the immediate subdermal space. The FaceTite applicator can be combined with synchronous volumization with micro fat grafting, or deep supraperiosteal hyaluronic acid or particulate stimulate fillers performed after or before the procedure. After the FaceTite procedure, synchronous Botox can be applied. In addition, once the FaceTite procedure is performed on the brow, under eye, cheek, and neck, fractional transepidermal ablative laser technology or fractional RF ablative technology can be used. Significant 1-step results have been achieved by the author by combining the FaceTite bipolar epidermal and subdermal RF skin-tightening applicator to the brow, under eye, cheek, and neck with synchronous, aggressive full-face and neck-fraction RF ablation (Fractora, Invasix), or fractional carbon dioxide resurfacing (Affirm CO2, Cynosure). The combination internal RF tightening combined with external RF (fractional or

Thermage™) can deliver very nice skin-rejuvenation results.

The small FaceTite applicator can also be used for skin tightening anywhere on the body. Good reports have been achieved by using FaceTite on the neck, either in the absence of a cervical facial rhytidectomy or for residual skin laxity after a facelift. The investigators[21–27] also use the FaceTite and NeckTite RF tightening devices to undermine skin flaps of the neck, lateral cheek, and brow before their surgical elevation as part of a rhytidectomy. Combined with BodyTite or traditional liposuction, the SkinTite applicator can be used for loose supra-umbilical skin, inner thigh skin, or arm skin, either alone or in combination with excisional or suctioning procedures.

The clinical results of internally delivered RF are significant and this opens the opportunities for plastic surgeons and cosmetic physicians to offer a nonexcisional, minimally invasive option for skin tightening in those patients who are not seeking a larger, more successful skin removal technique. The internal-external RF skin tightening can be combined with other currently successful minimally invasive techniques to optimize the nonexcisional results.

COMPLICATIONS

The complications from Thermage™ and the other devices that deliver nonablative transepidermal delivery of RF energy are negligible.[3] In patients properly selected for Thermage™ and external RF nonablative procedures, more than 90% of patients are happy with their treatment. Early disappointment with the original Thermage™ algorithms and tips with 50% of patients finding the treatment too painful and unacceptable levels of patient dissatisfaction have given rise to larger tips, modified algorithms, and technology with multiple passes where more than 90% of well-selected patients are quite happy with the modest skin tightening and rhytid reduction that they see. Other external RF nonablative technologies, with or without combination light-based energies, report similar high happiness indexes for properly selected patients for these nonablative procedures. The instances of transepidermal monopolar or bipolar, TriPollar, or octopolar burns has been reported to be far less than 0.1%. The dreaded complication of fat atrophy, which was a rare but unacceptable complication with the initial high-fluence Thermage™ algorithm, has fortunately been virtually eliminated.[3] The incidence of prolonged edema, swelling, scabbing, erythema, vesiculation, and scarification is again far less than 1%.[3]

The safety and efficacy of the transepidermal delivery of fractional ablative RF energy, or laser carbon dioxide and erbium yag ablative fractional energy has improved significantly over the full ablative complications and morbidity of a decade ago.[2–18] There is still risk of hypopigmentation if the fractional density fluence or pulse durations are too aggressive, and fractional ablative technologies, even fractional erbium yag, fractional carbon dioxide, and fractional RF, can lead to postinflammatory hyperpigmentation in those patients predisposed or prone to this complication.[2–18] The transepidermal fractional RF ablation, when used in appropriate settings, can be indicated in those patients in whom ablative technology may be contra indicated, specifically sun exposure and skin type 4 and occasionally 5.

The complications associated with the Invasix bipolar RF-assisted devices are clearly going to be higher and more substantive than the risks and complications associated with nonablative or minimally ablative transepidermal devices. In the hands of skilled plastic surgeons and cosmetic physicians, who are used to elevating the anatomic structures in the face, neck, and body and are able to apply local anesthesia and assess the epidermal-dermal junction, the Invasix technology can be very safe. There are many safety features built into the bipolar RF-assisted skin-tightening and liposuction devices. The epidermal external return electrode has impedance sensors (with automated high-impedance and low-impedance cutoffs) that greatly minimize the risks of "end dermal hit" burns and prevent eschar formation around the internal electrode. The external electrode has built-in epidermal temperature sensors and the physician can set the device to automatically cut off the RF energy at any epidermal temperature. This negative feedback loop allows the FaceTite, NeckTite, or BodyTite to be used and maintained at target epidermal temperatures of 40 to 42°C. In addition, when performing RF-assisted liposuction with the BodyTite device, the internal electrode-cannula constantly measures internal temperature and will also notify the physician when the internal temperature target has been met (usually 60 to 65°C). When performing superficial treatments, such as RF-assisted CelluTite, FaceTite, or NeckTite, because the distance between the internal electrode and moving epidermal electrode is so small, constant epidermal monitoring is all that is required to help avoid a thermal injury. When performing deeper techniques, such as RF liposuction, then an internal temperature monitor and feedback, as well as epidermal temperature–monitoring feedback and impedance safety measurements are provided to minimize the risks of overheating the structures internally, as well as creating epidermal-dermal thermal disruption. Reported incidents of a thermal injury using the Invasix RF internal and external device is less than 1%; however, there is a significant learning curve and the first 10 to 15 cases performed by any surgeon need greater care and attention. When a subdermal RF or laser energy results in a burn, it is full-thickness in nature and will often require surgical management when it has healed. Hyperpigmentation and hypopigmentation are not generally features of the internal and external RF devices. Excessive heating of the internal fat space and adipose tissue can lead to persistent subcutaneous nodules, which resolve with time and represent adipose tissue that was overheated and died, but was not removed with aspiration.[20–28,30,31] Although, with the advent of the internal thermistor on the cannula, the incidence of these soft tissue nodules is much lower.

Like all energy-assisted devices, such as ultrasound and laser, the instance of seroma when performing RF liposuction and internal RF skin tightening is increased over suction assisted lipoplasty alone. Although the complications of simultaneous internal and external delivery of RF energy are greater than those seen with nonablative Thermage™ devices, the advantages of up to 40% to 60% area contraction and the relatively low incidence of complications make the internal delivery of RF and the Invasix devices a very exciting area of growth for the plastic surgeon performing nonexcisional and excisional skin tightening. The advantage of being able to combine the internal and external RF energy with fractional ablative RF devices or fraction laser devices, Botox, and fillers adds to the armament of the plastic surgeon, providing yet another opportunity to keep patients in the practice, as they are seeing significant skin-tightening and skin-rejuvenation results without an excisional procedure.

NONINVASIVE AND MINIMALLY INVASIVE SKIN-TIGHTENING BUSINESS MODEL

Clearly, as plastic surgeons and as cosmetic surgeons interested in excisional procedures, there is great forethought, care, and attention to the business plan of nonexcisional skin-tightening devices before bringing noninvasive and minimally invasive technologies into one's practice. In general, each of these noninvasive and nonablative RF or nonablative laser devices will cost upwards of $100,000 or more. The lease payments alone on each of these devices can reach $2500 to $3000 per month, in addition to disposables and consumables. When adopting a nonexcisional skin-tightening technology into the practice of a plastic surgeon, whose livelihood is devoted to

excisional surgery, it is important that the right business model and expectations, both for the practice as well as the patient, are created.

As successful paradigm that the author has seen used in many plastic surgeons' offices is to add significant nonablative and minimally ablative facial technologies as an adjunct to the facial excisional practice. The marketing advantages of combining a minimally and noninvasive skin-tightening program with an excisional skin-tightening practice can be synergistic. If the plastic surgeon is committed to internal and external marketing and positions these technologies well, properly selected patients will be happy with their noninvasive and minimally invasive results, which can create an ongoing revenue stream that can be significant, and one day many of these patients will, in fact, move up to more excisional procedures.

NONINVASIVE AND MINIMALLY INVASIVE COMBINATION THERAPY

When patients present for facial rejuvenation, who are not quite sure exactly what procedure they may benefit from, seeking the advice of their plastic surgeon, it is wise to be armed with all the opportunities for skin rejuvenation. Many patients present for skin rejuvenation for primary facial or body skin laxity. Following excisional procedures with or without contouring, these individuals will be seeking some type of maintenance therapy that can be offered as well. Noninvasive and minimally invasive combinations that work well to generate good results include combinations of transepidermal monopolar RF, or bipolar and multipolar RF combined with intense pulse light, neurotoxin, and fillers. This basic combination delivers rhytid reduction skin tightening supported by neurotoxin, and soft tissue volumization of the midface and perioral region with color correction delivered by intense pulse light. It is quite common now with the combination therapy for the average individual who is 50 to 60 years old to look 5 years younger without an excisional procedure. Many patients are happy with this type of rejuvenation and enhancement and may never present for cervical facial rhytidectomy. For these patients and for the survival of plastic surgery, it is important that enough plastic surgeons become familiar with these therapies and become expert in the delivery of these therapies so that patients think of their plastic surgeon and not just their dermatologist or non–plastic surgery cosmetic physician for the delivery of these therapies. The disadvantage is that the business model can be expensive if not executed properly with proper patient selection and sound marketing and it can be an expense drag on practice profitability. Done well, howovor, with current and up-to-date marketing techniques, specifically Web site optimization; pay-per-click advertising; and basic, solid, good word-of-mouth referral, this can be an important adjunctive revenue stream that at least is expense and revenue neutral but can deliver significant patients for excision procedures as these minimally noninvasive patients stay in the practice.

SUMMARY

The nonablative Thermage™ RF device has evolved into a consistent, reproducible, and tolerable nonablative skin-tightening procedure with an abundance of clinical and basic science behind the current treatment algorithms. For more significant RF skin-tightening results, incorporating technology that can deliver subdermal and subcutaneous RF energy into the septofascial and fasciocutaneous hypodermal space of the face, neck, and body is more effective in achieving the desired result. With minimally invasive internal-external RF techniques, performed under local anesthesia, one can now begin to offer nonexcisional procedures to selective patients who would benefit from an augmented form of RF skin tightening. These patients can achieve skin-tightening results that are significant and impressive but do not replace traditional abdominoplasty, arm-lift, thigh-lift, neck-lift, or face-lift results. However, like the noninvasive facial business model, these individuals can be kept in the practice and can be offered noninvasive transepidermal nonablative RF Thermage™ maintenance treatments after their minimally invasive RF tightening results. One day, some patients will move up to the optimal skin-excisional procedures to give them the best possible result. Again, the goal is to ensure that safety and efficacy are maintained, that patient expectations are managed, and that patients who do not desire excisional procedures are given current and up-to-date, realistic optimal noninvasive or minimally invasive options.

THE FUTURE

It is an exciting time in skin tightening and the control of soft tissue laxity with nonexcisional techniques. Over the next few years, more published results will emerge that will help potentially turn the management of cellulite into a surgical disease, and plastic surgeons can continue to improve their ability to offer those patients who want significant skin tightening a minimally invasive nonexcisional, internal, and/or external RF

skin rejuvenation result that even traditional excisional plastic surgeons can be happy with.

REFERENCES

1. Selected characteristics of baby boomers 42 to 60 years old in 2006. US Census Bureau; 2006.
2. Moretti M, editor. Skin tightening: softening demand in a weak economy. Aliso Viejo (CA): Medical Insight Inc; 2008.
3. Sukal SA, Geronemus RG. Thermage: the nonablative radiofrequency for rejuvenation. Clin Dermatol 2008;26:602–7.
4. Fitzpatrick RE, Goldman MP, Satur NM, et al. Pulsed carbon dioxide laser resurfacing of photo-aged facial skin. Arch Dermatol 1996;132:395–402.
5. Fitzpatrick RE. CO2 laser resurfacing. Dermatol Clin 2001;19:443–51.
6. Sapijaszko MJ, Zachary CB. Er:YAG laser resurfacing. Dermatol Clin 2002;20:87–96.
7. Bruner E, Adamson PA, Harlock JN, et al. Laser facial resurfacing: patient survey of recovery and results. J Otolaryngol 2000;29:377–81.
8. Nanni CA, Alster TS. Complications of carbon dioxide laser resurfacing. An evaluation of 500 patients. Dermatol Surg 1998;24:315–20.
9. Goldberg DJ. Nonablative dermal remodeling: does it really work? Arch Dermatol 2002;138:1366–8.
10. Sadick NS. Update on non-ablative light therapy for rejuvenation: a review. Lasers Surg Med 2003;32:120–8.
11. Hardaway CA, Ross EV. Nonablative laser skin remodeling. Dermatol Clin 2002;20:97–111.
12. Bitter PJ, Mulholland SR. Report of a new technique for enhanced non-invasive skin rejuvenation using a dual mode pulsed light and radio-frequency energy source: selective radio-thermolysis. J Cosmet Dermatol 2002;1:142–3.
13. Fitzpatrick RE, Geronemus RG, Goldberg DJ, et al. Multicenter study of noninvasive radiofrequency for periorbital rejuvenation. Lasers Surg Med 2003;33:232–42.
14. Dover JS, Zelickson BD. Results of a survey of 5,700 patient monopolar radiofrequency facial skin tightening treatments: assessment of a low-energy multiple-pass technique leading to a clinical end point algorithm. Dermatol Surg 2007;33.900–7.
15. Sadick NS, Trelles MA. Nonablative wrinkle treatment of the face and neck using a combined diode laser and radiofrequency technology. Dermatol Surg 2005;31:1695–9.
16. Sadick NS. Combination radiofrequency and light energies: electro-optical synergy technology in esthetic medicine. Dermatol Surg 2005;31:1211–7.
17. Sadick HS, Sorhaindo L. The radiofrequency frontier: a review of radiofrequency and combined

radiofrequency pulsed-light technology in aesthetic medicine. Facial Plast Surg 2005;21:131–8.

18. Friedman DJ, Gilead LT. The use of a hybrid radio-frequency device for the treatment of rhytides and lax skin. Dermatol Surg 2007;33:543–51.

19. Kist D, Burns AJ, Sanner R, et al. Ultrastructural evaluation of multiple pass low energy versus single pass high energy radiofrequency treatment. Lasers Surg Med 2006;38:150–4.

20. DiBernardo B. The best of hot topics—lipo-transfer and SmartLipo. ASAPS, May 6, 2008.

21. Blugerman G, Shavelzon D, Paul M. A safety and feasibility study of a novel radiofrequency-assisted liposuction technique. Plast Reconstr Surg 2010; 125:998–1006.

22. Paul M, Mulholland RS. A new approach for adipose tissue treatment and body contouring using radiofrequency assisted liposuction. Aesthetic Plast Surg 2009;33(5):687–94.

23. Paul M, Blugerman G, Kreindel M, et al. Three-dimensional radiofrequency tissue tightening: a proposed mechanism and applications for body contouring. Aesthetic Plast Surg 2011;35(1):87–95.

24. Kreindel M, Mulholland RS. Radiofrequency energy. Body Language 2009;29:23–4.

25. Mulholland RS. An in-depth examination of radiofrequency assisted liposuction (RFAL). J of Cosmetic Surg and Medicine 2009;4:14–8.

26. Paul MD. Radiofrequency assisted liposuction comes of age: an emerging technology offers an exciting new vista in nonexcisional body contouring. Plastic Surgery Practice 2009;2:18–9.

27. Mulholland RS. The latest technologies to fight the bulge. Healthy Aging 2009;4:7–11.

28. Brightman L. RFAL Arm study Am Society Lasers Med and Surg annual meeting. Kissimmee (FL), June 2010.

29. Hruza G, Taub AF, Collier S, et al. Skin rejuvenation and wrinkle reduction using a fractional radiofrequency system. J Drugs Dermatol 2009;8(3): 259–65.

30. Goldman A. Submental Nd:YAG laser-assisted liposuction. Lasers Surg Med 2006;38:181–3.

31. Prado A, Andrades P, Danilla S, et al. A prospective, randomized, double-blind, controlled clinical trial comparing laser-assisted lipoplasty with suction-assisted lipoplasty. Plast Reconstr Surg 2006;118:1032–45.

Fractionation: A New Era in Laser Resurfacing

Nazanin Saedi, MD, Anthony Petelin, MD, Christopher Zachary, MBBS, FRCP*

KEYWORDS

- Fractional • Fraxel • Fractionation • Laser
- Resurfacing • Photothermolysis

KEY MESSAGES

- The development of fractionated laser technology, which creates a pixilated pattern of microscopic treatment zones and adjacent areas of sparing, is a milestone in the history of light-based rejuvenation.
- Treatment with the fractional ablative devices can approach results seen with the traditional carbon dioxide laser, with significantly less downtime and discomfort, and fewer complications.
- Although complications with fractionated lasers are rare, diligent patient management throughout the procedure and postoperative period remains critical in achieving optimal results.
- There are numerous fractional devices that use either ablative or nonablative treatment characteristics. These devices are not all made equal, and those who purchase such systems should make a careful determination about the relative efficacy of their proposed acquisition.

First used by Manstein and colleagues[1] in 2004, fractionated laser energy has quickly become an essential component of laser-based medical and aesthetic treatments. Although traditional full-face ablative laser resurfacing treats 100% of the skin, fractionated laser devices treat only a fraction of the skin and generally have the shape of vertically oriented cylinders of thermally damaged tissue. This design is unique in that each of these treatment areas is surrounded by normal, unaffected skin. Fractionated devices, with either thermal or ablative characteristics, are now produced by many laser companies. They are not all equal in their engineering or delivery capabilities, and thus potential buyers need to be cautious when choosing such a device for their practice. Although the gold standard remains the traditional CO_2 laser, these devices have approached this standard with much less downtime, and fewer side effects and complications.

HISTORY

Fully ablative laser skin resurfacing, with either the continuous-wave carbon dioxide (CO_2) or erbium:yttrium-aluminum-garnet (Er:YAG) lasers, gained popularity in the 1990s as the standard for facial rejuvenation.[2] The CO_2 laser emits light in the far infrared spectrum at 10,600-nm, and water is the major chromophore. When used, suprathreshold fluences result in rapid cellular heating and instant tissue vaporization known as ablation. Adjacent to the vaporized zone, subablative fluences induce tissue coagulation and protein denaturation through heat transfer.[3] This thermomechanical destruction generally extends 200 to 300 μm within the dermis, and is followed by a predictable and beneficial skin tightening phase through a process of heat-induced shrinkage of collagen and the initiation of new collagen formation.[1]

Disclosures: Christopher Zachary, MBBS, FRCP and Anthony Petelin, MD: none. Nazanin Saedi, MD: none.
Department of Dermatology, University of California at Irvine, Box 340 Medical Sciences, Irvine, CA 92697, USA
* Corresponding author.
E-mail address: czachary@uci.edu

Clin Plastic Surg 38 (2011) 449–461
doi:10.1016/j.cps.2011.02.008
0094-1298/11/$ – see front matter © 2011 Published by Elsevier Inc.

Operating at a wavelength of 2940-nm, the Er:YAG laser is 10 times better absorbed by water than the CO_2 laser, which has some fascinating sequelae including more superficial ablation, less collateral heating resulting in reduced hemostasis, absorption and ablation of the residual heated collagenous debris, and subsequent ability to drill deeply into the skin.

Minimization of thermal injury enhances healing and re-epithelialization, but it induces less dermal collagen contraction and remodeling than with the CO_2.[2]

Because of its dramatic results, traditional ablative laser resurfacing remains the gold standard in skin rejuvenation, but the significant postoperative morbidity and complications has led to a dramatic reduction in its use. Ablation of the entire epidermis is associated with copious oozing and crusting in the days following the procedure. Delayed healing can result in several weeks of uncomfortable dressing changes and debridement often requiring weeks off work or social activities. In many instances, erythema lasts 3 to 6 months.[3] The destroyed barrier protection increased significantly the risk of infection throughout the recovery period and required extensive care at home. Even with an experienced operator, the risk of scarring, delayed-onset permanent hypopigmentation, and demarcation lines was significant. For many patients (and physicians), this sequence of events was excessive, and consequently the early euphoria of laser skin resurfacing was met with a rapid decline in interest.

In an effort to overcome these problems, nonablative dermal remodeling became popular in the ensuing years. Using a variety of wavelengths, including near-infrared 1320-nm, 1450-nm, or 1540-nm lasers, radiofrequency or intense pulsed light, pulsed-dye laser, radiofrequency and focused ultrasound, selective injury of the dermis with relative or absolute sparing of the epidermis was developed and termed nonablative. The theory implied that bulk heating of the dermis without destruction of the epidermis may cause enough protein denaturation to stimulate collagen remodeling and synthesis. The maintenance of an intact epidermis using various cooling techniques prevented superficial wounds and lacked the side effects known to occur with the destruction of this layer. As a result of these mechanisms, gradual and tentative steps toward nonablative dermal remodeling were achieved. This technique was better tolerated than resurfacing with the CO_2 laser, and the downtime was minimal. However, the degree of benefit obtained often left both the patient and provider unimpressed.

The concept of fractionated laser surgery was first used, unbeknown to the researchers, in hair transplant surgery, where 1-mm holes were drilled in the bald scalp as recipient sites for hair transplants. Although the transplanted hairs took no better than in conventional hair transplantation, in retrospect the holes healed well, with limited scarring. This approach was incorporated into the work of Dr Manstein and Dr Anderson at the Wellman Center for Photomedicine, who first developed the functional concepts of fractionated laser surgery. It debuted in the literature in 2004 as the 1550-nm nonablative Fraxel laser, now called the Fraxel re:store (Solta Medical, Hayward, CA, USA).

MECHANISM

Fractional photothermolysis (FP) involves the application of very high-energy, narrow beams of light that create a pixilated appearance on the surface of the skin. With the ability to reach a depth of 1.5 mm, these focal zones of treatment, or microthermal zones (MTZs), are narrow cylinders of tissue destruction (**Fig. 1**). In comparison with both the traditional ablative and nonablative devices discussed previously, each fractionated laser beam is of extremely high fluence, sufficient to induce thermal damage or ablation of a very narrow tissue column surrounded by adjacent unaffected tissue. These surrounding areas of sparing act as reservoirs for healing, enabling the MTZs to resolve quickly with minimal discomfort by providing a foundation of structural and nutritional support and a reservoir for keratinocyte migration[1]; this is fundamental to all fractionated devices. It is the concept of focal destruction with islands of sparing that is paramount for the improved patient comfort and recovery time seen during the post operative period.

To further delineate the mechanism behind FP, Manstein and colleagues[1] performed the first lactate dehydrogenase (LDH) cell viability analysis on ex vivo tissue immediately after treatment with their prototype device. In this early study, they discovered microscopic areas of epidermal and dermal cell necrosis within the MTZs, which appeared to resolve rapidly within a few days.[1] No histologic or clinical evidence of persistence of the microthermal zones was present at 3 months.[1] Despite visible necrosis of the epidermis and dermis in the MTZs, the stratum corneum remained histologically and (to a large degree) functionally intact. Thus, rejuvenation with the prototype device was termed nonablative.[1]

The tissue injury created with FP stimulates the process of collagen remodeling and promotes

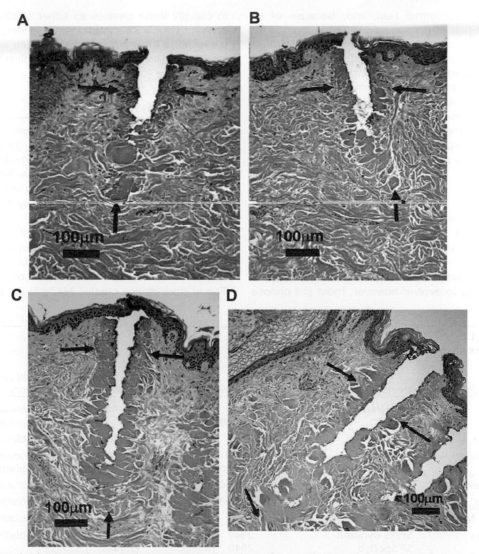

Fig. 1. Depth of ablation hematoxylin-eosin–stained sections of ex vivo human abdominal tissue treated with the 30-W, 10.6-mm, CO_2 laser at 9.2 mJ (*A*), 13.8 mJ (*B*), 18.0 mJ (*C*), and 23.3 mJ (*D*). The arrows outline the extent of denatured collagen zones. (*Adapted from* Hantash BM, Bedi VP, Chan KF, et al. Ex vivo histologic characterization of a novel ablative fractional resurfacing device. Lasers Surg Med 2007;39(2):89; with permission.)

elastic tissue formation, both of which are necessary for skin rejuvenation. New collagen and collagen remodeling markers such as heat shock proteins (47, 70, and 72), collagen III, proliferating cell nuclear antigen, and α-smooth muscle actin have been seen in treatment areas.[4] The expression of heat shock protein 47, which is required for collagen remodeling and maturation, has been detected within 1 week of treatment and persisted for nearly 3 months.[5] Additional benefits arise from the long-term wound healing response, which leads to replacement of photoaged dermal tissue with newly deposited collagen. These molecular changes are fundamental to the wound

healing response and are also believed to be responsible for the clinical improvements seen with fractional photothermolysis.[1]

Following treatment with a fractional photothermolysis device, the necrotic debris found at the level of the stratum corneum over each MTZ is quickly removed.[5,6] This material, now termed microscopic epidermal necrotic debris (MEND), has also been shown to contain an abundance of melanin on hematoxylin-eosin staining.[6] The repair of these epidermal defects causes extrusion and loss of the MEND at approximately 16 days.[6] This rapid exfoliation of the MEND therefore occurs simultaneously with the re-epithelialization of the irradiated epidermal field, and, because of its melanin-rich content, is said to be responsible for the efficacy of fractional photothermolysis in treating pigmentary disorders such as lentigines and melasma.[6] Intense pulsed light is more effective in removing epidermal pigmentation than the fractionated devices. It is more likely that the dramatically increased absorption of topical agents that occurs immediately after any fractionated treatment is responsible for the improvement in the appearance of the melasma in these subjects.

DEVICES

The success of fractional technology has spurred the recent development of many devices. **Table 1** provides a summary of the different types of devices currently available. Because technology advances rapidly, the terminology is continuing to evolve; however, most still choose

to classify these devices as either ablative fractional or nonablative fractional depending on the presence of an intact stratum corneum following treatment. This article follows this classification system.

Nonablative Systems

The prototype nonablative fractionated device developed by Reliant Technologies (now Solta Medical, Inc) was the 1550-nm erbium-fiber laser with a scanning headpiece, and is now known as Fraxel re:store. This device was used in the initial studies, and it is the most extensively evaluated device to date. It produces minimal to modest patient discomfort during treatment, although some patients may benefit from a topical anesthetic. Forced cold air is always used as an adjunctive safety and anesthetic complement. The re:store device creates MTZs in the order of

Table 1
Review of current fractionated laser systems

Manufacturer	Device	Wavelength (nm)	Medium	Ablative vs Nonablative
Alma	Pixel Harmony	2940	Er:YAG	Ablative
	Pixel CO$_2$	10,600	CO$_2$	Ablative
Cutera	Pearl	2790	YSGG	Ablative
Cynosure	Affirm	1440/1320	Nd:YAG	Nonablative
	Affirm CO$_2$	10,600	CO$_2$	Ablative
Eclipsemed	SmartXide DOT	10,600	CO$_2$	Ablative
Ellipse	Juvia	10,600	CO$_2$	Ablative
Focus Medical	NaturaLase Er	2940	Er:YAG	Ablative
Fotona	SP/XS Dynamis	2940	Er:YAG	Ablative
	SP Spectro	2940	Er:YAG	
Lasering	Mixto SX	10,600	CO$_2$	Ablative
Lumenis	Ultrapulse Active/Deep FX	10,600	CO$_2$	Ablative
Lutronic	eCO$_2$	10,600	CO$_2$	Ablative
Matrix	LS	10,600	CO$_2$	Ablative
Palomar	Lux 2940	2940	Er:YAG	Ablative
	Lux 1440	1440	Nd:YAG	Nonablative
	Lux 1540	1540	Er:glass	Nonablative
	Lux Deep IR	850–1350	Infrared	Nonablative
Quantel	ExelO$_2$	10,600	CO$_2$	Ablative
	Burane FX4/FX12	2940	Er:YAG	Ablative
Sciton	Profractional	2940	Er:YAG	Ablative
Sellas	Cis F1	10,600	CO$_2$	Ablative
	1550	1550	Er:fiber	Nonablative
Solta	Fraxel re:fine	1410	Er:fiber	Nonablative
	Fraxel re:store	1550	Er:fiber	Nonablative
	Fraxel re:store DUAL	1550/1927	Er:fiber/thulium	Nonablative
	Fraxel re:pair	10,600	CO$_2$	Ablative
Syneron	Matrix RF	Nonlaser	Bipolar RF	Nonablative

100 to 200 μm in width and 500 to 1400 μm in depth. Energy levels are adjustable from 4 to 70 mJ/MTZ. The original device used a blue optical dye to ensure accurate analysis of the scanning speed, which has now become unnecessary because of advancements in technology. It is generally a well-tolerated procedure, with erythema and edema routinely lasting 2 to 3 days after a standard treatment.

The Affirm (Cynosure, Westford, MA, USA) differed from the re:store in that it uses a 1440-nm laser operating through a complex array of lenses known proprietarily as Combined Apex Pulse (CAP) technology. The Affirm has been shown to be effective in many similar conditions as with the re:store, and it is US Food and Drug Administration approved for the treatment of periorbital and perioral rhytids. A recent advancement has been the addition of a 1320-nm wavelength stacked with the 1440-nm pulse, which seems to improve its efficacy.[7] The Affirm uses a stamping device to create zones of injury approximately 100 μm in width and 200 to 300 μm in depth. The procedure is generally well tolerated, with discomfort levels and postoperative erythema similar to those of other nonablative fractional devices.

Operating on its StarLux platform, Palomar Medical Technologies (Burlington, MA, USA) has 2 handpieces that use nonablative fractional technology with differing wavelengths. This platform allows the incorporation of various modalities, such as intense pulsed light (IPL) or fractionated lasers, to be attached to a single unit through the use of separate handpieces. The design is intended to add convenience and affordability, while enabling the physician to treat a variety of conditions. The platform also includes both the 1440-nm Nd:YAG and 1540-nm Er:glass handpieces to provide nonablative fractional technology.

Ablative Systems

Soon after the initial success of the original Fraxel device, work began on using the same technology with the CO_2 and Er:YAG lasers. Referred to initially as deep dermal ablation, the ablative fractional devices use very high energies to destroy columns of tissue that can reach depths of 1.5 mm. In contrast with the traditional devices, this not only creates a resurfacing effect but also causes a volumetric reduction of tissue and plumping of the dermis.

The Fraxel re:pair (Solta Medical, Hayward, CA, USA) was the first ablative fractional device to become available, in 2007. The device uses a 10,600-nm CO_2 laser that incorporates scanning handpiece technology in which both contact with the skin and speed of application are sensed and necessary for the laser to fire. Both energy and MTZ density can be adjusted. As described previously, in comparison with the nonablative fractional systems, there is more downtime associated with the ablative devices and pain control with topical anesthetics and anxiolytics is necessary for patient comfort, unless using very low-density, low-energy treatments.

Another well-studied ablative fractional device is the Active/Deep FX system (Lumenis Aesthetic, Santa Clara, CA, USA), which is part of the Ultra-Pulse platform. Also incorporating a CO_2 laser, this system uses both a large superficial spot treatment (Active FX) and a deeper, narrower true fractional treatment (Deep FX). The combination of both systems in one patient treatment is often referred to as Total FX. The Active FX creates a large superficial treatment zone with a beam diameter of 1.25 mm, and relies on a computer pattern generator (CPG) to create a random pattern of injury, which guards against bulk heating. The Deep FX portion uses a smaller spot size of 120 μm that can penetrate up to 1.5 mm.[8] The larger spot size of 1.25 mm is not fractional in the true sense of the word; it just separates one regular large pulse from another. However, the Deep FX 120 μm is indeed fractional, and emulates the Fraxel re:pair device. The main difference between these systems is the scanning (Fraxel) versus stamping (Deep FX) technology used to deliver the myriads of pulses to the skin. The Fraxel scanning device is faster and creates a more even delivery of pulses. In addition, the density of these devices is calculated differently, which is critically important. The calculation with the re:pair is based on the total area damaged (ablation and thermal coagulation) and the Deep FX density is based only on the area of vaporization. Thus, practitioners cannot use the same parameters of energy and density with both devices and hope to create similar wounds. However, these devices can be used to provide similar results, and purchase of a device depends on personal preferences, cost, maintenance, service, and so forth.

Several devices use fractional ablative technology using Er:YAG-based lasers, including the Sciton ProFractional (Sciton Inc, Palo Alto, CA, USA), the Alma Pixel (Alma Lasers, Buffalo Grove, IL, USA), and the Palomar StarLux2940 (Palomar Medical Technologies, Burlington, MA, USA). Each device has notable differences in its means of application, but each relies on a 2940-nm wavelength medium. This wavelength has a stronger affinity for water and, therefore, a single pulse creates a more superficial wound with less thermal damage than with CO_2-based systems.

Another popular fractional ablative device is the Pearl (Cutera, Inc, Brisbane, CA, USA), which uses a 2790-nm erbium:yttrium-scandium-gallium-garnet (Er:YSGG) laser. The Er:YSGG has less water absorption than the 2940-nm Er:YAG, allowing for more heat transfer to surrounding tissue and subsequent collagen stimulation. The device comes equipped with both a nonfractional handpiece for 100% coverage and a fractional handpiece. The combination of the two has been shown to provide results equivalent to the Fraxel re:pair and the Lumenis Deep FX.

A recent addition to the fractional world is the thulium 1927-nm laser by Solta Medical Inc. For reasons currently not well understood, this device is effective at removing widespread actinic keratoses. We have shown that focal injury can produce generalized improvement, in the same way that lawn aeration produces a uniform improvement in the appearance of the grass. Roy Geronemus (Geronemus, personal communication, 2010 with CBZ) now prefers this device rather than the use of photodynamic therapy for extensive facial precancers. The thulium device has a nonlinear depth-to-energy profile, unlike the 1550-nm nonablative devices. Thus, the maximum depth of penetration is achieved at around 20 mJ per pulse. At that energy, the dermal thermal injury profile is similar to a superficial CO_2 laser, the difference being that there is no epidermal loss with the thulium, and thus no exudation or bleeding. This difference is a major advance both from a treatment and outcome point of view. These patients have improvements in their numbers of precancers, and also a considerable improvement in their cosmetic outcomes. Care should be taken to avoid using densities of more than 50%; although some have used 75% (Fitzpatrick, personal communication, 2010 to CBZ), others are using 25% to 30% density.

There is emerging technology that applies the concept of fractionation to radiofrequency (RF) with the recent development of the Matrix RF (Syneron Medical Ltd, Yokneam, Israel). The device uses bipolar RF in a fractionated manner through an applicator using an array of multielectrode pins that cause heating in the areas of pin contact and subsequent sparing of those areas in between. The device is tunable ,in that the relative proportion of ablation versus coagulation can be adjusted depending on the treatment indications. The Matrix RF works, but is not as versatile as many of the fractionated laser devices. However, this represents the first RF device capable of inducing skin ablation and heat transfer in a fractionated manner.

INDICATIONS

Fractional photothermolysis can be applied to all the usual indications, including photoaging, pigmentation, superficial or deep rhytids, and scar revision. The benefits are the reduction in downtime, the lack of discomfort in the healing period, and the relative lack of side effects. The major indications for fractional photothermolysis are similar to traditional skin rejuvenation and include photoaging, skin pigmentation, skin tightening, and scar revision.

Photoaging

In the initial studies using the 1550-nm nonablative device, Manstein and colleagues[1] reported significant improvements in periorbital rhytids and skin texture after treatment with their prototype. These studies showed mild improvement in 12% of patients, noticeable improvement in 30% of patients, and moderate to significant improvement in 54% of patients after 1 to 4 treatments. The investigators found a linear pattern of shrinkage related to the thermal injury.[1] The initial tissue shrinkage was followed by an apparent relaxation after 1 month, with retightening seen at 3 months.[1] This pattern of injury and healing is seen clinically with tissue contraction up to 12 months, and a subsequent 10% relaxation thereafter.[9]

We reported the prototype device used for ablative fractionated photothermolysis,[5] which showed greater degrees of improvement in photoaging with fractionated CO_2 laser technology compared with the original nonablative device. Although further studies are welcomed to directly compare the effectiveness of the ablative versus nonablative fractionated devices for photoaging and rejuvenation, it is generally considered (and is the opinion of these authors) that the increased downtime and invasiveness of the ablative devices reaps greater rewards.

Since these initial studies, several others have also shown improvements in photo-damaged skin with both ablative and nonablative FP, including improvement of mild to moderate rhytids (**Fig. 2**), photoaging of the hand,[10] and photoaging of nonfacial skin.[3] Fractionation has also been shown to be effective in the treatment of poikiloderma of Civatte.[11] The MTZs of thermal injury induced with a nonablative FP device resulted in rapid healing and clinical improvement in pigmentation and texture variation associated with this condition.[12]

Acne Scarring

The initial studies of fractionated lasers on acne scaring were done with nonablative devices. In

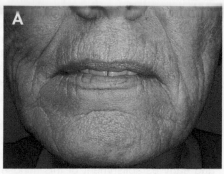
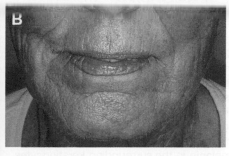

Fig. 2. Ablative fractional resurfacing for the treatment of perioral rhytids. (*A*) Appearance of perioral rhytids before treatment. Settings used for this treatment: 70 mJ, level 8, and 30%. (*B*) Compared with (*A*), there is significant improvement in the appearance of perioral rhytids after 2 treatments. Settings used for this treatment: 70 mJ, level 8, and 30%. (*Courtesy of* Christopher Zachary, FRCP.)

one study, patients with ice-pick to boxcar scars underwent a series of 5 FP treatments at 1-week to 3-week intervals.[3] Mean clinical improvement ranged from 25% to 50% and was assessed using digital photography. The nonablative devices have also shown efficacy in atrophic-type acne scars. In another study consisting of 53 patients with atrophic scarring, patients received a series of 3 monthly FP treatments (Fraxel re:store, Solta Medical, Hayward, CA, USA), with mean clinical improvement ranging from 51% to 75%.[13]

Ablative fractional resurfacing has not only shown significant efficacy in the treatment of acne scarring but it also seems to be superior to the nonablative modalities. A study of 30 patients with moderate to severe acne scarring underwent 1 to 3 treatments with the Fraxel re:pair (Solta Medical, Hayward, CA, USA). Mild to moderate overall improvement was noted with energies ranging from 20 to 100 mJ and densities of 600 to 1600 MTZ/cm.[14] When treating acne scarring, very high energy (70 mJ) in combination with very high density (70%) has shown more efficacy than low energy and low density.

Fractional photothermolysis is becoming increasingly popular in the treatment of dark-skinned patients (Fitzpatrick skin types III–VI) with acne scarring.[15] In a study of 27 Korean patients (Fitzpatrick skin types IV–V) with moderate to severe scarring, the patients' self-assessed degrees of improvement ranged from excellent improvement in 30%, significant improvement in 59%, and moderate improvement in 11%.[16] This was accomplished after 3 to 5 treatments with the Fraxel re:store (Solta Medical, Hayward, CA, USA).

Improvement of postinflammatory erythema associated with acne has also been described with the use of nonablative FP lasers.[17] It is speculated that the 1550-nm wavelength targets tissue water and may lead to thermally induced destruction of dermal blood vessels, resulting in improvement of erythema.[17]

Other Forms of Scars

The 1550-nm Fraxel re:store has been shown to be effective in the treatment of hypopigmented facial scars.[18] In these patients, additional improvements were also noted in the overall texture of the scar and surrounding skin.[18] Another study comparing the efficacy of nonablative FP with that of the pulsed dye laser (PDL) for the improvement of surgical scars noted greater improvement with the fractionated device.[19] After a series of 4 treatments, the portion of surgical scars treated with FP showed a mean improvement of 75.6%, versus the PDL, which had a mean improvement of 53.9%.[19] Furthermore, the scars with significant hypopigmentation showed more repigmentation after treatment with the fractional device. These investigators postulate that the greater depth of penetration and focal microthermal zones of injury with nonablative fractional photothermolysis, inducing collagenolysis and subsequent neocollagenesis, accounted for its superiority in scar remodeling.[19]

Pigmentary Disorders

In the initial reports on the efficacy of nonablative FP in treating melasma, 10 female patients (Fitzpatrick skin types III–V) were treated at 1-week to 2-week intervals with the Fraxel re:store (Solta Medical, Hayward, CA, USA).[20] Parameters consisted of fluences ranging from 6 to 12 mJ and densities between 2000 and 3500 MTZ/cm[2].[20] Following 4 to 6 sessions, physician evaluation confirmed that 60% of patients achieved 75% to 100% clearance.[20] In another study, 10 patients with melasma (Fitzpatrick skin types III–IV) were treated with a nonablative FP device (Fraxel re:store, Solta Medical, Hayward, CA, USA), and the histology was examined.[21] Patients received a total of 4 treatments at 2-week intervals, and biopsies were obtained from all subjects both before and 3 months following treatment. Histologically, post-treatment specimens showed a relative decrease in melanocyte quantity compared with pretreatment samples on light microscopy.[21] Furthermore, post-treatment electron microscopy revealed fewer melanocytes and less melanin in the surrounding keratinocytes than in the pretreatment specimens.[21] Clinical improvements in melasma were less extensive in patients with progressively darker skin types.

Although these initial studies showed promise for the treatment of melasma with FP, more recent reports have suggested limitations in its efficacy because of the high recurrence rates after treatment, especially in those patients with darker skin types.[15]

Other conditions that have been successfully treated using FP technology include residual hemangioma,[22] minocycline-induced hyperpigmentation,[23] granuloma annulare,[24] disseminated superficial actinic porokeratosis,[25] and colloid millium.[26] There is also developing research in treating burn injuries with these devices.

PREPROCEDURE AND POSTPROCEDURE CONSIDERATIONS
Patient Selection

First, a thorough history and physical is essential to understanding each patient's unique medical condition. Careful attention should be paid to history of prior laser procedures and response, any history of delayed healing or hypertrophic scarring, patient skin type, current and past medications, level of apparent anxiety, history of infections (especially herpes simplex [HSV]), and any evidence of an immunocompromised status. Special consideration should be given to patients with any active local or systemic infections or keloid scarring. Patients with a history of connective tissue disease, diabetes, and drug, alcohol, or tobacco abuse should be treated cautiously because their wound healing may be impaired. Avoid treating patients with a personal or family history of vitiligo. Patients who have used isotretinoin in the past 6 months (or up to a year by some clinicians' standards) may also be at increased risk for impaired healing.

In this authors' opinion, one of the most important considerations regarding patient selection begins during the initial consultation with the establishment of patient expectations. It is paramount that the patient and physician identify the problem to be treated together and work to establish a reasonable level of expectation for improvement. The patient must understand that often only one treatment with an ablative fractionated device may achieve marked improvement; however, the patient will have significantly more downtime than the several treatments generally required to achieve similar results with a nonablative system. Most importantly, the patient must understand that individual responses always vary, and early establishment of this mindset helps to ensure patient satisfaction.

Preoperative Considerations

Once patient selection with appropriate expectations and a thorough explanation of risks is complete, the perioperative period is crucial to help avoid many of the potential pitfalls and complications associated with laser resurfacing. Careful planning, the development of a consistent routine, and close follow-up with the patient are all important in this regard. Although many of the recommendations mentioned here might be standard procedure for some laser surgeons, or omitted in the practices of others, they deserve mention only as 1 method among many that these authors have found particularly useful.

All patients receive HSV prophylaxis using either acyclovir 400 mg orally three times daily or the often better-tolerated valacyclovir 500 mg orally twice daily, regardless of documented history of an outbreak. This therapy is initiated on the morning of the procedure and continued for 7 to 10 days following the treatment. When patients arrive on the day of the procedure, they are first instructed to cleanse their faces thoroughly for 5 minutes with soap, water, and a terry towel. For patients undergoing low-energy, low-density, nonablative fractional resurfacing, often there is no preprocedure anesthesia and the treatment can be initiated. However, for patients undergoing ablative fractional resurfacing, it is our practice to apply a 23%/7% lidocaine/tetracaine topical emulsion to the treatment sites for 1 hour. Thirty minutes before ablative resurfacing, patients may also receive an intramuscular injection of meperidine (Demerol) 50 mg, hydroxyzine (Vistaril) 25 mg, and ketorolac (Toradol) 60 mg, depending on weight and tolerance. Be careful to monitor these patients and to avoid excessive dosing. In our experience, patients tolerate this combination of sedation, analgesia, and anti-inflammatory agent well because it allows for excellent patient comfort throughout the treatment and may contribute to decreased postprocedure inflammation and edema. When needed, local nerve blocks have been used in instances of persistent patient discomfort caused by aggressive energy settings or a patient with low pain tolerance. One hour following the application of topical anesthesia, the topical anesthesia is removed and the procedure is initiated.

Postoperative Considerations

Throughout the procedure and immediately following, the skin is evaluated for any signs of adverse reaction such as dramatic vasospasm (skin whitening), blistering, or sloughing. **Figs. 3** and **4** show the appropriate response during the treatment. An assessment is also made regarding the patient's level of discomfort. In our experience, pain, whether immediate or delayed after surgery, is a poor prognostic indicator and often represents the first clue to an adverse reaction. Although some investigators advocate oral or intramuscular steroids in the postoperative phase, we use a potent topical steroid, such as fluocinonide 0.05% ointment, which is applied generously to the face immediately following treatment. The patient is given explicit verbal and written care instructions that call for consistent application of either a petrolatum-based or zinc oxide–based emollient. A dilute acetic acid solution is also

recommended to cleanse the area periodically throughout the day as well as to aid in decreasing colonization of microbes and to help avoid crusting. Although many investigators debate the prudence of postoperative antibiotics and/or antifungals, given the low incidence of impetigo and candidiasis shown to date, this author does not routinely prescribe them.

Consideration is also given for darker skin types or in those who suffer from melasma. In these instances, a 4% hydroquinone cream is initiated as soon as the exudative phase of the recovery has stopped and the patient can tolerate a topical application. Sun protection and avoidance remains standard for all patients after surgery.

Arguably, the most important component to postoperative care of a laser patient is close follow-up. Most adverse reactions occur between days 2 and 7 following the procedure,[27] and it is only through open lines of communication and timely reevaluation with patients that the early signs of trouble can be recognized, with the hope of an early intervention.

COMPLICATIONS

To date, both nonablative and ablative fractional lasers have shown fewer complications than traditional ablative lasers. The following list represents

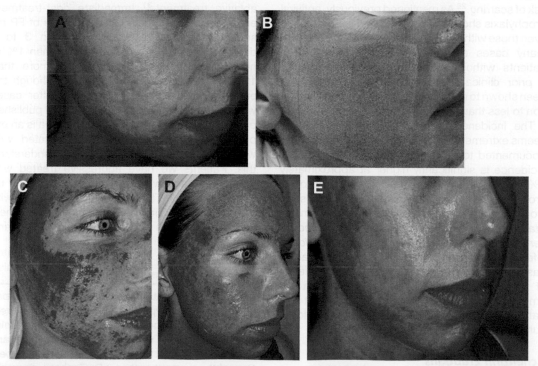

Fig. 3. Improvement of acne scarring. (*A*) Pretreatment photograph. (*B*) Midtreatment. (*C*) Immediately after treatment. During surgery, MTZs are evident with pinpoint bleeding. (*D*) Four days after surgery. (*E*) One month after treatment. (*Courtesy of* Christopher Zachary, FRCP.)

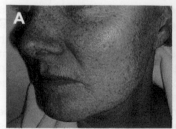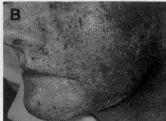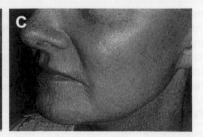

Fig. 4. Treatment of photoaging with fractionated CO_2 laser. (*A*) Pretreatment. (*B*) Midtreatment. Pinpoint bleeding from MTZs is characteristic. (*C*) After treatment. (*Courtesy of* Christopher Zachary, FRCP.)

complications seen to date. However, as fractional devices continue to gain in popularity and as more procedures are performed by inexperienced operators, the list of complications will grow.

Infections

The most common infection after fractional laser skin resurfacing is related to the herpes simplex virus, with reported rates ranging from 0.3% to 2%.[28,29] The infection rates with traditional (nonfractionated) ablative laser resurfacing were much higher, with 2% to 7% of cases developing HSV reactivation.[30] Infected patients often develop superficial erosions in the first week after treatment and the occurrence can dramatically increase the risk of scarring.[28] As mentioned previously, antiviral prophylaxis should be administered to all patients, even those without a documented history, because many cases of reactivation have occurred in patients without evidence or remembrance of a prior clinical outbreak.[31] This approach has been shown to minimize the rate of patient reactivation to less than 0.5% in healthy individuals.[28]

The incidence of bacterial infection after FP seems extremely low, with 0.1% of all treated cases documented to develop impetigo,[28] although our incidence is significantly higher at approximately 1% to 2%. A potential cause of pathogen overgrowth during the postoperative period is excessive wound occlusion leading to growth of primarily *Staphylococcus aureus* and *Pseudomonas aeruginosa*.[31] A case of *Mycobacterium chelonae* infection after fractionated CO_2 facial resurfacing has recently been reported.[32] Given the prevalence of methicillin-resistant *S aureus* (MRSA) in the ambulatory setting today, it is prudent that any patient failing to progress as expected should be cultured to rule out this infectious agent.

Acneiform Eruptions

The rates of acneiform eruptions are significantly lower (2%–10%) with fractional skin resurfacing compared with tradition skin resurfacing.[28] Milia development has been reported in as many as 19% of treated patients.[28] Since occlusive moisturizers and dressings can exacerbate these eruptions, such agents can be changed to noncomedogenic equivalents when appropriate.[33] With moderate to severe acne flares, a short course of oral tetracycline-based antibiotics is often helpful and can even be used before subsequent treatments to prevent future outbreaks.[13]

Prolonged Erythema

Prolonged erythema is defined as post-treatment redness that persists longer than 4 days with nonablative resurfacing and beyond 1 month with ablative treatment.[31] Immediate post-treatment erythema is an expected consequence of FP resurfacing that usually resolves within 3 to 4 days.[34] It has been reported in less than 1% of nonablative-treated patients,[28] and more than 12.5% of ablative-treated patients, although the erythema typically resolved in the latter cases within 3 months.[35] Despite all these published opinions concerning erythema, erythema is an expected and necessary event associated with wound healing, and clinicians should understand this. Patients we have aggressive treated with fractionated ablative laser surgery are red for up to 4 to 6 weeks. This redness is associated with heat shock protein persistence indicating new collagen formation and collagen remodeling, and is not a problem.

Changes in Pigmentation

It is well known that patients with darker skin types (Fitzpatrick skin types III–VI) have a higher likelihood of developing postinflammatory hyperpigmentation (PIH), which occurs following any inflammatory insult to the skin in darker skin types. One of the present authors, Dr Zachary, does not worry about PIH following laser surgery; he guarantees it! Unless, that is, the necessary steps are taken to prevent it. In general, PIH occurs less frequently with FP laser skin resurfacing compared with traditional resurfacing. But the incidence seems dependent on the system used, the parameters applied, and skin types treated. To minimize the risk, patients should avoid sun exposure at least 2 weeks before and after FP, and the application of a topical 4% hydroquinone early in the recovery phase can assist dramatically.[36]

Compared with traditional full-face CO_2 laser resurfacing, delayed-onset, permanent hypopigmentation seems an extremely uncommon complication of fractional laser skin resurfacing. To date, there is one reported case involving transient hypopigmentation 15 days after treatment, attributed to the prophylactic use of topical tretinoin and hydroquinone, which resolved after discontinuation of these medications.[37] Because hypopigmentation can occur several months after treatment, there remains a need for close long-term follow-up to evaluate its occurrence. However, these devices have been in use for more than 4 years, and even long-term complications would be expected to have surfaced by now.

Scarring

Hypertrophic scarring has been reported as an adverse effect of traditional rejuvenating devices, but there have been several recent reports of scarring being associated with fractionated devices. Both vertical and horizontal hypertrophic bands have been described on the neck.[27] These are all likely related to technical problems with excessive and repeated stamping or scanning in the same area. The skin is surprisingly resilient, even at higher densities if the treated zones are allowed to cool down between passes. Despite this, the use of excessively high-energy densities in underprivileged areas, such as the neck, chest, or any other area with fewer adnexal structures, may be associated with complications. If these areas become infected, scarring may occur.[38] Other scar-prone anatomic locations that also require more conservative treatment protocols include the periorbital and mandibular regions. Early treatment of hypertrophic scarring consists of the use of topical corticosteroids or silicone gel products, intralesional corticosteroid injections, and PDL therapy.[39] Counterintuitively, the same laser that might have induced scarring could be used to improve the scarring. Ample evidence exists to support the use of either nonablative or ablative fractionated devices at low energies and low densities in the treatment of scarring.

Although other complications of FP devices, such as ectropion,[27] eruptive keratoacanthomas,[40,41]

heat recall phenomena,[42] delayed pinpoint purpura,[43] and cold-induced urticaria, have all been seen, the side effect profile of fractional photothermolysis is considerably less than those experienced with CO_2 and Er:YAG resurfacing. Although further long-term studies are warranted in this regard, the early results seem promising.

SUMMARY

The development of fractional photothermolysis is a milestone in the history of laser technology and cutaneous resurfacing. The fractionated laser is a novel concept that produces only a focal destruction of skin, in which undamaged surrounding regions can rapidly participate in wound healing. The science, although still in its infancy, has already shown clear efficacy in the treatment of skin surface and textural abnormalities, scarring, rhytids, laxity, and numerous other conditions. Although adverse reactions seem minimal to date, the prepared clinician is still most likely to yield the fewest complications. With the increase in popularity of this procedure, there will continue to be an influx of new devices to the market. Any new technology needs to be studied carefully before it becomes generally adopted. Conversely, any new device that works can generally be manipulated to improve its efficacy by a factor of 10. Continued scientific scrutiny by the academic community and use of new parameters are guaranteed to result in better outcomes for patients. It is fascinating that fractionation began with nonablative devices and evolved into the ablative wavelengths, and yet nonablative is still preferred for certain conditions. Fractional photothermolysis has so far withstood the test of time, and we consider it inevitable that this same technology will soon be available as a home-use device.

REFERENCES

1. Manstein D, Herron GS, Sink RK, et al. Fractional photothermolysis: a new concept for cutaneous remodeling using microscopic patterns of thermal injury. Lasers Surg Med 2004;34:426–38.
2. Gold MH. Update on fractional laser technology. J Clin Aesthet Dermatol 2010;3(1):42–50.
3. Geronemus R. Fractional photothermolysis: current and future applications. Lasers Surg Med 2006;38:169–76.
4. Jih MH, Kimyai-Asadi A. Fractional photothermolysis: a review and update. Semin Cutan Med Surg 2008;27(1):63–71.
5. Hantash BM, Bedi VP, Kapadia B, et al. In vivo histological evaluation of a novel ablative fractional resurfacing device. Lasers Surg Med 2007;39(2):96–107.

6. Hantash BM, Bedi VP, Sudireddy V, et al. Laser-induced transepidermal elimination of dermal content by fractional photothermolysis. J Biomed Opt 2006;11:041115.

7. Weiss RA, Gold MH, Bene N, et al. Prospective clinical evaluation of 1440-nm laser delivered by microarray for treatment of photoaging and scars. J Drugs Dermatol 2006;5(8):740–4.

8. Berlin AL, Hussain M, Phelps R, et al. A prospective study of fractional scanned nonsequential carbon dioxide laser resurfacing: a clinical and histopathologic evaluation. Dermatol Surg 2009;35(2):222–8.

9. Ortiz A, Tremaine AM, Zachary CB. Long term efficacy of a fractional resurfacing device. Abstract presented at American Society for Laser Medicine and Surgery Conference. National Harbor (MD), April 1–5, 2009.

10. Jih MH, Goldberg LH, Kimyai-Asadi A. Fractional photothermolysis for photoaging of hands. Dermatol Surg 2008;34:73–8.

11. Behroozan DS, Goldberg LH, Glaich AS, et al. Fractional photothermolysis for treatment of poikiloderma of Civatte. Dermatol Surg 2006;32:298–301.

12. Rahman Z, Alam M, Dover JS. Fractional laser treatment for pigmentation and texture improvement. Skin Therapy Lett 2006;11:7–11.

13. Alster TS, Tanzi EL, Lazarus M. The use of fractional laser photothermolysis for the treatment of atrophic scars. Dermatol Surg 2007;33:295–9.

14. Walgrave SE, Ortiz AE, MacFalls HT, et al. Evaluation of a novel fractional resurfacing device for treatment of acne scarring. Lasers Surg Med 2009;41(2):122–7.

15. Tierney EP, Kouba DJ, Hanke W. Review of fractional photothermolysis: treatment indications and efficacy. Dermatol Surg 2009;35:1445–61.

16. Lee HS, Lee JH, Ahn GY, et al. Fractional photothermolysis for the treatment of acne scars: a report of 27 Korean patients. J Dermatolog Treat 2008;19:45–9.

17. Glaich AS, Goldberg LH, Friedman RH, et al. Fractional photothermolysis for the treatment of postinflammatory erythema resulting from acne vulgaris. Dermatol Surg 2007;33:842–6.

18. Glaich AS, Rahman Z, Goldberg LH, et al. Fractional resurfacing for the treatment of hypopigmented scars: a pilot study. Dermatol Surg 2007;33:289–94.

19. Tierney E, Mahmoud B, Srivastava D, et al. Treatment of surgical scars with fractional photothermolysis versus pulse dye laser: randomized control trial. Dermatol Surg 2009;35:1172–80.

20. Rokhsar CK, Fitzpatrick RE. The treatment of melasma with fractional photothermolysis: a pilot study. Dermatol Surg 2005;31:1645–50.

21. Goldberg DJ, Berlin AL, Phelps R. Histologic and ultrastructural analysis of melasma after fractional resurfacing. Lasers Surg Med 2008;40:134–8.

22. Blankenship TM, Alster TS. Fractional photothermolysis of residual hemangioma. Dermatol Surg 2008;34:1112–4.

23. Izikson L, Anderson RR. Resolution of blue minocycline pigmentation of the face after fractional photothermolysis. Lasers Surg Med 2008;40:399–401.

24. Karsai S, Hammes S, Rutten A, et al. Fractional photothermolysis for the treatment of granuloma annulare: a case report. Lasers Surg Med 2008;40:319–22.

25. Chrastil B, Glaich AS, Goldberg LH, et al. Fractional photothermolysis: a novel treatment for disseminated superficial actinic porokeratosis. Arch Dermatol 2007;143:1450–2.

26. Marra DE, Pourrabbani S, Fincher EF, et al. Fractional photothermolysis for the treatment of adult colloid milium. Arch Dermatol 2007;143:572–4.

27. Fife DJ, Fitzpatrick RE, Zachary CB. Complications of fractional CO_2 laser resurfacing: four cases. Lasers Surg Med 2009;41:179–84.

28. Graber EM, Tanzi EL, Alster TS. Side effects and complications of fractional laser photothermolysis: experience with 961 treatments. Dermatol Surg 2008;34:301–5.

29. Setyadi HG, Jacobs AA, Markus RF. Infectious complications after nonablative fractional resurfacing treatment. Dermatol Surg 2008;34:1595–8.

30. Nanni CA, Alster TS. Complications of carbon dioxide laser resurfacing. An evaluation of 500 patients. Dermatol Surg 1998;24:315–20.

31. Metelitsa AI, Alster T. Fractionated laser skin resurfacing treatment complications: a review. Dermatol Surg 2010;36(3):299–306.

32. Palm MD, Butterwick KJ, Goldman MP. *Mycobacterium chelonae* infection after fractionated carbon dioxide facial resurfacing (presenting as an atypical acneiform eruption): case report and literature review. Dermatol Surg 2010;36(9):1473–81.

33. Tanzi EL, Wanitphakdeedecha R, Alster TS. Fraxel laser indications and long-term follow-up. Aesthet Surg J 2008;28:675–8.

34. Fisher GH, Geronemus RG. Short-term side effects of fractional photothermolysis. Dermatol Surg 2005;31:1245–9.

35. Rahman Z, MacFalls H, Jiang K, et al. Fractional deep dermal ablation induces tissue tightening. Lasers Surg Med 2009;41:78–86.

36. Chan HH, Manstein D, Yu CS, et al. The prevalence and risk factors of post-inflammatory hyperpigmentation after fractional resurfacing in Asians. Lasers Surg Med 2007;39:381–5.

37. Tan KL, Kurniawati C, Gold MH. Low risk of post-inflammatory hyperpigmentation in skin types 4 and 5 after treatment with fractional CO_2 laser device. J Drugs Dermatol 2008;7:774–7.

38. Goldman MP, Fitzpatrick RE, Manuskiatti W. Laser resurfacing of the neck with the erbium:YAG laser. Dermatol Surg 1999;25:164–7.

39. Alster T, Zaulyanov L. Laser scar revision: a review. Dermatol Surg 2007;33:131–40.

40. Gewirtzman A, Meirson DH, Rabinovitz H. Eruptive keratoacanthomas following carbon dioxide laser resurfacing. Dermatol Surg 1999;25:666–8.

41. Mamelak AJ, Goldberg LH, Marquez D, et al. Eruptive keratoacanthomas on the legs after fractional photothermolysis: report of two cases. Dermatol Surg 2009;35:513–8.

42. Foster KW, Fincher EF, Moy RL. Heat-induced "recall" of treatment zone erythema following fractional resurfacing with a combination laser (1320 nm/1440 nm). Arch Dermatol 2008;144:1398–9.

43. Fife DJ, Zachary CB. Delayed pinpoint purpura after fractionated carbon dioxide treatment in a patient taking ibuprofen in the postoperative period. Dermatol Surg 2009;35:553.

Laser, Light, and Energy Devices for Cellulite and Lipodystrophy

Jennifer D. Peterson, MD*, Mitchel P. Goldman, MD

KEYWORDS

• Cellulite • Radiofrequency • Laser • Energy devices

KEY POINTS

1. Cellulite is a difficult to treat and nearly unpreventable anatomic state with multifactorial exacerbating factors. It affects primarily women on the lateral thighs and buttocks.
2. Multiple devices using radiofrequency (RF), laser, and light-based energies, alone or in combination and coupled frequently with tissue manipulation, are currently used for the improvement of cellulite.
3. Patients who wish to lessen cellulite may combine treatments with other procedures, such as liposuction. Results with devices alone are usually moderate in benefit and are short lived; therefore, frequent touch-up treatments may be required.
4. Patients should understand that these energy devices are not without risk; adverse events such as bruising, pain, and hyperpigmentation are more common, but blistering and even scarring are infrequent but possible adverse effects.

Historically a sign of beauty and wealth, the presence of cellulite is now considered aesthetically objectionable. The term cellulite is used in modern times to describe the dimpled or puckered skin of the posterior and lateral thighs and buttocks seen in many trim and overweight women. The appearance is often described to resemble the surface of an orange peel or that of cottage cheese. It affects all races, and it is estimated that 85% of women older than 20 years have some degree of cellulite.[1] Cellulite is known medically as liposclerosis, gynoid dystrophy, edematofibrosclerosis, or dermopanniculitis.[2] Goldman[3] describes cellulite as a normal physiologic state in postadolescent women that serves to ensure adequate caloric availability for pregnancy and lactation by maximizing adipose deposits. Adipose tissue is also essential for nutrition, energy, support, protection, and thermal insulation.[4]

PREDISPOSING FACTORS

There are many predisposing factors that contribute to cellulite:

1. Gender: due to the underlying structure of fat and connective tissue, described later, women are more likely to develop cellulite
2. Heredity: the degree and presence of cellulite, as with body habitus, is often similar between women within the same family
3. Race: cellulite is more common in White women than Asian or African American women[5]
4. Increased subcutaneous fat: due to the unique histology of cellulite-affected skin, more adipose tissue in the subcutaneous layer enhances the appearance of cellulite on the skin surface[6]

Dr Peterson has no disclosures.
Dr Goldman has conducted research trials for Cynosure, Eleme, Syneron, CoolTouch, and Deka.
Goldman, Butterwick, and Associates Cosmetic Laser Dermatology, 9339 Genesee Avenue, Suite 300, San Diego, CA 92121, USA
* Corresponding author.
E-mail address: Jdd4920@hotmail.com

Clin Plastic Surg 38 (2011) 463–474
doi:10.1016/j.cps.2011.02.003
0094-1298/11/$ – see front matter © 2011 Elsevier Inc. All rights reserved.

5. Age: after puberty, women begin to develop cellulite as a part of normal anatomic and physiologic development. With advancing age, cellulite increases in severity as a reflection of thinning of the epidermis.

Unfortunately, these predisposing factors are difficult if not impossible to alter, thus cellulite prevention is not attainable at present.

HISTOLOGY

Histologically, cellulite is the result of localized adipose deposits and edema within the subcutaneous tissue. In women, fascial bands of connective tissue are oriented longitudinally and extend from the dermis to the deep fascia. These bands form fibrous septa that segregate fat into channels resembling a down quilt or mattress, and the subcutaneous fat is projected superficially into the reticular and papillary dermis. As the fat layer expands, the perpendicular connective tissue remains fixed and anchored to the underlying tissue, creating a superficial puckered appearance of the skin.[4,7,8] Ultrasonographic studies of cellulite have shown the striking feature of herniation of the subcutaneous fat into the reticular and papillary dermis (**Fig. 1**).[9]

It is thought that fatty acids are modified through peroxidation by free radicals. These events are hypothesized to contribute to the worsening of local microcirculation by disrupting venous and lymphatic drainage. This skin phenomenon is rarely found in men because the connective tissue in men is not normally arranged vertically but in a crisscross pattern that is gender typical for the skin of the thighs and buttocks (**Fig. 2**).[4,7]

PATHOPHYSIOLOGIC MECHANISMS OF CELLULITE

The pathophysiology of cellulite is multifactorial. Adipose tissue is vascular, leading to the theory that cellulite may worsen in predisposed areas where circulation and lymphatic drainage have been decreased, possibly because of local injury or inflammation. Under normal conditions, fat cells are embedded in a network of reticular fibers. In cellulite, interstitial edema results from an increased permeability in the local microvasculature. As a result, a chronic inflammatory process ensues around the reticular fiber network. Subsequently, the reticular fibers increase in number (hyperplasia) and thickness (hypertrophy), worsening the compromised microcirculation,[3] which is evident clinically as the classic orange peel appearance of overlying skin and as reduced blood perfusion.

The formation of cellulite is also under hormonal influence. Estrogen is known to stimulate

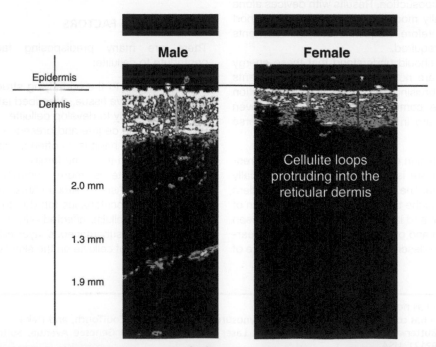

Fig. 1. High-resolution ultrasonographic images of subcutaneous fat in men and women. Note that the fat herniations into the dermis for the female are absent in the male. (*Courtesy of* Drs Agustina Vila Echague and Avram; and *reproduced from* Goldman MP, Hexsel D, editors. Cellulite: pathophysiology and treatment. 2nd edition. New York: Informa Healthcare; 2010. p. 28; with permission.)

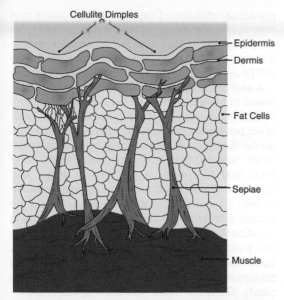

Cellulite Dimples

Epidermis

Dermis

Fat Cells

Sepiae

Muscle

Fig. 2. The organization of the adipocytes between the fibrous septa (in a crisscross pattern) results in the dimpling of the skin, a characteristic of cellulite. (*Reproduced from* Goldman MP, Hexsel D, editors. Cellulite: pathophysiology and treatment. 2nd edition. New York: Informa Healthcare; 2010. p. 25.)

lipogenesis and inhibit lipolysis, resulting in adipocyte hypertrophy. This hormonal function may explain the onset of cellulite at puberty, the condition being more prevalent in women, and the exacerbation of cellulite with pregnancy, nursing, menstruation, and estrogen therapy (oral contraceptive use and hormone replacement).[10] The opposite seems true for men. Although there are a limited number of studies involving men, it is hypothesized that the combination of gender-specific soft tissue histology at the cellulite-prone anatomic sites, with a relatively lower circulating estrogen level, may be responsible for the lower incidence of cellulite in men.[3,4] Although not proven, it is possible that circulating androgens may have an inhibitory effect on cellulite development by contributing to a different pattern of adipose tissue storage (ie, more truncal than on the buttocks and thighs).

CLASSIFICATION

Nurnberger and Muller developed a classification system for grading cellulite severity. For this method, the physician accentuates cellulite dimpling by gently pinching an area of tissue between the fingers and the thumb. For larger areas, the skin of the thigh can be compressed between 2 hands. This technique is referred to as the mattress phenomenon because the dimpled

pinched skin resembles a bed mattress. Cellulite may be graded for severity on a scale of I to IV (**Box 1**).[3,5,6]

ENERGY-BASED TREATMENT: OVERVIEW

Many currently accepted cellulite therapies target deficiencies in lymphatic drainage and microvascular circulation. Based on the understanding of the cause and nature of this condition, several treatment modalities have been developed and can be divided into 5 main categories: attenuation of aggravating factors, physical and mechanical methods, pharmacologic agents, RF energy, and laser energy.[5] Treatments such as application of topical creams and lotions, ultrasound, electrolipolysis, iontophoresis, and mesotherapy have all been tried; although these treatments are effective for temporary, mild improvement,[11] none have been proven to provide long-term resolution of cellulite.[2] The following sections describe the development of multiple devices using RF, laser, and light-based energies, alone or in combination and coupled frequently with tissue manipulation, for the improvement of cellulite. Two other technologies, an externally applied low-level laser (Zerona, Erchonia, McKinney, TX, USA), which is US Food and Drug Administration (FDA) cleared for noninvasive body contouring, and a unipolar RF device (Thermage™ Solta Medical, Hayward, CA, USA), which is FDA cleared for the temporary improvement in the appearance of cellulite, are

---

Box 1
Nurnberger-Muller cellulite classification scale

Grade I

No or minimal cellulite based on observation when standing, the pinch test, or gluteal muscle contraction

Grade II

Irregular skin topography on observation. Cellulite is enhanced by pinching or gluteal contraction. Subjects may have skin pallor or decreased temperature and sensation

Grade III

Skin exhibits the classic orange peel dimpling, peau d'orange, at rest. Small subcutaneous nodularities may be palpated

Grade IV

In addition to the characteristics described in grades I to III, there is more severe puckering and palpable nodules

discussed elsewhere in this issue and will not be discussed further in this article. Laser-assisted liposuction for the improvement of cellulite is also reviewed later.

TriActive

TriActive (Cynosure, Inc, Westford, MA, USA) has the capability to treat cellulite and postliposuction fibrosis with a tri-fold treatment approach using diode laser, contact cooling, and massage to work synergistically to restore the body's normal homeostatic environment. The TriActive laser energy is emitted through six 808-nm diode lasers to target the endothelial cells to enhance arterial, venous, and lymphatic flow and promote neovascularization. The contact cooling system can manually be adjusted from 10°C to 25°C and it aids in decreasing edema by causing an initial vasoconstriction followed by a compensatory vasodilatation allowing for the pooled fluid to remobilize. The rhythmic massage, which can be selected as either single or dual phase, counteracts circulatory stasis, thereby mobilizing fluids by stimulating lymphatic drainage. In addition, the massage stretches the connective tissue, thus smoothing the interface between the dermis and epidermis.

The parameters of the TriActive system can be manipulated to optimize patient results. The depth and intensity of the rhythmic massage can be controlled by the frequency (0.1–5.0 Hz) and duty cycle (20%–80%). The frequency (hertz) measures the number of aspirations per second. At higher frequencies, a superficial mechanical action is achieved, whereas lower repetition rates stimulate deeper tissue. The duty cycle is the percentage of time for which the aspiration is active between one aspiration and the next. For example, a duty cycle of 70% indicates that the aspiration is active 70% of the time between the 2 aspirations. The higher the value, the stronger the action. Thus, by manipulating the duty cycle and frequency, the intensity and depth of the message can be increased or decreased.

For Fitzpatrick skin types I through III, it is recommend to start at 30 W and then adjusting for patient discomfort and erythema. The frequency should initially be set at 3 Hz with a duty cycle of 60%; the former may be increased to 4 or 5 Hz, but the latter needs to be decreased to 50%. The dual mode is advised for the massage setting. When treating darker skin types, Fitzpatrick skin types IV through VI, energy should be adjusted down to an initial fluence of 20 W. The fluence should be adjusted based on patient discomfort and the level of erythema. The

previously mentioned repetition rates (hertz) and duty cycles can be used for skin types I to III. No matter what the skin type is, the contact cooling function should be on and set at the coolest level (10°C) and can be adjusted during the treatment.

A seal of the applicator should always be chambered to the skin; when air is heard to be sucked into the chamber, it indicates that the applicator is not positioned properly for ideal vacuum suction on the skin. Five minutes should be spent on each major surface, that is, the posterior thigh, outer thigh and hip, inner thigh, anterior thigh, and buttocks. Each treatment should last approximately 30 minutes, and each zone should be treated with 3 to 5 passes, with the end point being significant erythema and warmth radiating from the treated skin. The TriActive device has also been used before, during, and after other surgical procedures including liposuction and abdominoplasty. Goldman[12] has noted a marked improvement in irregularities when TriActive is performed after liposculpture. This improvement may be because of the redistribution of dystrophic adipose cells.

The experimental studies in Europe regarding the efficacy of TriActive were conducted by Zerbinati,[13] in which 10 patients were enrolled and each was treated with 20-minute sessions 3 times a week. To evaluate the efficacy of the technique, all the patients were requested not to change habits such as diet, physical activity, and lifestyle in general. Clinical observation, circumference of the thighs and hips, plicometry, skin elasticity, and thermography were recorded. All patients noted an increase in skin tone and a reduction in the circumference of the areas treated.[13]

A similar study to those presented earlier to evaluate the efficacy of the TriActive system without the lymphatic drainage protocol confirmed the importance of lymphatic drainage. A total of 13 healthy women aged 19 to 51 years, with a mean age of 36.6 years and a mean body mass index of 22.26 (19.2–29.3; calculated as the weight in kilograms divided by height in meters squared), were included in the study. Mean starting percentage body fat of the subjects was 22.18% (16.46%–31.02%). Subjects underwent biweekly treatments for 6 weeks. Treatments were administered locally only on the hips and thighs. Efficacy was measured via waist, hip, and thigh circumferences; elasticity; and thermography. Analysis of the results included a subjective evaluation of pretreatment and posttreatment photos by 5 blinded evaluators. An overall improvement of 21% was noted among the treated patients. The most notable improvement was in the appearance of cellulite (23%), skin texture (16%), size (15%), and skin tone (14%). The results of thermography evaluated in this study showed neither changes of mean temperature nor variations in uniformity of temperature distribution in the treated areas. The results revealed a trend toward modest improvement, with steady improvements in hip and thigh circumferences. Comparison to pre-treatment photos also suggests modest improvements in the appearance of cellulite and overall appearance, with those subjects starting with the least symptoms showing the greatest degree of improvement. Comparing these results to those of the previous studies suggests the importance of considering the entire system and method as a whole concept to be diligently performed for maximizing results.[14]

Gold[15] evaluated TriActive on 10 women with cellulite who were treated with 15 biweekly sessions. Of the 10 subjects, 9 completed the study and the 1-month follow-up period. There were no significant changes in the subject's weight. An approximate 50% improvement in the visual grading scale was noted in 80% of subjects.

Nootheti and colleagues[16] performed the first comparative study to determine the relative efficacy of treatment of cellulite using 2 novel modalities, TriActive and VelaSmooth (Syneron Medical Ltd, Yokneam Illit, Israel). VelaSmooth is based on a combination of 2 different ranges of electromagnetic energy, which produces heat, infrared (IR) light and RF combined with mechanical manipulation of the skin and it also has been demonstrated to improve the appearance of cellulite (see later discussion). Patients were treated twice a week for 6 weeks, with randomization of TriActive on one side and VelaSmooth on the other side. A total of 12 treatments per leg were performed. Cellulite grading was determined using the 4-stage Nurnberger-Muller scale, and measurements of thigh circumference were taken before treatment and after the final treatment. Visual inspection and photographic grading were quantified and statistically examined.

In comparing efficacy of treatment between VelaSmooth and TriActive, 28% versus 30% improvement was calculated in the upper-thigh circumference measurements, whereas 56% versus 37% improvement was observed in the lower-thigh circumference measurements. These differences in treatment efficacy, based on the thigh circumference measurements, were not found to be significant ($P > .05$). Based on before and after blinded photographic evaluation, 25% (19 of 20) of the subjects showed improvement in cellulite appearance for both TriActive and VelaSmooth. Based on random photographic

grading from a scale of 1 to 5 (1, no improvement; 5, most improvement), the average percentages of improvement for VelaSmooth and TriActive are 7% and 25%, respectively. This difference was also not found to be significant ($P = .091$). Perceived change grade was also calculated based on random side-by-side comparisons of before and after photographs. About 75% (15 of 19) subjects showed improvement in the VelaSmooth-treated leg, whereas 55% (11 of 19) showed improvement in the TriActive-treated leg. The average mean percentage of improvement was roughly the same for both the treatments (22% [VelaSmooth] and 20% [TriActive]) and showed no statistically significant difference ($P > .05$).

Bruising was reported in 60% of the subjects. Incidence and intensity of bruising was 30% higher in the VelaSmooth-treated leg than in the TriActive-treated leg. Of the 20 subjects, 7 reported bruising with VelaSmooth, 1 reported bruising with TriActive, and 3 reported bruising with both VelaSmooth and TriActive. Extent of bruising ranged from minor purpura to larger and diffused bruises, which lasted for a week on average with no intervention. This study revealed that both treatments effectively reduced the appearance of cellulite; however, with a P value of .05, no statistically significant difference was observed between TriActive and VelaSmooth in the reduction of cellulite. TriActive provides low-energy diode laser, contact cooling, suction, and massage, whereas VelaSmooth provides a combination of 2 different ranges of electromagnetic energy, IR light and RF, combined with mechanical manipulation of the skin. After a biweekly treatment for 6 weeks, there was no statistical significance between the 2 units in the upper- or lower-thigh circumference measurements, randomized photographic evaluations, or perceived change in before and after photographic evaluations.[16]

VelaSmooth

VelaSmooth is based on a combination of 2 different ranges of electromagnetic energy, which produces heat, IR light and RF, known as ELOS (Syneron Medical Ltd, Yokneam Illit, Israel). VelaSmooth is a device that combines controlled IR light (700–2000 nm, in the most current model) and conducted bipolar RF energies with mechanical manipulation of the skin to improve the appearance of cellulite.[17–19] In the most current model, the VelaSmooth peak optical energy is 35 W and the peak RF energy is 60 W. Prior models had a peak optical energy of 12.5 to 20 W and a peak RF energy of 20 to 50 W.

By combining RF energy with optical energy, the required amount of optical energy may be reduced. As a result, most skin types can be successfully treated because RF does not target melanin, and therefore, epidermal heating is reduced. Manipulation is provided via vacuum suction and mechanical rollers in a 40 × 40-mm applicator head.

Before initiating treatment, the skin should be cleaned. Conductive lotion is applied to the treatment area, gel should never be used. Once rehydrated, the skin does not need constant reapplication of conductive lotion even if it appears dry, the electrode rollers remain coupled to the skin as long as proper pressure and contact is made by the operator. However, additional lotion should be applied during treatment if it becomes difficult to move the applicator across the treatment area. Proper applicator seal to the skin surface is indicated by the lack of hearing air being sucked into the chamber in addition to a non-flashing light indicator on the applicator. For the effective and safe delivery of RF energy, it is ensured that the RF rollers maintain equal compression and contact with the skin surface.

Each treatment area (ie, posterior thigh, anterior thigh, inner thigh, outer thigh and hip, buttocks) should be treated for 5 minutes with 3 to 6 passes of the VelaSmooth applicator. The targeted end point is significant erythema and warmth (40°C–42°C, which is maintained for 5–10 minutes) in the treatment area. The time for each treatment session is approximately 20 to 30 minutes per side of the body. With the most current model of VelaSmooth, the manufacturer recommends treatments once a week for 4 to 6 weeks; however, most studies have been performed using earlier, less-powerful models and included biweekly treatments for 4 weeks.[17–20]

All 3 parameters on this device can be independently adjusted to tailor treatment to each patient's needs. The treatment levels on all 3 components range from 1 to 3. To maximize the effectiveness of the device for the treatment of cellulite, areas should be treated with the highest levels of IR light and RF (as tolerated by the patient), with a vacuum level of 1 to 2. However, the following exceptions apply: (1) all treatments levels should never be simultaneously set at maximum parameters; (2) in skin types IV to VI or tanned skin, the IR light should be set to 1 to 2. If the patient does not experience lasting erythema or excessive heat, the level may be increased to 2 to 3 and the skin response should be reevaluated; and (3) to increase the degree of patient comfort in sensitive areas, such as the inner thighs and abdomen, the vacuum can be adjusted to

a level 1 or 2. Adverse events include erythema, pain, edema, bullae formation, scabbing, ecchymoses, postinflammatory hyperpigmentation, and scarring.[17,18,20,21]

A total of 35 female patients with cellulite of the thighs and/or buttocks were treated in a 2-arm, multicenter study by Sadick and Mulholland.[18] The first group (n = 20) received biweekly treatments for 4 weeks, whereas the second group (n = 15) received biweekly treatments for 8 weeks. All patients were treated with maximum tolerance parameters for all energies (RF maximum energy, 20 W and optical maximum energy, 20 W). Two patients developed crusting, which resolved within 3 days. All patients were evaluated on a quartile scale for percentile improvement from baseline to 3 to 4 weeks after the last treatment session. All patients demonstrated some improvement in the appearance of cellulite. However, patients treated with 16 treatments achieved higher levels of physician-graded improvement, corresponding to a 50% to 75% or 75% to 100% improvement.

Alster and Tanzi[17] investigated 20 patients with moderate thigh and buttock cellulite using biweekly VelaSmooth (20 W RF, 20 W IR) treatments for 4 weeks. This study was conducted in a randomized, split-leg manner, with the untreated leg serving as the control. Physician-graded improvement was based on a quartile scale, similar to the study by Sadick and Mulholland. About 10% of patients experienced ecchymoses, and 90% experienced improvement in the appearance of cellulite on the treated leg, with a mean improvement of nearly 50% at 1 month after the last treatment. All but one of these subjects were interested in receiving treatments to the control leg. Of note, at 3 and 6 months after the last treatment, the physician-graded improvement scale decreased to approximately 35% and 25%, respectively.

Sixteen patients were treated with biweekly treatments for thigh cellulite for 4 weeks in a study by Kulick.[20] All patients were treated with maximal machine parameters, using a RF energy of 20 W and an optical energy of 12.5 W. All patients were followed up for 6 months after their last treatment. Transient erythema occurred after treatment in all patients. Bruising occurred in 32.25% of subjects, but resolved within a week. A single patient sustained a second-degree burn. At 3 and 6 months after the last treatment, the mean investigator-graded improvement scores were 62% and 50%, respectively. At both time points, all patients graded their cellulite improvement to be more than 25%.

In a study by Boey,[21] 17 women received VelaSmooth (using the earlier low-energy model) treatments for mild to moderate cellulite on the thighs, buttocks, and abdomen. The mean investigator-graded improvement from baseline was 32.9%, whereas the mean subject-graded improvement from baseline was 30.6%. Follow-up times and a description of the treatment regimen were not provided. Bruising was reported in 58.8% of patients, but no crusting was reported. Most patients experienced temporary erythema and edema.

In a study by Sadick and Magro,[19] 20 patients with thigh and buttock cellulite were randomized to receive 12 biweekly VelaSmooth treatments in a split-leg fashion. Of the 16 patients who completed the study, 31.25% experienced bruising at some point during the study. At 4 and 8 weeks after the last treatment, as graded by the investigator's quartile-based scale, 50% (at both time points) of subjects and by an independent investigator-evaluated quartile-based scale, 50% and 68.75% (respectively) of subjects had more than 25% improvement in the appearance of cellulite in the treated leg. At 8 weeks' follow-up, 31.25% of patients had more than 51% improvement in the appearance of cellulite in the treated leg as graded by the independent investigator.

Similar, split-anatomic controlled studies with the 20 W RF and 20 W IR VelaSmooth have continued to show improvement in the appearance of cellulite as rated by investigator[22,23] and subject-based[22] grading scales. Many investigators have recommended monthly maintenance treatments to help sustain the clinical improvements.[17,22]

VelaShape

VelaShape (Syneron Medical Ltd, Yokneam Illit, Israel) is an FDA-cleared device for the noninvasive temporary circumferential reduction in thigh size and temporary cellulite reduction, based on the same combination of bipolar RF, IR light (700–2000 nm), vacuum, and mechanical tissue manipulation as the original VelaSmooth device. Vela-Shape combines the previous VelaSmooth treatment head along with a smaller (30 × 30 mm) treatment head, the VelaContour (Syneron Medical Ltd, Yokneam Illit, Israel).

VelaShape II is a newer version of the original VelaShape, with 20% more power allowing for shorter treatment sessions, as well as an improved interface terminal to optimize treatments and facilitate device maintenance. The applicator heads have different energy and vacuum parameters. On the VelaShape II platform, the VelaContour is able to achieve up to 440 mbar negative pressure,

20 W peak IR energy, and 23 W peak RF energy, whereas VelaSmooth is able to achieve up to 380 mbar negative pressure, 35 W IR energy, and 60 W RF energy. Instructions for the use of VelaShape are similar to those listed in the previous section. Additional instructions for Vela-Shape are as follows: large areas (such as the waist, hips, and thighs) are treated with the VelaSmooth applicator for most of the treatment session. In curved small areas, such as the lower abdomen and the periumbilical area, and/or over local fatty deposits, the VelaContour applicator is used instead. The VelaContour treatment is identical to that of VelaSmooth; however, a 20% overlap is recommended with VelaContour. With the new higher-energy VelaShape II, treatments are delivered at weekly intervals (VelaShape II User Manual, 2009). Clinical studies with these newer devices are presently underway. In the authors' office, they have noted a significant improvement over the use of VelaSmooth.

SmoothShapes

SmoothShapes (Eleme Medical, Inc, Merrimack, NH, USA) is an FDA-cleared device for the temporary improvement in the appearance of cellulite that involves the application of dual wavelengths of laser energy (650 and 915 nm) along with vacuum and massage.

Neira and colleagues[24] investigated the effects of low-level laser energy on adipose tissue. This group demonstrated when adipocytes were exposed to a 635-nm wavelength, a transitory pore was produced within the adipocyte membrane, releasing fat into the intracellular space. Pore formation in the adipocyte membrane was repeated in another controlled study.[25] As a result, the 650-nm wavelength was chosen for its action in enhancing adipocyte membrane permeability and fat emulsification. Of note, the 650-nm wavelength is absorbed minimally in the epidermis and dermis, which allows for enhanced penetration to the subcutaneous tissue. The 915-nm wavelength scatters less than the 650-nm wavelength and is preferentially absorbed by the lipids in fat cells. A temperature increase within the adipocytes results in fat liquefaction. Both the wavelengths are reported to stimulate neocollagenesis and improve blood and lymphatic circulation. Tissue manipulation, using vacuum and massage, enhances the transfer of the liquefied fat within the adipocytes into the intracellular spaces along with improving circulation of blood and lymphatic fluid.

The most current SmoothShapes treatment head (also known as the Photomology module) consists of 2 rollers, a vacuum chamber, four

650-nm light-emitting diodes (LEDs) (1 W), and eight 915-nm laser diodes (15 W) in a 90 × 90 mm dimension. Prior models delivered maximum energies of 1 W from the 650-nm LED and 10 W from the 915-nm diodes. Subcutaneous tissue up to 10 mm depth is heated via the dual laser energy with surface temperatures remaining less than 40°C.

Ecchymoses, erythema, edema, pain, burn, abrasions, scaling, infection, dyspigmentation, and scarring are potential adverse effects from SmoothShapes.

The suction level is recommended not to exceed 500 mbar (375 mm Hg). When initiating treatment, the treatment head is placed on the skin surface and then moved across the treatment area. Each treatment area (eg, posterior, lateral, and anterior thighs) is approximately 8.5 × 11 in. The duration of each treatment area can be selected with a maximum treatment time of 30 minutes, with a default time of 10 minutes (SmoothShapes XV User Manual, 2010).

To date, most SmoothShapes clinical trials have investigated the volumetric effects of Smooth-Shapes in patients with cellulite, as graded by circumferential reduction and magnetic resonance imaging (MRI), but not the improvement in the appearance of cellulite itself.[26–28] In the study by Lach,[26] 88.9% of subjects who completed the study reported they were "somewhat" or "definitely" pleased with the results of their treatment. In an abstract presented by Fournier and colleagues,[29] 8 to 12 biweekly treatments were performed using the 915-nm (10 W) and 650-nm (1 W) SmoothShapes device to evaluate the effects on cellulite. Thirty female patients, with Fitzpatrick skin types I to V and with mild to moderate cellulite of the thighs were enrolled in this split-leg study, using the untreated leg as the control. The group reported that a high level of patient satisfaction was achieved.

SmoothShapes was performed on 20 women, with skin types II to VI and with mild to moderate lateral thigh cellulite in a study by Kulick.[30] Patients received biweekly treatments for 4 weeks, with the application of Photomology treatment head for 15 minutes per lateral thigh. Energy was delivered at the maximum settings (1 W for 650 nm, 10 W for 915 nm). Photographic evaluations were performed with standard digital photography and 3-dimensional digital photography at baseline and 1, 3, and 6 months after the final treatment. Textural images for all patients were developed from the 3-dimensional digital photography computer database.[30]

Improved resolution of textural changes was reported with the 3-dimensional digital photography

system. Physician-rated improvement was seen in 82% of subjects at 1 month and in 76% at both 3 and 6 months posttreatment. Seventeen patients completed the study, and no adverse events were reported. Textural images showed elevations of depressed areas and reduction of surface bulges. Computer-generated volumetric analysis demonstrated a decrease in thigh volume. At 6 months after the final treatment, 94% of subjects reported sustained improvement in the appearance of cellulite. Percentile improvements based on quartile scales or a similar grading system were not evaluated.[30] Further studies evaluating the clinical appearance of cellulite are necessitated.

Accent

The Accent XL (Alma Lasers Ltd, Caesarea, Israel) platform consists of 2 treatment heads, one using unipolar RF and the other bipolar RF, which is FDA-cleared for the treatment of wrinkles and rhytides. As compared with bipolar RF, unipolar RF is able to affect deeper structures (up to 15–20 mm).[31–33] The Accent XL UniPolar treatment head emits electromagnetic radiation, and heat is generated through high-frequency (40.68 MHz) oscillations within water molecules. Heat is then subsequently transferred into neighboring tissues.[32,33] Because of the increased depth of penetration, the unipolar treatment head has been investigated for the improvement of the appearance of cellulite.[31,32]

Because of the lack of melanin absorption by RF energy, all skin types can be successfully treated.[33] The Accent XL UniPolar treatment head has an integrated cooled treatment tip to increase patient comfort. The unipolar RF energy is delivered up to 200 W. Before initiation of treatment, mineral oil is applied to the treatment area. The operator moves the handpiece across the treatment (6 × 10 in gridded) area in 30-second passes in a circular fashion. Consecutive passes are applied to the gridded area until the treatment end point (40°C–43°C, measured via IR thermometer) is achieved.[34]

Treatment sessions are performed every other week for up to 3 to 4 months.[34] Transient erythema is common and expected. Crusting, blistering, scarring, dyspigmentation, pain, and ecchymoses are potential adverse events associated with unipolar RF treatment.[31–33]

Alexiades-Armenakas and colleagues[31] assessed 10 female patients with cellulite distributed over the thighs using a novel cellulite grading scale (0–4), which reflected the appearance of contours and dimple depth, density, and distribution. In a randomized split-leg manner, all patients received a mean of 4.22 (range, 3–6) treatments (administered every other week) to the investigational limb, with the untreated leg serving as a control. Unipolar RF energy was emitted at 150 to 200 W per 30-second pass. Photographs were assessed by 2 blinded physicians at each treatment and at 1 and 3 months after the last treatment. At 3 months after the final treatment, dimple density, distribution, and depth improved by 11.25%, 10.75%, and 1.75% to 2.5%, respectively. Overall, an average 7.83% improvement in the appearance of cellulite was reported on the treated leg; however, statistical significance was not obtained. Although most patients demonstrated transient erythema, there were no episodes of scarring, crusting, or dyspigmentation.[31]

A total of 30 patients with moderate to severe thigh cellulite were treated every other week for 3 months with 150 to 170 W of unipolar RF. All areas were treated with 3 passes and 30 seconds per pass. Patients were evaluated 6 months after the final treatment via photography, MRI, estimation of plasma lipid concentrations, and skin biopsy. No changes in plasma lipid levels or blistering, dyspigmentation, or scarring were observed. MRI evaluations at the conclusion of the study failed to reveal a change in the subcutaneous tissue. Fibroplasia of the dermis was noted on histologic examination at 6 months after the final treatment. No changes were present in the subcutaneous tissue on histology. Using standardized digital photography, performed at baseline and 6 months after the final treatment, the mean cellulite improvement was 2.9 (as graded on a 4-point scale). It was concluded that the longevity of results in this study was because of the induction of dermal fibroplasias.[32] Although studies have revealed a good safety profile with unipolar RF, there is a general lack of consensus regarding the efficacy in the improvement of the clinical appearance of cellulite.[31,32]

Exilis

Exilis (BTL Industries, Inc, Prague, Czech Republic), a device that combines monopolar RF and ultrasonic energy, has recently been introduced to the market with an FDA clearance for the noninvasive treatment of wrinkles and rhytides. Animal studies in porcine tissue have demonstrated that a penetration depth of 30 mm is safely obtainable. The Exilis body treatment head has a cooling tip, an integrated IR thermometer for constant temperature monitoring of the skin surface, and an adjustable RF (watt) energy control. Peak monopolar RF energy and ultrasonic energy are 120 W and 3 W/cm^2, respectively. The integrated Energy Flow Control system eliminates peaks of RF energy. A unique feature of this device, as compared with other RF devices, is the sensor monitors for constant contact between the skin surface and applicator. If the treatment head is removed from the skin surface during treatment, arcing, pain, blistering, or a burn will not result.

Anecdotally, this device has been used off-label for improvement in the appearance of cellulite; however, randomized clinical trials are lacking. For the treatment of cellulite, the treatment area is divided into 20 × 10-cm sections. The grounding electrode is placed adjacent to the zone of treatment, and mineral oil is applied to the skin surface within the gridded area. The cooling tip is adjusted to 10°C, and the treatment head is moved continuously in a circular array within the 200-cm^2 grid. The recommended starting RF energy is 50 W and it should be increased over 1 minute until a surface temperature of 40°C to 41°C is reached. Once the target temperature is attained, treatment is continued for an additional 3 minutes to maintain the skin surface at 40°C to 41°C while the RF energy is simultaneously decreased. The average treatment time per grid is 6 minutes, with a total treatment time of 30 minutes per session. Treatments are administered weekly for 3 to 4 weeks. For the following 48 hours after treatment, patients are encouraged to increase their fluid intake, which enhances treatment efficacy by allowing degraded adipose tissue by-products to be eliminated (Exilis User Manual, 2009). Further studies are necessitated to investigate the effects of Exilis on the appearance of cellulite.

TriPollar

TriPollar (Pollogen, Tel Aviv, Israel) combined 3 RF electrodes to deliver low-level (5–30 W) RF energy into the dermis and subcutaneous tissues at a depth of up to 20 mm to produce volumetric heating for immediate collagen contraction and neocollagenesis. The depth of heating is roughly equivalent to the mean difference between the spacing of the RF electrodes. The polarity of the 3 electrodes is in constant alternating rotation between all electrodes (ie, all electrodes have the capability to act as positive or negative, although 1 is always positive and 2 are negative) to avoid overheating of the positive electrode. Cutaneous cooling is not required with this device.[35] As of October, 2010, this product has not received FDA clearance yet.

Before treatment, the skin surface is cleansed and dried. Glycerin oil is applied to the treatment area and then the applicator head is glided across the skin surface in either circular or linear strokes. Erythema and warmth during treatment are expected. Skin temperature should be monitored with an IR thermometer to prevent surface temperatures increasing above 40°C to 42°C, and once the target temperature is obtained,[35] treatment is continued for an additional 2 minutes.[36] Treatments are administered weekly for 6 to 8 weeks, and monthly maintenance treatments are encouraged. Adverse events include erythema (although expected and transient), burns, bruising, and mild discomfort during treatment.[35]

The only cellulite study was performed by Manuskiatti and colleagues[36] on 39 patients with mild to severe cellulite involving the arms, abdomen, buttocks, or thighs. Treatments were administered weekly for 8 treatments using 20.0 to 28.5 W total per treatment. Thirty-seven patients (81 anatomic sites) completed the study. One month after the final treatment session, nearly a 50% mean improvement in the clinical appearance of cellulite, as graded by a blinded investigator, was observed.

Laser-Assisted Lipolysis for the Treatment of Cellulite

Laser-assisted lipolysis (LAL) is indicated for body contouring.[37] Although some physicians use LAL exclusively without liposuction, others think it is best served as an adjunct to liposuction.[38,39] With traditional liposuction, the improvement in appearance of cellulite is modest, and in certain instances, it may exacerbate cellulite.[40] Because of the simultaneous capabilities of LAL to emulsify fat and stimulate neocollagenesis, resulting in skin shrinkage and tightening,[37,38,41–43] it was extrapolated that this technology may have a role in the treatment of cellulite.

Goldman and colleagues[40] investigated a combination approach of laser lipolysis using a pulsed 1064-nm Nd:YAG laser (SmartLipo, Deka, Calenzo, Italy) and autologous fat transplant in 52 women with moderate to severe cellulite of the hips, buttocks, thighs, flanks, and/or abdomen. Fat was manually harvested via syringe aspiration from a site distant to the areas treated with LAL. An average volume of 240 cm³ of centrifuged adipose tissue was then transferred to the depressed areas with a 10% to 15% overcorrection. Ecchymoses and edema were common, but no burns or infections occurred. At 1 year posttreatment, patient evaluation of improvement was greater than 75% in 30.8% of patients and 51% to 75% in 53.8% of patients. Although patient satisfaction was high, the isolated effect of the laser was unknown.

In a small study by Palm and Goldman,[44] 9 patients (11 sites) received treatment with either LAL (CoolLipo, CoolTouch Inc, Roseville, CA, USA) or mechanical disruption with a liposuction microcannula. At the conclusion of the study, there was no difference in the efficacy between the 2 treatment regimens, with both groups improving by 1 point on a 4-point investigator-evaluated scale. Patient-evaluated improvement did not differ between the 2 regimens.[44] Further larger studies are needed to investigate the effects of LAL alone in the management of cellulite.

SUMMARY

Cellulite is a normal female sexual characteristic that cannot be "cured." It has only been brought to the attention of the female population by the mass media as a condition to be treated. However, cosmetic dermatologists have developed a variety of methods to improve the appearance of cellulite. Although this improvement is temporary, it may last several months. Thus, patients who wish to have smoother skin with less visible cellulite can undergo a series of treatments and then return for additional treatments as necessary. Future research will try and extend both treatment efficacy and duration. The extent of research will be stimulated by the public's demand for treatment.

REFERENCES

1. Draelos ZD, Marenus KD. Cellulite – etiology and purported treatment. Dermatol Surg 1997;23:1177–81.
2. Avram MM. Cellulite: a review of its physiology and treatment. J Cosmet Laser Ther 2004;6:181–5.
3. Goldman MP. Cellulite: a review of current treatments. Cosmet Derm 2002;15:17–20.
4. Querleux B, Cornillon C, Jolivet O, et al. Anatomy and physiology of subcutaneous adipose tissue by in vivo magnetic resonance imaging and spectroscopy: relationships with sex and presence of cellulite. Skin Res Technol 2002;8:118–24.
5. Rossi AB, Vergnanini AL. Cellulite: a review. J Eur Acad Dermatol Venereol 2000;14:251–62.
6. Nurnberger F, Muller G. So-called cellulite: an invented disease. J Dermatol Surg Oncol 1978;4:221–9.
7. Pierard GE, Nizet JL, Pierard-Franchimont C. Cellulite: from standing fat herniation to hypodermal stretch marks. Am J Dermatopathol 2000;22:34–47.
8. Pellicier F, Andre P, Schnebert S. [The adipocyte in the history of slimming agents]. Pathol Biol 2003;51:244–7 [in French].
9. Salter DC, Hanley M, Tynan A, et al. In-vivo high-definition ultrasound studies of subdermal fat

lobules associated with cellulite. J Invest Dermatol 1990;29:272–4.

10. Sainio EL, Rantanen T, Kanerva L. Ingredients and safety of cellulite creams. Eur J Dermatol 2000;10: 596–603.

11. Rao J, Goldman MP. A double-blinded randomized trial testing the tolerability and efficacy of a novel topical agent with and without occlusion for the treatment of cellulite: a study and review of the literature. J Drugs Dermatol 2004;3:417–27.

12. Goldman MP. The use of Tri-Active in the treatment of cellulite. In: Goldman MP, Hexsel D, editors. Cellulite: pathophysiology and treatment. 2nd edition. New York: Informa Healthcare; 2010. p. 99.

13. Zerbinati N. The Triactive system; a simple and effective way of combating cellulite. 2002 (Internal study conducted by Deka).

14. Boyce S, Pabby A, Chuchaltkaren P, et al. Clinical evaluation of a device for the treatment of cellulite: Triactive. Am J Cosmet Surg 2005;22:233–7.

15. Gold M. The use of rhythmic suction massage, low level laser irradiation, and superficial cooling to effect changes in adipose tissue/cellulite. Lasers Surg Med 2006;38(Suppl 18):65.

16. Nootheti PK, Magpantay A, Yosowitz G, et al. A single center, randomized, comparative, prospective clinical study to determine the efficacy of the Velasmooth system versus the Triactive system for the treatment of cellulite. Lasers Surg Med 2006;38: 908–12.

17. Alster TS, Tanzi EL. Cellulite treatment using a novel combination radiofrequency, infrared light, and mechanical tissue manipulation device. J Cosmet Laser Ther 2005;7:81–5.

18. Sadick NS, Mulholland RS. A prospective clinical study to evaluate the efficacy and safety of cellulite treatment using the combination of optical and RF energies for subcutaneous tissue heating. J Cosmet Laser Ther 2004;6:187–90.

19. Sadick N, Magro C. A study evaluating the safety and efficacy of the VelaSmooth system in the treatment of cellulite. J Cosmet Laser Ther 2007; 9:15–20.

20. Kulick M. Evaluation of the combination of radio frequency, infrared energy, and mechanical rollers with suction to improve skin surface irregularities (cellulite) in a limited treatment area. J Cosmet Laser Ther 2006;8:185–90.

21. Boey G. Cellulite treatment with a radiofrequency, infrared light, and tissue manipulation device. The American Society of Dermatologic Surgery Annual Meeting. Palm Desert (CA), October 28, 2006.

22. Romero C, Caballero N, Herrero M, et al. Effects of cellulite treatment with RF, IR light, mechanical massage and suction treating one buttock with the contralateral as a control. J Cosmet Laser Ther 2008;10:193–201.

23. Wanitphakdeedecha R, Manuskiatti W. Treatment of cellulite with a bipolar radiofrequency, infrared heat, and pulsatile suction device: a pilot study. J Cosmet Dermatol 2006;5:284–8.

24. Neira R, Arroyave J, Ramirez H, et al. Fat liquefaction: effect of low-level laser energy on adipose tissue. Plast Reconstr Surg 2002;110(3):912–22.

25. Smalls LK, Hicks M, Passeretti D, et al. Effect of weight loss on cellulite: gynoid lypodystrophy. Plast Reconstr Surg 2006;118(2):510–6.

26. Lach E. Reduction of subcutaneous fat and improvement in cellulite appearance by dual-wavelength, low-level laser energy combined with vacuum and massage. J Cosmet Laser Ther 2008; 10:202–9.

27. Pankratov MM, Morton S. SmoothShapes treatment of cellulite and thigh circumference reduction: when less is more. In: Goldman MP, Hexsel D, editors. Cellulite: pathophysiology and treatment. 2nd edition. New York: Informa Healthcare; 2010. p. 126.

28. Gold MH, Khatri KA, Hails K, et al. Reduction in thigh circumference and improvement in the appearance of cellulite with dual-wavelength, low-level laser energy and massage. J Cosmet Laser Ther 2011; 13(1):13–20.

29. Fournier N, Pankratov M, Aubree AS, et al. Cellulite treatment with Photomology technology. American Society for Laser Medicine and Surgery Meeting. National Harbor (MD), January 5, 2009.

30. Kulick MI. Evaluation of a noninvasive, dual-wavelength laser-suction and massage device for the regional treatment of cellulite. Plast Reconstr Surg 2010;125:1788–96.

31. Alexiades-Armenakas M, Dover JS, Arndt KA. Unipolar radiofrequency treatment to improve the appearance of cellulite. J Cosmet Laser Ther 2008; 10:148–53.

32. Goldberg DJ, Fazeli A, Berlin AL. Clinical, laboratory, and MRI analysis of cellulite treatment with a unipolar radiofrequency device. Dermatol Surg 2008;34:204–9.

33. Del Pino ME, Rosado RH, Azulea A, et al. Effect of controlled volumetric tissue heating with radiofrequency on cellulite and the subcutaneous tissue of the buttocks and thighs. J Drugs Dermatol 2006;5: 709–17.

34. Unaeze J, Goldberg DJ. Accent unipolar radiofrequency. In: Goldman MP, Hexsel D, editors. Cellulite: pathophysiology and treatment. 2nd edition. New York: Informa Healthcare; 2010. p. 115.

35. Manuskiatti W. TriPollar radiofrequency. In: Goldman MP, Hexsel D, editors. Cellulite: pathophysiology and treatment. 2nd edition. New York: Informa Healthcare; 2010. p. 158.

36. Manuskiatti W, Wachirakaphan C, Lektrakul N, et al. Circumference reduction and cellulite treatment with

a TriPollar radiofrequency device: a pilot study. J Eur Acad Dermatol Venereol 2009;23:820–7.

37. Goldman A, Gotkin RH. Laser-assisted liposuction. Clin Plast Surg 2009;36:241–53.

38. Badin AZ, Moraes LM, Gondek L, et al. Laser lipolysis: flaccidity under control. Aesthetic Plast Surg 2002;26:335–9.

39. Kim KH, Geronemus RG. Laser lipolysis using a novel 1064 nm Nd:YAG laser. Dermatol Surg 2006;32:241–8.

40. Goldman A, Gotkin RH, Sarnoff DS, et al. Cellulite: a new treatment approach combining subdermal Nd:YAG laser lipolysis and autologous fat transplantation. Aesthet Surg J 2008;28: 656–62.

41. Katz B, McBean J. The new laser liposuction for men. Dermatol Ther 2007;20:448–51.

42. Katz B, McBean J. Laser-assisted lipolysis: a report on complications. J Cosmet Laser Ther 2008;10:231–3.

43. DiBernardo BE. Randomized, blinded split abdomen study evaluating skin shrinkage and skin tightening in laser-assisted liposuction versus liposuction control. Aesthet Surg J 2010;30(4):593–602.

44. Palm MD, Woodhall K, Goldman MP. Single-Center, Randomized, Prospective Clinical Study comparing CoolLipo 1320 nm Nd:YA6 laser lipolysis to traditional liposculpture in the treatment of cellulite. Presented at the American Society of Dermatologic Surgery National Meeting. Phoenix (AZ), October 4, 2009.

Sclerotherapy: It Is Back and Better

Margaret W. Mann, MD

KEYWORDS

- Spider veins • Sclerotherapy • Varicose veins

KEY POINTS

1. Sclerotherapy is the gold standard treatment of spider and reticular veins.
2. Sodium tetradecyl sulfate (STS, sodium-1 iso-butyl-4-ethyloctyl sulfate in 2% benzoyl alcohol) and polidocanol (hydroxyl polyethoxy-dodecane) are the safest and most efficacious US Food and Drug Administration (FDA)-approved sclerosing agents currently in the market.
3. To maximize outcome and minimize side effects, it is essential to use proper technique and chose the right concentration, volume, and type of sclerosant for each vessel size.
4. The treatment of leg veins should follow a logical algorithmic approach. Incompetent perforators and venous reflux should be treated before treatment of spider and reticular veins.

Varicose, reticular, and telangiectatic veins are a common complaint, appearing in one-third of patients before the age of 25 years. It is estimated that up to 55% of women and 40% to 55% of men will develop spider veins by the age of 50 years.[1] Although most patients present with cosmetic concerns, up to 50% of patients with varicose veins and even spider veins can develop significant symptoms. These symptoms include pain, burning, aching, heaviness, itching, swelling, and restless leg. Patients with severe varicose veins and truncal venous insufficiency can go on to develop adverse sequelae, including superficial thrombophlebitis, stasis dermatitis, leg ulceration, and lipodermatosclerosis.

Sclerotherapy was described as a treatment of varicosities as early as the 1830s. Fegan, in 1963, popularized the technique of sclerotherapy. The aim of sclerotherapy is the fibrous occlusion of the vessel lumen. Rather than merely thrombosing a vessel that may be amenable to recanalization, sclerosing a vessel transforms it into a fibrous cord, which cannot be recanalized.[2,3] In principle, all types and calibers of varicose veins can be treated with sclerotherapy. However, surgery is the mainstay of treatment for larger and truncal varicosities, whereas sclerotherapy remains the gold standard for small-caliber varicose veins, including reticular and spider veins.[4] The goal of surgery and sclerotherapy is to improve venous hemodynamics to achieve a good functional and aesthetic outcome.

VENOUS ANATOMY AND TERMINOLOGY

The venous system is complex and variable; varicose, reticular, and telangiectatic veins may communicate with the great saphenous and short saphenous veins of the superficial system. Likewise, the superficial and deep venous systems are interconnected by perforator veins. Therefore, recognition and treatment of the most proximal point of reflux is required to ensure successful outcome. Treatment should follow an algorithmic approach—the incompetent great saphenous, short saphenous, or perforator vein should be treated first, followed by varicosities, reticular veins, and then finally telangiectasias (Fig. 1).

Venulectasias and varicose, reticular, and telangiectatic leg veins are defined by their size (Table 1). By convention, varicose veins are tortuous veins more than 4 mm in diameter. Reticular veins are bluish veins measuring between 2 and 4 mm in diameter. Venulectasias are superficial bluish vessels less than 2 mm in diameter. Telangiectasias or spider veins are flat red vessels less than 1 mm in diameter (Fig. 2).

The author has nothing to disclose.
Department of Dermatology, University of California, C340 Medical Sciences I, Irvine, CA 92697, USA
E-mail address: margaret.mann@gmail.com

plasticsurgery.theclinics.com

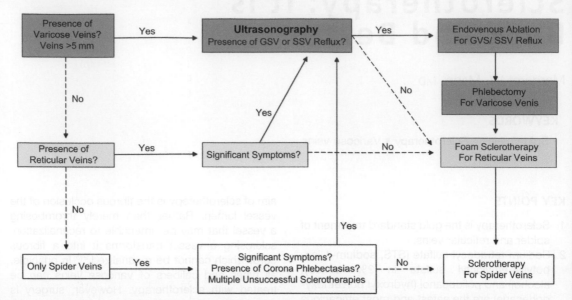

Fig. 1. Evaluation and treatment of leg veins should follow an algorithmic approach. Incompetent perforators and venous reflux should be treated before treatment of spider and reticular veins. GSV, great saphenous vein; SSV, short saphenous vein.

SELECTING THE IDEAL PATIENT FOR SCLEROTHERAPY

As with most cosmetic procedures, choosing the ideal patient is paramount to success. A proper evaluation should be performed before sclerotherapy. Evaluation includes history taking, clinical examination and, if necessary, Doppler or duplex ultrasonographic investigation. Patients with isolated spider and reticular veins will be effectively

treated with sclerotherapy. Similarly, reticular and telangiectatic veins distributed on the lateral thigh are amenable to sclerotherapy alone. This lateral subdermic plexus is considered to be an embryonic remnant and is not associated with incompetence in the superficial or deep venous system (see **Fig. 2**).

The presence of palpable varicosities, veins greater than 5 mm, or prominent spider veins along the medial malleolus (a sign called corona phlebectasia, **Fig. 3**) are signs of possible truncal

Table 1
A guide to selective effective concentration of sclerosant by vessel size

Vessel Size (mm)	Recommended Effective Concentration (%)					
	Liquid Sclerosant				Foam Sclerosant	
	Sotradecol	Polidocanol	Hypertonic Saline	Glycerin	Foam Sotradecol	Foam Polidocanol
Matting	—	—	—	40–50	—	—
<1 Telangiectasia/ Spider Veins	0.1–0.2	0.25–0.5	11.7	50–72	—	—
1.0–2.0 Venulectasia	0.2–0.3	0.5–1.0	11.7–23.4	—	—	—
2.0–4.0 Reticular Veins	0.33–0.5	1.0–2.0	23.4	—	0.2–0.5	0.5–1
>4 mm Varicose Veins	0.5–1.0	2.0–5.0	—	—	0.5–1.0	0.75–2.5

Adapted from Mann WM, Berk DR, Popkin DL, et al. Handbook of dermatology: a practical manual. Oxford (UK): Wiley-Blackwell Publishing; 2009. p. 234–6.

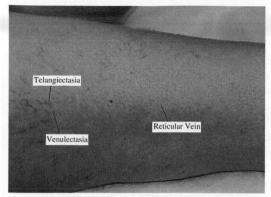

Fig. 2. The lateral subdermic plexus responds well to sclerotherapy. The largest-diameter vessel should be treated first; reticular veins are treated with 0.2% STS foam, followed by venulectasias with 0.2% STS, and finally, spider veins with 0.1% STS.

insufficiency. Likewise, spider veins that are refractory to multiple sclerotherapy treatments may be associated with incompetent perforators. Even in the absence of palpable veins, patients with significant symptoms (such as cramping, aching, fatigue, stasis dermatitis, or swelling) may have reflux disease. These patients should undergo diagnostic duplex ultrasonography to evaluate for valvular incompetence (see **Fig. 1**).

Great or short saphenous vein incompetence is best managed with endovenous laser or radio frequency ablation. With the use of local tumescent anesthesia, these minimally invasive techniques have outperformed traditional ligation and stripping, which were historically associated with higher morbidity. Patients can ambulate immediately after the endovenous ablation procedure, and most patients can resume normal activities within 24 to 48 hours. Varicose veins, especially elevated

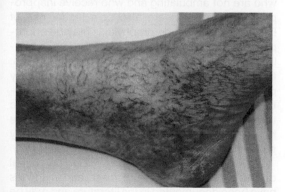

Fig. 3. The presence of corona phlebectasia and stasis dermatitis along the medial malleolus suggests possible venous insufficiency along the great saphenous vein. Before treatment of these spider veins, this patient should undergo ultrasonography to evaluate for valvular incompetence.

vessels more than 4 mm in diameter, can be treated using ambulatory microphlebectomy.[5] Veins are permanently removed using a vein hook through small incisions (1–2 mm in length). Unless the source of incompetence is addressed first, sclerotherapy in these patients is often ineffective and frustrating.

PATIENT CONSENT, COMPLICATIONS, AND RISKS

When performed properly, sclerotherapy is associated with a low incidence of complications. Proper patient education including pretreatment and posttreatment instructions will help ensure patient understanding and compliance. Physicians should review potential risk of sclerotherapy (**Table 2**). Patients should be reminded that several treatment sessions are usually required and that final results may not be apparent for weeks to months. Maintenance treatment is usually necessary over time. This information should be explained by written consent and information sheet.

Pigmentation, matting, and more uncommonly, thrombophlebitis and skin ulceration may occur. The risk of these complications depends on the sclerosant used, its concentration, the volume injected, and the technique of the injector. The risk of pigmentation ranges from 0.3% to 10% and is related to hemosiderin deposition and/or melanogenesis from excessive inflammation.[6] Pigmentation can be reduced by using the lowest effective sclerosant concentration and volume necessary (see **Table 1**). The use of compression stockings for 1 to 3 weeks after treatment may reduce the risk of pigmentation[7] and improve clinical outcome. Intravascular coagulum may occur, especially after treatment of larger-caliber vessels; prompt evacuation with a No. 11 blade stab incision reduces the development of hyperpigmentation and thrombophlebitis. When pigmentation occurs, it can take months to resolve. Superficial thrombophlebitis can be treated with compression and nonsteroidal antiinflammatory drugs. Most recently, a rare phenomenon of localized hypertrichosis after sclerotherapy has been reported.[8]

Telangiectatic matting, which occurs in 2% to 4% of cases, is the result of neovascularization likely related to excessive volume or concentration of sclerosant. Matting usually responds to gentle sclerotherapy with low sclerosant concentration. This is one instance when laser therapy may be superior to sclerotherapy for treating telangiectatic matting. If significant matting occurs, ultrasonography may reveal underlying reflux disease. If matting persists despite treatment, it should be

Table 2
Possible complications in sclerotherapy, and how to avoid them

Possible Complications	Methods to Avoid Them
Hyperpigmentation	Use lowest concentration and volume possible Use compression bandage post sclerotherapy
Matting	Use lowest concentration and volume possible Consider laser therapy instead
Bruising	Use compression bandage post sclerotherapy
Blister	Usually from ill-fitting compression stockings and bandages
Skin ulceration and necrosis	Use lowest concentration and volume possible
Allergic reaction	More common in patients with marked allergic diathesis Consider using only hypertonic saline in these patients

Neurologic symptoms:
  transient migrainelike
  symptom/scintillating
  scotomas/TIA/stroke
	Avoid foam sclerotherapy in patients with a history of PFO
	Use low volume of foam

Thrombophlebitis	Compression after treatment Avoid treatment of larger-diameter vessels (consider phlebectomy instead)
DVT/thromboembolism	Avoid large volume of foam sclerosant Encourage patient to ambulate after sclerotherapy

Abbreviations: DVT, deep venous thrombosis; PFO, patent foramen ovale; TIA, transient ischemic attack.

left alone because it generally resolves spontaneously over several months.

Skin necrosis may occur with extravasation of a high concentration of sclerosant into the perivascular tissue. It is most commonly associated with hypertonic saline. The ankle, popliteal fossa, and pretibial areas are more prone to ulceration. Rarely, extensive skin necroses have been reported after properly performed intravascular injection. In these cases, the presence of aberrant arteriovenous anastomoses from chronic venous hypertension may allow the sclerosant to pass from the veins directly into the arterial circulation, inadvertently causing arterial thrombosis.[6,9] The development of a porcelain-white blanching is typically an early sign of an arteriolar injection and impending skin necrosis. Recommended treatments include the use of massage; injection of normal saline, lidocaine, or hyaluronidase; as well as the use of topical 2% nitroglycerin paste.[10]

Although rare, reports of visual disturbance, chest tightness, deep venous thrombosis (DVT), and coughing have been associated with both liquid and foam sclerotherapies, but they are more frequently reported after using foam sclerosants. According to the French multicenter registry, of 12,173 sessions, the rate of serious complication per session with liquid sclerosant is 0.22% and with foam sclerosant is 0.58%.[11] Most serious complications occur immediately after treatment (51%) or within 4 weeks of treatment (23.5%). Three cases

of delayed adverse reaction (more than 4 weeks since treatment) were reported in the French registry; 1 case was related to pigmentation and 2 were related to muscular vein thrombosis.[12]

Prospective studies have shown that the risk of DVT is higher in patients with a previous history of thromboembolism or thrombophilia and when larger volumes of foam sclerosant are used[13] in treating perforator and truncal veins. The incidence of DVT ranges from 0.09% in the French registry[14] (reviewed >10,000 patients) to 1.8% in a smaller series (reviewed 332 patients).[15] Patients who are not ambulating and who receive inappropriate compression are also at a higher risk of DVTs. Anticoagulation prophylaxis may be appropriate in patients with a high risk of thromboembolism and known thrombophilia.[4] In most cases, thromboembolic events diagnosed in routinely performed duplex ultrasonography after sclerotherapy are asymptomatic.[14,16] Therefore, specific tests for thrombophilia before sclerotherapy are not considered necessary unless clinical history suggests further investigation.

Neurosensory complications including visual disturbances, headaches, dizziness, and migraines have been documented in the literature and may be dose-related. Whereas isolated cases of transient ischemic attacks (TIAs) and strokes have been reported, in the large French registry of 12,173 sessions, no stroke or TIAs were observed.[12] Transient visual disturbances, such as scotoma, are the most commonly reported complication; incidence ranges from 0.25% to 1.75% with foam sclerosants and 0.05% to 0.07% with liquid sclerosants.[11] This disturbance generally resolves within 30 minutes in most patients and is likely to recur with subsequent sessions.[17]

Recent reports have focused on the association of patent foramen ovale (PFO) and neurologic adverse events during foam sclerotherapy.[18,19] Morrison and colleagues[20] studied 20 patients who described visual or respiratory symptoms after foam sclerotherapy. A transthoracic echocardiogram of these patients during foam sclerotherapy showed the presence of foam sclerosant in the left atrium in 65% of these patients. Of 9 patients who then underwent transcranial Doppler during foam sclerotherapy, 5 had evidence of foam in the middle cerebral artery. The investigators concluded that PFO may allow gas bubbles injected during sclerotherapy to reach the arterial cerebral circulation, although most cases are benign and resolve quickly. In cases of known PFO or a history of neurologic symptoms with sclerotherapy, only low volumes of foam should be used. These patients should remain lying down for 30 minutes to avoid any calf muscle contraction or Valsalva maneuvers, which may allow the foam to migrate to the cerebral circulation.[17] Whereas the prevalence of PFO has been estimated at 27% of the general population,[21] the incidence of neurologic complications associated with foam sclerotherapy is very rare given that millions of injections have been administered over the years. Considering the transient nature and infrequency of adverse events, the European consensus meeting does not advocate PFO screening before foam sclerotherapy.[22]

Severe allergy is very uncommon; urticaria, asthma, hay fever, and anaphylactic shock have been reported after sclerotherapy. The incidence of an allergic reaction is 0.3%, and such reaction may occur with any sclerosant agent.[10] An allergic reaction is the least likely with hypertonic saline. The highest incidence is with ethanolamine oleate. Patients with a history of multiple allergies and asthma may be at a higher risk of allergic complications.

CONTRAINDICATIONS

Absolute and relative contraindications to treatment by sclerotherapy[2,4,17,23] are listed in the following sections.

Relative Contraindications

- Marked allergic diathesis/severe bronchial asthma
- Poor general health/severe concomitant disease (malignancy and cardiovascular and respiratory tract diseases)
- Immobility
- Known thrombophilia or hypercoagulable state
- Needle phobia
- Known asymptomatic PFO (especially with foam sclerotherapy)
- Leg edema
- Very large varices (increased risk of thrombophlebitis, may be more amenable to surgery)
- Arteriovenous malformation (more difficult to treat and higher risk of necrosis).

Absolute Contraindications to Treatment

- Known allergy to the sclerosant
- History of extensive DVT with obliteration of the deep venous system
- Acute superficial or deep vein thrombosis
- Local infection in the area of sclerotherapy, cellulitis, or severe systemic infection
- Pregnancy
- Advanced peripheral arterial occlusive disease (stage 3 or 4)
- Advanced collagen vascular disease.

SCLEROSING AGENTS

At present, there is no perfect sclerosant that is 100% effective and free of complications. All sclerosing agents used in the literature have varying efficacy and toxicity; in general, the more potent agents have greater efficacy and concomitant side effects.[24] These agents fall into 3 categories: detergents, osmotic agents, and chemical irritants (**Table 3**). The most commonly used sclerosants are STS, polidocanol, hypertonic saline, and chromated glycerin.

Detergent sclerosants were first introduced in the 1920s and are still the most popular sclerosants used worldwide. Compared with older agents, detergent sclerosants have a more favorable benefit-to-risk ratio as well as the added ability to create bubbles when agitated for foam sclerotherapy. As of 2010, there are 2 FDA-approved sclerotherapy solutions STS (Sotradecol) and polidocanol (Asclera). STS has been approved for use in the United States since 2004. Polidocanol was recently FDA approved in April 2010 but has been used extensively in Europe for decades. Because both agents are commercially available in the market, physicians should avoid using compound pharmacy for equivalent products. A sampling of 3 compounding formulations showed the presence

Table 3
Commonly used sclerosing agents

Sclerosing Agent	Brand Name	FDA Approval	Maximum Dosage	Pain	Necrosis	Pigmentation	Other
Detergent: cause protein theft denaturing resulting in the loss of cell surface lipids and disruption of endothelial cell membrane							
STS	Sotradecol Fibro-vein	Yes, 1946	10 mL of 3% solution	Minimal	Occasional, at concentration >1%	Moderate risk	0.1%–0.3% anaphylaxis
Polidocanol	Asclera Aethoxy sclerol	Yes, 2010	10 mL of 3% solution	Minimal	Rare	Low risk at high concentrations	0.2% anaphylaxis
Sodium morrhuate	Scleromate	Yes, 1930	10 mL	Moderate	Frequent	Moderate risk	3%–10% cases of anaphylaxis (highest risk)
Ethanolamine oleate	Ethamolin	Off-label use; for esophageal varices only	10 mL	Mild	Occasional	Moderate risk	Risk of hemolytic reaction, renal failure, pleural effusion, allergic reaction
Osmotic agents: damage the cell wall by dehydration of endothelial cells through osmotic gradient							
Hypertonic saline 23.4% (NaCl)	Hypertonic saline	Off-label use FDA approved it as an abortifacient	10–20 mL	Painful, muscle cramps	Significant if extravasated	Low risk	No allergic reaction
10% Saline + 5% dextrose	Sclerodex	No	10–20 mL	Painful	Significant if extravasated	Minimal risk	Low risk of allergic reaction
Chemical irritants: act as corrosive agents that induce damage by direct caustic destruction of endothelial cells							
Glycerin	Chromex Scleremo	No	5–10 mL	Moderate	Rare	Least likely	Viscous solution, rare allergic reaction with chromated glycerin
Polyiodine iodine	Varigloban, Variglobin, Sclerodine	No	3 mL of 6%	Painful	Occasional	Low risk	Viscous solution, rare allergic reaction to iodine Renal insufficiency

Adapted from Mann WM, Berk DR, Popkin DL, et al. Handbook of dermatology: a practical manual. Oxford (UK): Wiley-Blackwell Publishing; 2009. p. 234–6.

of contaminants and inconsistency between labeled concentration and actual composition.[25]

STS is a synthetic surfactant used since the 1940s. Although the recommended maximum dose varies with investigators, the current product insert recommends a maximum of 10 mL of a 3% solution.[24] STS is commercially available in 1% and 3% concentrations but is commonly diluted with normal saline to the desired concentration. Unlike injections of hypertonic saline, STS injections are relatively painless, unless extravasation occurs. STS is associated with a higher risk of pigmentation, especially when higher concentrations are used. Tissue necrosis is rare and is associated with the concentration used; an intradermal injection of 1% STS resulted in immediate tissue ulceration but a similar volume of 0.5% STS injection did not.[24]

Polidocanol was first marketed as a topical and local anesthetic in 1930s then used as a sclerosing agent in the 1960s. Polidocanol has an anesthetic effect, which makes it less painful than other sclerosants. The maximum recommended dose varies in the literature; the range varies from 10 to 20 mL of 3% solution[26] to the European guidelines of 2 mg/kg (10 mL 1% solution for a 50-kg individual).[27] At near maximum dosage, patients have reported perioral paresthesia or strange taste sensation, which may be related to the anesthetic property of polidocanol. Toxic levels can produce cardiotoxicity, much like lidocaine toxicity, resulting in bradycardia and hypotension. Polidocanol is reported to cause less pigmentation than STS, although this may be related to the concentration used rather than to the intrinsic property of polidocanol.[24]

Hypertonic saline 23.4% is approved by the FDA as an abortifacient; its use in sclerotherapy is off label. As a naturally occurring molecule in the human body, hypertonic saline has a low risk of toxicity and lacks allergenicity, making it ideal for patients with marked allergic diathesis. The drug is also readily available and inexpensive. Unlike STS and polidocanol, hypertonic saline causes burning discomfort and cramping on injection. There is a higher risk of skin ulceration and hyperpigmentation.

Glycerin is a chemical irritant that induces direct injury to endothelial cells through a heavy metal cauterizing effect. It is not FDA approved for use in the United States, although it is commonly used in Europe. The maximum recommended dose per session is 10 mL (glycerin 72% and chromium alum 0.8%).[28] Glycerin is ideal for small telangiectatic veins. It has a low risk of hyperpigmentation and telangiectatic matting. However, glycerin is more painful on injection and difficult to work with because it is viscous. The addition of lidocaine minimizes discomfort and reduces its viscosity. In the past, chromium alum was added to glycerin (chromated glycerin) to augment its sclerosing effects and to prevent hematuria induced by pure glycerin alone.[24] Because of the high risk of allergy to chromium, however, most phlebologists use only pure glycerin solutions.

COMPARISON OF SCLEROSING AGENTS

Because clinically equivalent concentrations have not been clearly established between polidocanol and STS, it is difficult to compare the efficacy and rates of complications between these 2 agents. Furthermore, whereas it is common practice to dilute STS to reduce the side effects, clinical studies generally use STS in 1% solution as per FDA-approved indications. Nevertheless, several studies have compared various concentrations of polidocanol and STS and concluded similar efficacy between the 2 agents. Polidocanol has been shown in some studies to cause fewer side effects, but this may be because of the higher equivalent concentration used with STS in the comparison arm. In general, STS is approximately 3 times as potent as polidocanol.[24]

A recently published double-blinded, randomized study compared polidocanol, STS, and isotonic saline (placebo). In the polidocanol group, patients were treated with 0.5% polidocanol for telangiectatic veins and 1% polidocanol for reticular veins. In the STS group, all patients were treated with 1%. In the placebo group, all patients were treated with isotonic saline. Patients were then evaluated at weeks 12 and 26. The vessel clearance rates for the polidocanol and STS groups were significantly higher than that for the placebo group at week 12 (polidocanol 96%; STS 92%) and week 26 (polidocanol 95%; STS 91%). The difference in vessel clearance rates between STS and polidocanol was not statistically significant. There were significantly more side effects in the STS group, including local irritation, hyperpigmentation, necrosis, ulcer, hematoma, and matting. Patient satisfaction was significantly lower with STS (64%) than with polidocanol (88%).[29]

At lower concentrations, STS and polidocanol showed similar efficacy, side effects, tolerability, and patient satisfaction. Rao and colleagues[30] treated 20 subjects with varying concentrations of either polidocanol (0.5%, 1%, or 1% foam) or STS (0.25%, 0.5%, or 0.5% foam) depending on the size of their veins (>1 mm, 1–3 mm, or 3–6 mm). Adverse events, including ecchymosis, hyperpigmentation, coagulum formation, and telangiectatic matting, were similar between the 2 groups. Goldman[31] also stratified treatment of 129 patients with either polidocanol (0.5%, 1%, or 3%) or STS (0.25%, 0.5%, or 1.5%) based on vessel size. Both agents were equally effective, with a similar side effect profile. There was an increase in skin necrosis with STS[31]; this could likely be due to the selection of 1.5% STS, which is known to cause skin necrosis at concentrations greater than 1%.

In a single-blinded randomized study, 72% chromated glycerin was more effective at vessel clearance of telangiectasias and reticular veins than polidocanol 0.25% solution and foam.[32] The lower efficacy of polidocanol may be because of the relatively low concentration selected. Nevertheless, the investigators found an increased incidence of matting and hyperpigmentation with polidocanol than with chromated glycerin. Similarly, in a small nonblinded study, 72% glycerin was found to be more efficacious than 0.25% STS for treating telangiectatic veins 0.2 to 0.4 mm in size.[33] Glycerin also demonstrated a lower risk of hyperpigmentation (3%–5%), telangiectatic matting (5%–10%), and tissue necrosis (1%–3%)[33,34] than STS.

FOAM SCLEROTHERAPY

Foam sclerotherapy is more efficacious in sclerosing larger-diameter vessels because the bubbles mechanically displace blood, thereby maximizing the contact time and surface area between the sclerosant and the vein endothelium. In comparison to liquid sclerotherapy, lower concentration and volume are needed to effectively sclerose veins using foam. Foam sclerotherapy was first described in the literature by Foote[35] in 1944 and Orbach[36] in 1950. In the 1990s, Cabrera Garrido and colleagues[37] and Monfreux[38] published methods for producing foam, which was used for the treatment of great saphenous veins and vascular malformation under ultrasound guidance. Cabrera Garrido and colleagues[37] reported that foam greatly extended the range of vein diameter that could be treated by sclerotherapy.

Many investigators have described methods of foam preparation; the most widely used method was first described by Tessari, commonly called the double syringe technique, in which 2 disposable syringes are connected using a 3-way stopcock. A mixture of sclerosant and room air is pumped back and forth approximately 10 to 20 times between the 2 syringes to produce foam.[17] The preferred ratio of liquid sclerosant and air is usually 1 part sclerosant to 3 or 4 parts air.

Whereas the use of foam sclerotherapy has been widely documented in the published literature as a standard procedure, the transformation of liquid sclerosant into foam is an off-label use; patients should be adequately informed of the potential side effects. Compared with liquid sclerosant, foam sclerosants have been associated with a higher risk of pigmentation, thrombophlebitis, and ulceration. More importantly, the risk of serious adverse events such as neurologic and pulmonary complications is higher when a high volume of foam is injected into larger-caliber varicosities. To minimize these complications, the European consensus meeting in 2003 initially recommended a maximum volume of 6 to 8 mL of foam injected per session.[2,39] The maximum volume was increased to 10 mL per session during the 2006 European consensus meeting.[4,22] Larger volumes (up to 45 mL) have been used in the treatment of reticular veins with no major sequelae.[40] Nevertheless, experienced phlebologists recommend no more than 0.5 mL of foam per injection into telangiectasias and reticular veins[39] and no more than 1 to 2 mL per injection into larger varicosities.[17]

Foam sclerotherapy is best used for reticular and varicose veins. According to the European consensus meeting, most experts use foam for the treatment of veins between 3 and 6 mm (96% of participants), 6 and 8 mm (84%), and up to 15 mm (60%) in size. In contrast, a minority of participants use foam to treat telangiectatic veins less than 1 mm (29%) or larger than 18 mm (25%).[39]

A higher concentration of sclerosant produces more viscous foam, which is more powerful and suitable for use in larger-caliber veins. On the other hand, liquid foam created by using a lower concentration of sclerosant should be used for smaller vessels to reduce adverse events.[39] The foam created is stable for about 1 to 2 minutes, thus it is usually injected immediately. One study noted that the use of a 5-μm filter hub with the double syringe technique increased foam stability by 47 seconds when compared with using the hub with the standard 2-way connector.[41] Most experts treat feeding reticular veins first, then proceeding with liquid sclerotherapy to treat telangiectasias. To ensure proper placement of the foam sclerosant, aspiration of a small amount of blood should be visualized before injection. During treatment of larger veins, some investigators advocate leg elevation during treatment[2,17,39] to impede movement of the foam into the deep venous circulation. In addition, ultrasound guidance should be used with injection of larger varicosities.[39]

SELECTION OF THE PROPER SCLEROSANT CONCENTRATION

Choosing the right concentration, volume, and type of sclerosant for each type of vein is essential for good outcome from sclerotherapy. Lack of efficacy can arise if not enough scloersant is injected. Insufficient damage to the endothelium leads to thrombosis rather than fibrosis, and recanalization often occurs. Conversely, complications such as hyperpigmentation, telangiectatic matting, and ulcerations may occur if excessive concentrations or volumes are used. In most cases, complications are related to the injection technique, volume, and concentration used rather than to a function of the specific sclerosant. Thus, the lowest effective concentration and volume should be used to optimize outcome and minimize adverse effects.

The selection of concentration and volume is based on vessel size. The recommended maximum effective concentrations for various sclerosants are outlined in **Table 1**. Dilution tables should be readily available for staff to avoid mistakes in preparation of sclerosants. Diluted solutions should be clearly labeled.

MY SCLEROTHERAPY TECHNIQUE

Numerous techniques have been described in performing traditional liquid sclerotherapy. The following is my general approach to sclerotherapy.

1. The procedure is generally performed with the physician comfortably seated and the patient in the supine position. Loupes can be useful for visualizing small vessels.
2. A sclerotherapy tray should be set up with the following (**Fig. 4**) equipments:
   - A few 3-mL syringes with 30-gauge ½-inch needles. These syringes should be clearly labeled with the concentration. I prefer 2 mL of sclerosing agent in each 3-mL syringe to allow for better manual control and dexterity.
   - Cotton balls
   - Paper tape
   - Isopropyl alcohol in a small basin
   - A 3-way stopcock.

3. The sclerosant concentration should be selected based on the size of vessels, using the lowest effective concentration needed (see **Table 1**). For most patients with telangiectasias and reticular veins, I use 0.1% and 0.2% STS.
4. The largest-diameter vessel should be treated first. For example, reticular veins should be treated first, followed by venulectasias, and finally, the associated telangiectatic web (see **Figs. 1** and **2**). An entire vessel array should be treated in a given session. When treating larger veins with foam, treatment should proceed from the distal veins and progress proximally.
5. The skin is first cleansed with cotton balls soaked with isopropyl alcohol.
6. I have found that swabbing the skin with alcohol and placing a small drop of sclerosant on the skin before injection reduce light scatter and glare, improving visibility and clarity of the vessels.
7. Apply countertraction with your nondominant hand; this will allow for better visualization. I often rest the fifth finger of my dominant hand on the skin for better stability with cannulation (**Fig. 5**).
8. A 30-gauge needle, bent at a 45° angle, is injected with the bevel up to help facilitate superficial injections. Insert the needle in a superficial plane (nearly parallel to the skin); the vessels are often more superficial than they appear (**Fig. 6**).
9. Injection should be performed slowly with light pressure. You should see the flow of the sclerosant temporarily displacing the blood in the vessel. The presence of a raised wheal or

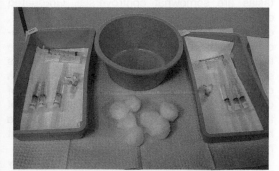

Fig. 4. Typical sclerotherapy tray setup. Note syringes clearly labeled with concentration and separated, center basin for 70% isopropyl alcohol, and cotton balls.

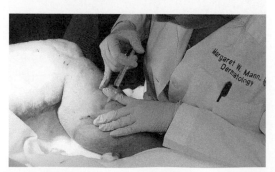

Fig. 5. The use of countertraction with the nondominant hand will allow for better visualization. The fifth finger of the dominant hand should be rested on the patient for better stability.

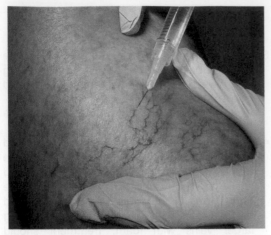

Fig. 6. Bending the needle at a 45° angle, insert the needle nearly parallel to the skin. Telangiectasias are often much more superficial than they appear.

severe pain during injection indicates perivascular extravasation.

10. Avoid injecting over the medial and lateral malleolus because these areas are more prone to ulcerations.
11. When treating reticular or larger veins, it is essential to aspirate and visualize a small amount of venous blood before injection to ensure proper placement into the vasculature (**Fig. 7**). No more than 0.5 mL of foam sclerosant should be used per injection of reticular vein and 1 to 2 mL per injection of varicose veins.
12. Foam is created with a 2- or 3-way stopcock and 2 syringes, one with 1 mL of sclerosant and the other with 3 mL of room air. The 2

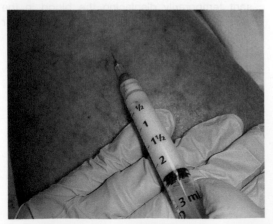

Fig. 7. When treating reticular veins, be sure to aspirate before injection of the sclerosant to ensure proper placement into the vasculature. Telangiectasias are too small and do not require aspiration.

syringes are then pumped quickly 10 to 20 times. Closing the aperture of the stopcock slightly helps create longer-lasting foam. Injection should be made within 1 to 2 minutes (**Fig. 8**).

13. Once the feeding reticular veins are treated with foam sclerosant, the remaining telangiectasias and venulectasias are treated with liquid sclerosant. Because of the small caliber of these vessels, aspiration before injection is not necessary. Usually, 0.1 to 0.3 mL of sclerosant is injected per injection.
14. Local compression with paper tape and cotton ball should be performed along the course of the sclerosed veins.
15. Graduated compression hose (20–30 mm Hg) is used to reduce complications such as thrombophlebitis and to improve clinical outcome. Thigh-high or pantyhose stockings rather than knee-length stockings are preferred, because full-leg stockings better protect against venous thrombosis and compress along the entire length of treatment.
16. In the first few days after treatment, patients should be encouraged to ambulate to reduce the risk of thrombotic events and to avoid intense exercise, hot baths, tanning beds, and sauna.
17. In most cases, patients generally require 2 to 4 treatment sessions. Repeated treatment of the same area should be spaced 6 to 8 weeks apart to allow adequate time for fibrosis of the treated vessels and resolution of inflammation.

POSTSCLEROTHERAPY CARE

Although most phlebologists advocate the use of compression after treatment of large varicose veins, the duration and degree of compression after sclerotherapy of reticular veins and telangiectasias are somewhat controversial. Graduated compression therapy reduces the risk of DVT, edema, and superficial thrombophlebitis. Immediate compression allows for more direct apposition of treated vein walls, which in turn enhances sclerosis and decreases thrombus formation.[7] A controlled study demonstrated that the use of compression stockings after sclerotherapy of telangiectasias enhances outcome and reduces hyperpigmentation in a statistically significant manner.[7]

The duration of compression after sclerotherapy was addressed by several controlled studies. One study showed that the duration of compression directly correlates with the degree of improvement. Three weeks of continuous compression

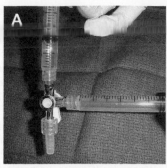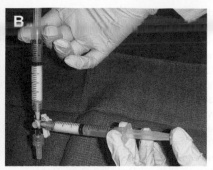

Fig. 8. The double syringe method for creating sclerosant foam. (*A*) One syringe with 1 mL of 0.2% STS and a second syringe with 3 mL of room air connected by a 3-way stopcock. (*B*) The 2 syringes are then pumped quickly 10 to 20 times. The injection should be made within 1 to 2 minutes.

resulted in the most improvement and the least amount of hyperpigmentation, although even 3 days of compression was better than no compression.[7] On the other hand, another study found that prolonged compression (6 weeks) was not superior to short-term therapy. Patients undergoing prolonged compression were more likely to complain of discomfort, foot swelling, and bandage intolerance. Two studies found no difference in superficial thrombophlebitis with short-term (3–7 days) versus prolonged (6 weeks) compression.[42,43] Another study showed no statistically significant difference in cosmetic appearance and symptomatic improvement between short-term (8 hours) and prolonged (6 weeks) compression.[44]

Several studies assessed the strength of compression and outcome. Although high compression is necessary >20 mm Hg), these studies suggest that class I (20–30 mm Hg) and class II (30–40 mm Hg) stockings were equally effective in improving the symptoms of venous insufficiency.[45,46] Furthermore, the incidence of hyperpigmentation and superficial thrombophlebitis were no different between the 2 groups.[42,45] Given identical improvements, class I stockings are preferred because patient compliance is higher.

There are several options for compression including nonelastic and elastic bandages and compression stockings; most phlebologists and patients prefer the convenience of compression stockings. Patients should continue low-impact exercises, such as walking after treatment, but heavy aerobic exercises to the legs should be avoided for 1 week.

SUMMARY

The treatment of leg veins should follow a logical algorithmic approach. Before treatment of small

vessels, incompetent perforators and venous reflux disease should be addressed first. Sclerotherapy remains the gold standard for treatment of spider and reticular veins. Although no perfect sclerosant exists, STS and polidocanol are both FDA-approved agents with superior efficacy and safety profile. Using a proper technique and choosing the right concentration, volume, and type of sclerosant for each type of vein are essential to good outcome and minimizing side effects. When performed properly, sclerotherapy provides a satisfying outcome for both the patient and the physician.

ACKNOWLEDGMENTS

The author would like to acknowledge Daniel Popkin MD, Anthony Petelin MD, and Suzanne Wolffer for their assistance with this manuscript.

REFERENCES

1. Callam MJ. Epidemiology of varicose veins. Br J Surg 1994;81(2):167–73.
2. Rabe E, Pannier-Fischer F, Gerlach H, et al. Guidelines for sclerotherapy of varicose veins. Dermatol Surg 2004;30:687–93.
3. Drake LA, Dinehart SM, Goltz RW, et al. Guidelines of care for sclerotherapy treatment of varicose and telangiectatic leg veins. J Am Acad Dermatol 1996;34:523–8.
4. Rabe E, Pannier F. Sclerotherapy of varicose veins with polidocanol based on the guidelines of the German Society of Phlebology. Dermatol Surg 2010;36:968–75.
5. Sadick NS. Choosing the appropriate sclerosing concentration for vessel diameter. Dermatol Surg 2010;36:976–81.
6. Goldman MP, Sadick NS, Weiss RA. Cutaneous necrosis, telangiectatic matting and hyperpigmentation following sclerotherapy. Dermatol Surg 1995;21:19–29.

7. Weiss RA, Sadick NS, Goldman MP, et al. Post-sclerotherapy compression: controlled comparative study of duration of compression and its effects on clinical outcome. Dermatol Surg 1999;25:105–8.

8. Oh TS, Kim YJ, Song HJ. Localized hypertrichosis after sclerotherapy. Dermatol Surg 2010;36:1064–5.

9. Bergan JJ, Weiss RA, Goldman MP. Extensive tissue necrosis following high concentration sclerotherapy for varicose veins. Dermatol Surg 2000;26:535–42.

10. Zimmet SE. The prevention of cutaneous necrosis following extravasation of hypertonic saline and sodium tetradecyl sulfate. J Dermatol Surg Oncol 1993;19(7):641–6.

11. Guex JJ. Complications of sclerotherapy: an update. Dermatol Surg 2010;36:1056–63.

12. Guex JJ, Schliephake DE, Otto J, et al. The French polidocanol study on long term side effects: a survey covering 3357 patients years. Dermatol Surg 2010;36:993–1003.

13. Myers KA, Jolley D. Factors affecting the risk of deep venous occlusion after ultrasound-guided sclerotherapy for varicose vein. Eur J Vasc Endovasc Surg 2008;36:602–5.

14. Guex JJ, Allaert FA, Gillet JL, et al. Immediate and midterm complications of sclerotherapy: report of a prospective multicenter registry of 12,173 sclerotherapy sessions. Dermatol Surg 2005;31:123–8.

15. Bergan J, Pascarella L, Mekenas L. Venous disorders: treatment with sclerosant foam. J Cardiovasc Surg 2006;47:9–18.

16. Gillet JL, Guedes JM, Guex JJ, et al. Side effects and complications of foam sclerotherapy of the great and small saphenous veins: a controlled multicentre prospective study including 1025 patients. Phlebology 2009;24:131–8.

17. Smith PC. Foam and liquid sclerotherapy for varicose veins. Phlebology 2009;24(Suppl 1):62–72.

18. Bush RG, Derrick M, Manjoney D. Major neurological events following foam sclerotherapy. Phlebology 2008;23:189–92.

19. Ceulen RP, Sommer A, Vernooy K, et al. Microembolism during foam sclerotherapy of varicose veins. N Engl J Med 2008;358:14.

20. Morrison N, Neuhardt DL, Rogers CR, et al. Comparisons of side effects using air and carbon dioxide foam for endovenous chemical ablation. J Vasc Surg 2008;47:830–6.

21. Hagen PT, Scholz DG, Edwards WD. Incidence and size of patent foramen ovale during the first 10 decades of life: an autopsy study of 965 normal hearts. Mayo Clin Proc 1984;59:17–20.

22. Breu FX, Guggenbichler S, Wollmann JC. 2nd European Consensus Meeting on foam sclerotherapy 2006, Tegernsee, Germany. Vasa 2008;37(Suppl 71):1–30.

23. Sadick N, Li C. Small vessel sclerotherapy. Dermatol Clin 2001;19:473–81.

24. Duffy DM. Sclerosants: a comparative review. Dermatol Surg 2010;36:1010–25.

25. Goldman MP. Sodium tetradecyl sulfate for sclerotherapy treatment of veins: is compounding pharmacy solution safe? Dermatol Surg 2004;30:1454–6.

26. Duffy DM, Hsu JT, Alam M, et al, editors. Procedures in cosmetic dermatology series. The Netherlands: Elsevier; 2006. p. 71–106.

27. Kreussler: Fachinformationen Aethoxysklerol 0,25%/0,5%/1%/2% Stand 06/2005, Aethoxysklerol 3%/4%, Stand 09/2005 [package insert]. Rheingaustraße, Wiesbaden (Germany): Chemische Fabrik Kreussler & Co. GmbH; 2005.

28. Duffy DM. Varicose veins and telangiectasias diagnosis and treatment. In: Goldman MP, Weiss RA, Bergan JJ, editors. Techniques of small vessel sclerotherapy. St Louis (MO): Quality Medical Publishing; 1999. p. 518–47.

29. Rabe E, Schliephake D, Otto J, et al. Sclerotherapy of telangiectases and reticular veins: a double-blind, randomized, comparative clinical trial of polidocanol, sodium tetradecyl sulphate and isotonic saline (EASI study). Phlebology 2010;25:124–31.

30. Rao J, Wildermore JK, Goldman MP. Double-blind prospective comparative trial between foamed and liquid polidocanol and sodium tetradecyl sulfate in the treatment of varicose and telangiectatic leg veins. Dermatol Surg 2005;31:631–5.

31. Goldman MP. Treatment of varicose and telangiectatic leg veins: double-blind prospective comparative trial between aethoxyskerol and sotradecol. Dermatol Surg 2002;28:52–5.

32. Kern P, Ramelet AA, Wutschert R, et al. Single-blind, randomized study comparing chromated glycerin, polidocanol solution, and polidocanol foam for treatment of telangiectatic leg veins. Dermatol Surg 2004;30:367–72.

33. Leach BC, Goldman MP. Comparative trial between sodium tetradecyl sulfate and glycerin in the treatment of telangiectatic leg veins. Dermatol Surg 2003;29:612–5.

34. Martin DE, Goldman MP. A comparison of sclerosing agents: clinical and histologic effects of intravascular sodium tetradecyl sulfate and chromated glycerin in the dorsal rabbit ear vein. J Dermatol Surg Oncol 1990;16:18–22.

35. Foote RR. Varicose veins. London: Butterworth & Co; 1949. p. 1–225.

36. Orbach EJ. The thrombogenic activity of foam of a synthetic anionic detergent (sodium tetradecyl sulfate NNR). Angiology 1950;1:237–43.

37. Cabrera Garrido JR, Cabrera Garcia-Olmedo JR, Garcia-Olmedo Dominguez MA. Elargissement des limites de la schleotherapie: noveaux produits sclerosants. Phlebologie 1997;50:181–8 [in French].

38. Monfreux A. Traitement sclérosant des troncs saphéniens et leurscollatérales de gros calibre par

la méthode mus. Phlebologie 1997;50;351–3 [in French].

39. Breu FX, Guggenbichler S. European consensus meeting on foam sclerotherapy, April 4–6 2003, Tegernsee Germany. Dermatol Surg 2004;30:709–17.

40. Palm MD, Guiha IC, Goldman MP. Foam sclerotherapy for reticular veins and nontruncal varicose veins of the legs: a retrospective review of outcomes and adverse effects. Dermatol Surg 2010;36:1026–33.

41. Shirazi AR, Goldman M. The use of a 5-μm filter hub increases foam stability when using the double-syringe technique. Dermatol Surg 2008;34:91–2.

42. Fraser IA, Perry EP, Hatton M, et al. Prolonged bandaging is not required following sclerotherapy of varicose veins. Br J Surg 1985;72(6):488–90.

43. Moody AP, Nicklin S, Wilcox A, et al. Prospectively randomised trial of 1 versus 6 weeks of compression after sclerotherapy for varicose veins. Br J Surg 1996;83(Suppl 1):48.

44. Raj TB, Makin GS. A random controlled trial of two forms of compression bandaging in outpatient sclerotherapy of varicose veins. J Surg Res 1981;31(5):440–5.

45. Shouler PJ, Runchman PC. Varicose veins: optimum compression after surgery and sclerotherapy. Ann R Coll Surg Engl 1989;71:402–4.

46. Veraart JC, Neumann HA. Effects of medical elastic compression stockings on interface pressure and edema prevention. Dermatol Surg 1996;22:867–71.

Injectable Therapies for Localized Fat Loss: State of the Art

Diane Duncan, MD[a], Adam M. Rotunda, MD[b],*

KEYWORDS

- Phosphatidylcholine • Deoxycholate • Injection lipolysis
- Adipolysis • Lipodissolve

KEY POINTS

1. The US Food and Drug Administration (FDA) or any regulatory body worldwide has not approved injectable therapies to remove small quantities of fat.
2. Lipodissolve and mesotherapy are unapproved combinations of unregulated compounded medication associated with adverse events and controversy.
3. An adipolytic medication, sodium deoxycholate, is in registration trials for the reduction of submental fat.
4. A lipolytic medication, a combination of a beta agonist (solmeterol xinafoate) and a steroid (fluticasone propionate), is in registration trials for the reduction of abdominal fat.
5. The clinical applications of the (currently) unapproved medications presented in this review represent the authors experiences and a summary of the literature, not the outcome of clinical data generated through the ongoing pharmaceutical development of adipolytic or lipolytic formulations.

Since Rittes developed the procedure of injecting subcutaneous fat for localized reduction, a decade of erratic progress and setbacks in the use and understanding of injectable therapies for fat has passed. After being received with initial enthusiasm earlier in the decade, by 2007 mesotherapy and injectable methods for fat loss (termed most often as Lipodissolve, injection lipolysis, and injection adipolysis) were the subjects of critical scrutiny by the media and the US Food and Drug Administration. Despite the fact that the process of liposuction developed in much the same way (first tried on patients and then studied in the laboratory), the reputation of injectable fat loss therapies remains tarnished whereas, liposuction is the second most popular aesthetic procedure in the United States.

Liposuction removes fat by mechanical avulsion. The process has been enhanced by ultrasound, vibration, laser assistance, and radiofrequency heating. Nonsurgical fat reduction options include cryolipolysis, various types of external radiofrequency and ultrasound, low-level light therapy, and various injection methods. Although traditional mesotherapy remains unproven as a fat reducer, multiple researchers have confirmed the efficacy of injecting deoxycholate-based compounds, with recent focus on clarifying the exact mechanism of action as well as optimizing safety. The two most commonly used injectable formulas are phosphatidylcholine/deoxycholate (PC/DC) and deoxycholate (DC) alone. The use of additives or cocktail-type formulas, which defined traditional mesotherapy, has become less and less popular as proof of their lack of therapeutic efficacy and the presence of side effects has become well

Disclosure: Dr Duncan has no conflict of interest or commercial interests regarding the topic presented.
Disclosure: Dr Rotunda is the co-inventor of several patents that describe methods to reduce subcutaneous fat with deoxycholate.
[a] Private Practice, 1701 East Prospect Road, Fort Collins, CO 80525, USA
[b] 1100 Quail Street, Suite 102, Newport Beach, CA 92660, USA
* Corresponding author.
E-mail address: arotunda@hotmail.com

Clin Plastic Surg 38 (2011) 489–501
doi:10.1016/j.cps.2011.02.005
0094-1298/11/$ – see front matter © 2011 Elsevier Inc. All rights reserved

known. Therefore, the focus of this article rests primarily on injectable PC/DC and DC as methods to locally reduce fat.

Despite nonapproval by any regulatory body worldwide for the purpose of localized fat loss, practitioners have been using approved PC/DC combinations, such as Lipostabil (Aventis; Frankfurt, Germany) or Lipobean (Amipharm; Seoul, Korea), off-label for subcutaneous fat reduction in Europe and Korea, respectively. Clinicians using PC/DC combination or DC alone elsewhere, including the United States, obtain their medications from compounding pharmacies. Over the past decade, clinical practice has changed in that PC/DC or DC formulas have been replaced with more dilute solutions in an effort to increase safety and reduce side effects. Furthermore, although US users tend to treat small areas, such as the neck and jawline, lipomas, and bra rolls, other high-volume users, such as Korean physicians, treat larger areas, such as the abdomen, arms, and thighs. Low treatment costs and the availability of a standard, pharmaceutical-grade formula make injection lipolysis a popular fat reduction treatment in Korea, although the rest of the world has not seen a similar rise in popularity.

MECHANISM OF ACTION
Membrane Disintegration

The mechanism of adipocyte lysis following injection of phosphatidylcholine or deoxycholate has been the subject of debate for many years. Several aspects of the controversy persist.

The mechanics of adipocyte lysis, the lytic agent, and the role of phosphatidylcholine, if any, are still conjecture to many practitioners, despite publication of scientifically proven illustrations of mechanism of action over a 5-year period.[1,2] Speculation spoken as truth has led many clinicians to think and propagate the notion that rather than fat cell lysis caused by disintegration of cell membrane by detergent (DC), the scientifically proven mechanism, that adipocyte lysis following PC/DC or DC injections is induced by apoptosis,[3] stimulation of hormone sensitive lipase,[4] or the beta-adrenergic-stimulated egress of glycerol and fatty acids,[5] all unsubstantiated theories.

The process of oncosis reveals the mechanism of action of detergent substrates on fatty tissue.[6] Oncosis differs from the term *necrosis* as the method of cell death in that necrosis describes what happens to cells only after death. The process of oncosis, a term revived by cellular pathologists in 1995, was originally described by von Recklinghausen in 1910. The term *oncosis* is based on the Greek word for swelling, *onkos*. This process is usually seen after an anoxic event, which can be precipitated by an infarct or by a sudden cutoff of cellular oxygen. Clinically, the process is usually a regional one, localized to the affected tissue. It is characterized by sudden onset of profound cellular swelling and subsequent formation of blebs or mechanical insults in the cell wall, which cause an increase in membrane permeability. A sharp drop in regional pH is seen in the region caused by cellular oxygen deprivation. There is a subsequent shift to anaerobic glycogen metabolism. Glycolysis produces lactic acid, which in severely ischemic tissues is unable to be removed because of the lack of local circulation. If local circulation is restored at this point, cell death does not occur. If cellular respiration is not restored, lysosomes leak hydrolase into the favorable acid environment, causing further damage to the cell membrane. Irreversible cell destruction continues as the cell wall undergoes lysis. The detergent effect of sodium deoxycholate histologically creates the appearance of moth eaten holes in the adipocyte membranes[7] immediately upon injection, perhaps promoting the lysosome hydrolase activity. Although the cells can repair small areas of membrane injury, larger areas of damage create an irreparable cascade of events leading to cell death.[8]

Subsequent loss of mitochondria function, with subsequent insufficient adenosine triphosphate reduces cell functioning, sodium-potassium ion pump activity, and further regional swelling. Cellular and soft-tissue swelling reduce local circulation, with closing pressure of venules leading to the no-reflow phenomenon, as is seen in tissue affected by the sudden failure of venous circulation in a free flaps.[9] Profound localized swelling creates an opportunity for extensive fat necrosis and even overlying skin loss is at risk (see later discussion).

Apoptosis

Claims of an apoptotic mechanism of cell death following PC/DC injections began with Peckitt in 2006,[3] who describes a complex caspase cascade. Apoptosis is an important means of regulating cell populations and is characterized by noninflammatory cell shrinkage followed by phagocytosis. Studies performed in Regensburg[10] tested tissue injected with a phosphatidylcholine/deoxycholate formula for apoptotic markers, which were found to be present. The process of apoptosis, characterized by noninflammatory shrinkage of affected cells, does not clinically or histologically correlate with the tissue reaction generated by deoxycholate injection. Furthermore, as of this writing (Bechara FG, unpublished data, 2011) there is unpublished experimental data to support a lytic, nonapoptotic mechanism of PC/DC induced cell death.

Two types of cell death can be seen following a single subcutaneous injection of a toxic substance.[11] Histologically, the region that stains pink under a hematoxylin and eosin (H&E) preparation indicates death by oncosis. Karyolytic nuclei are another oncotic marker. At the periphery of the region of coagulation necrosis, along the margin of live and dead cells, the occasional histologic presence of half moon nuclei marking apoptotic cell death is observed. These cells are few, and are only noted at the edge of the much larger region of oncotic tissue. If an apoptotic index (ratio of counted oncolytic dead cells vs apoptotic dead cells per hundred dead cells) is counted, the index is quite low (0 to 3 cells per 100) depending entirely on the region counted. Apoptosis is, by definition, a nonmassive reaction. The only current reproducible method of generating large regions of apoptosis is the repeated freezing and thawing of regional tissue, as is seen in cryolipolysis.

Although causative factors may vary, oncosis is generally induced by situations producing anoxia; whereas, apoptosis is either programmed because of cell signaling or by thermal shock. Histologic evaluation of detergent injected fat can clearly define both. Along with swelling, oncosis is accompanied by the presence of inflammation, specifically a neutrophilic infiltrate, and a later migration of macrophages in to the region.

IDENTIFICATION OF LYTIC AGENT

Deoxycholate was initially isolated from PC in 2004 and identified as the predominant lytic agent in the PC/DC formulation.[1] Early literature supporting the role of DC as the lytic agent has been independently supported by a stem cell study performed by numerous studies.[12] Occasionally, publications persist the notions that phosphatidylcholine is the active agent in PC/DC treatments.[13,14] The difficulty in identifying the true lytic agent is that phosphatidylcholine is not significantly water soluble and therefore isolation of PC in water-based cell lysis experimental models have been technically difficult to reproduce.[15–22] This problem was solved by identifying an inert solvent that was used to isolate PC as a single agent.[23] The study performed at the McGowan research institute in Pittsburgh isolated PC, as well as other common constituents of Lipostabil and compounded PC/DC mixtures, to determine cytotoxicity and lipolytic activity of each constituent, using cultured adipocytes derived from stem cells. Cytotoxicity was calculated using lactate dehydrogenase and oil red O. Lipolytic activity (as opposed to cell lysis,

lipolysis maintains cell integrity) was measured using a glycerol and triglyceride assay. The measure of permanent destruction of adipocytes is important, as many lipolytic agents only cause temporary egress of glycerol and triglyceride, and therefore only temporary results can be achieved. **Table 1** shows the absence of any lytic activity by isolated PC and the results of the lysis assays. The only agent that causes adipolysis in a standard Lipostabil formula, or compounded PC/DC formulation, is sodium deoxycholate.

UTILITY OF DC ALONE VERSUS PC/DC

Phosphatidylcholine, a phospholipid comprising a significant percentage of mammalian cell membranes, lacks detergent or adipolytic activity, as previously discussed; it would be counterintuitive to think that a substance that comprises most of the biphospholipid structure of a cell membrane could induce membrane disintegration.

There is great variation in the degree of tissue response, the dispersion of adipocyte lysis, and the onset of cell reaction between PC/DC and DC formulations. Previous studies have demonstrated that subcutaneous injection of deoxycholate and PC/DC both produce localized inflammatory reactions, with DC (**Fig. 1**) appearing to produce more inflammation and cell lysis compared with PC/DC mixtures. Much if not all of these differences can be accounted for the fact that PC has an apparent buffering effect upon DC, thereby minimizing inflammation/tissue

Table 1
Qualitative levels of adipolysis after incubation with various agents

Test Solution	Adipocyte Cell Lysis Obtained with this Solution
PC50/DC42	++
Deoxycholate 1.0%	+++
Deoxycholate 2.4%	+++
Phosphatidylcholine 5.0% in mineral oil	0
Isuprel 0.08% injectable	0
Local anesthetic 5.0%	0
Saline 0.9% (control)	0
Benzyl alcohol	0

PC in isolation from DC does not cause adipolysis (fat cell lysis) or lipolysis (triglyceride breakdown). These data are the first to experimentally confirm prior deductions that PC will not reduce fat without DC.

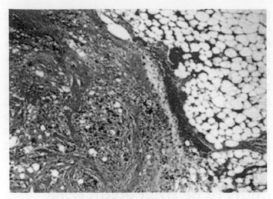

Fig. 1. Histologic findings of an excised lipoma 48 hours after subcutaneous infiltration with DC (1%), revealing a well-demarcated area of acute inflammation, extravasated erythrocytes, and necrosis adjacent to unaffected adipose tissue (hematoxylin and eosin, original magnification x10).

damage. This theory has been supported by recent experimental data, which demonstrates attenuation of DC LD_{50} (the concentration of a substance at which 50% of cells die) by the addition of PC. Additional studies reveal that PC/DC combinations produce more dispersion (**Figs. 2, 3**) relative to DC alone. As increasing concentrations of deoxycholate are introduced into PC/DC combinations, the onset of adipocyte lysis is hastened.

Isolated deoxycholate as well as PC/DC combinations reduce localized fat, and when injected with correct technique, are safe and efficacious. Clinical indications should direct which one of these compounds should be used for each condition. When a small, localized fatty deposit is present and near total removal is the desired outcome, DC alone (at 1% or less) would be indicated. The best illustration of this would be treatment of submental fat (**Fig. 4**), bra strap fat, and lipomas. When a broader region is the target, some clinicians add PC thinking that it permits a more even dispersion of the solution. If a large, broad, or thick region of fat is the desired treatment region, some clinicians increase the PC/DC ratio to 1:<1 to minimize the PC-induced cholinergic side effects or significantly dilute PC/DC solutions. The thought that PC is inert, or perhaps even a buffer that inhibits the lytic

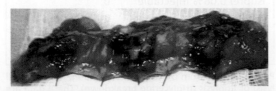

Fig. 2. Dispersion pattern, sodium deoxycholate 42 mg/mL at 10 minutes.

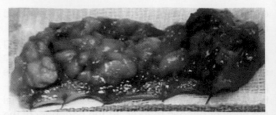

Fig. 3. Dispersion pattern, PC 50 mg/mL and DC 42 mg/mL at 10 minutes.

activity of DC motivates most clinicians to consider using DC formula without PC, at low concentrations.

TISSUE SPECIFICITY OF DEOXYCHOLATE

In cell cultures, a significant, dose-dependent nonspecific toxic effect of deoxycholate, as well as formulas containing PC/DC, has been reported (**Fig. 5**). Adipocytes, melanoma cells, skeletal muscle cells, keratinocytes, and fibroblasts are more or less uniformly destroyed with DC, although keratinocytes appear to be more susceptible to DC relative to the others.

In an effort to track the body's processing of injected DC radioisotope-labeled DC was injected into the fat pads of mice. Almost half of the DC injected was transported to the intestinal tract within 24 hours of injection into fat tissue. A peak accumulation in the small intestine was noted at 4 hours, and at 5 days, the remaining DC was eliminated in the feces.[21]

Several mechanisms are theorized to account for why DC injections (and similarly PC/DC) are not completely ablative to all surrounding tissue. It has been determined, using albumin in the experimental model, that protein is protective of adipocytes to the cell lytic effects of DC. Investigators demonstrated that albumin neutralizes or binds DC in nonadipose tissue, given the lack of tissue damage seen by endogenous DC (ie, present in the gut and circulatory system).[21] Nevertheless, skin necrosis following direct dermal or superficial subcutaneous injections with PC/DC has been reported and is attributable to deoxycholate because no other active ingredients in the formula have been identified.

Another group of investigators tested the effect of intra-neural injections of 0.1 mL of Lipostabil into the left posterior tibial nerve of 10 rats.[24] Ten other rats were injected with a saline control in the same region. The rats were observed on a walking track for 21 days. No statistically significant clinical signs of nerve damage were noted. At 21 days the animals were sacrificed and the treated and control nerves were subjected to

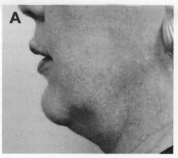
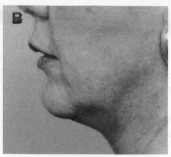

Fig. 4. Patient profile (*A*) before and (*B*) 2 months after 5 monthly injection sessions with 1.0 mL of DC (1%) into the submental fat.

histologic examination and also to electron microscopy. Grossly and histologically (including H&E as well as electron microscopy), the treated and nontreated nerves looked similar with surprisingly minimal inflammation.

One of the early studies of the detergent effects of sodium deoxycholate showed that in vitro, porcine fat and muscle was ablated by high-dose (5%) DC, as well as PC/DC (5.0%/2.5%) injection.[1] Further, Thuangtong and colleagues[21] showed a cytotoxic response in cell culture by 4 different cell types to PC/DC. Jancke[24] also found that Lipostabil had dose-related cytolytic effects on adipose tissue, vascular smooth muscle cells, renal epithelial cells, and myocytes. Schuller-Petrovic[25] found that injection of subcutaneous fat in rats caused fibrosis in cutaneous muscle, with partial muscle loss. Changes were reported to be dose related. Cytotoxic necrosis was noted in both adipose tissue and in the walls of adjacent blood vessels. The visible histologic progression of events that occurs following detergent injections is well documented.[26,27] Depending on the

agent used, gradually inflammation and subsequent cell membrane rupture, or immediate cell wall lysis (with deoxycholate) can be seen. The presence of foamy macrophages is noted with both DC and PC/DC.

The takeaway lesson from all studies should be that when injecting PC/DC or DC alone for the purpose of fat reduction, the injector should be keenly aware of the location of the tip of the needle. Only subcutaneous injections not adjacent to skin or muscle will be safely tolerated. As DC effects are clearly dose related, a lower dose (concentration and volume) of DC per injection site will reduce the risk of undesired sequelae.

CELL SIGNALING AND CYTOKINES

Not only is there signaling within the damaged adipocytes but also messages among cells. Bechara[28] has studied the influence of TNF-A and cytokines. Seven subjects with lipomas were treated with Lipostabil. Analysis of biopsy specimens noted upregulated levels of tumor necrosis factor (TNF)-a, as well as interleukin (IL)-4, IL-6, and IL-10, which are proinflammatory cytokines, in the early postinjection phase. TNF-a is cited as the mediator of the immediate and visible histamine response, noted as immediate and sometimes profound swelling, erythema, and regional warmth and discomfort. No increase in IL-2, IL-5, and eosinophilic granulocytes was noted. Occasionally, macrophages can become killer cells when appropriately signaled. The elevated TNF-a levels signal macrophages to bind to receptors on a target adipocyte, and will induce apoptosis. As macrophages are also involved in phagocytosis of necrotic cells, the presence of apoptotic fat cells along the periphery of the lipolytic reaction can be explained as TNF-a generated.[29]

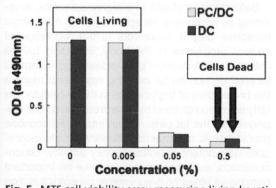

Fig. 5. MTS cell viability assay measuring living keratinocytes exposed to phosphatidylcholine/deoxycholate and deoxycholate. Absorbance (OD) is directly related to cell viability. Increasing concentration of either PC/DC or DC alone produces cell death. DC alone profoundly reduces cell viability, with PC producing minimal effect.

REGULATORY ISSUES

The development of new technologies is usually begun as an in vitro process in the laboratory, followed by animal testing, and then by FDA submission and subsequent clinical trials. Although the time from research initiation to FDA approval is usually 3 to 5 years for devices (or less), depending on their regulatory path, drugs have a much longer (5–10+ years) and more costly testing and approval process. Although the FDA has approved many fillers as devices, review by the FDA[30] has clearly designated phosphatidylcholine and deoxycholate as drugs. According to the FDA a substance is considered a drug if the purpose of the substance is to change the structure or function of an animal or human.[29] The chemical, even though found in endogenous tissue, is also considered a drug if administered exogenously. According to Rittes, personal communications, August 2010, Sanofi Aventis, the manufacturers of Lipostabil in Brazil, declined to seek National Health Surveillance Agency (ANVISA, the Brazilian equivalent of the FDA) approval for use of their formula for reducing subcutaneous fat. In fact, the company issued a statement that it did not support the use of the drug for this purpose. Moreover, use of Lipostabil is off-label *only* in countries where Lipostabil is approved for other indications (ie, for dyslipidemia, angina). Any combination of PC with DC or DC alone is *not off-label* in the United States, because these have not been approved for any other indication.

Currently, almost all of PC/DC, the most popular injected formula worldwide, is being compounded in the United States and, in select European countries, compounded or used in the form of Lipostabil, the pharmaceutical medication. However, according to its package insert, the manufacturer does not support the use of subcutaneous injections of Lipostabil.[31] Because of the extremely high cost of new drug development and lack of patent protection, existing phosphatidylcholine/deoxycholate combinations have not found a pharmaceutical developer.

KYTHERA Biopharmaceuticals (Calabasas, California), is currently seeking approval for a deoxycholate-based fat-reducing formula for submental fat; as of this writing, they are entering phase III (the last phase of clinical drug development) outside the United States and entering phase IIb (dose and tolerability testing) in the United States. KYTHERA Biopharmaceutical is seeking regulatory approval in the United States and worldwide for a low-dose (1% or less DC) formulation called ATX-101. This strategy is consistent with the experiences of experienced injectors, which suggests that low-dose formulations of PC/DC or DC alone is a prudent approach to yield gratifying results while minimizing risks. The company has sublicensed the sale and marketing of ATX-101 to Intendis (Berlin, Germany, a subsidiary of Bayer HealthCare) outside the United States. As previously noted, the results of registration studies will ultimately determine the fate of ATX-101.

Lithera, Inc (San Diego, CA, USA) is developing a novel injectable combination of a steroid plus a beta-adrenergic agent, also for fat localized (see details later). Completion of rigorous clinical testing and regulatory approval will determine if any of these companies are successful at marketing their products and making it into clinics throughout the world.

LIPOLYSIS

LIPO-102 is a novel injectable treatment created by Lithera, Inc and currently in registration trials to achieve local, selective fat-tissue reduction (termed according to the company "injection lipoplasty").[32] Using FDA-registered drugs proven safe and effective in other indications, LIPO-102 targets and stimulates natural fat metabolism to produce nonablative, nonsurgical fat-tissue reduction in specific locations. In clinical testing, using sophisticated imaging technology (Canfield Vectra analysis) weekly injections of LIPO-102 for 4 to 8 weeks produce significant reductions in abdominal circumference and volume.

LIPO-102 is a combination of salmeterol xinafoate and fluticasone propionate. Salmeterol xinafoate is a highly selective, long-acting β_2-adrenergic receptor agonist. Fluticasone propionate is a synthetic trifluorinated glucocorticoid. The two drug products currently under development are formulated as either sterile solutions or as separate lyophiles. The single-use, sterile, preservative-free solutions will be mixed and diluted with saline if necessary, to form LIPO-102.

Salmeterol xinafoate is a highly selective, long-acting β_2-adrenergic receptor agonist. Adrenergic receptors play a major role in the regulation of several processes in the body, including fat-cell metabolism. Activation of β_2-adrenergic receptors located on human fat cells by salmeterol triggers the breakdown of triglycerides in these cells to free fatty acids and glycerol by means of lipolysis (no adipolysis, as the fat cells remain intact). Fluticasone propionate is a synthetic trifluorinated glucocorticoid with potent antiinflammatory activity. Glucocorticoids, such as fluticasone, have an important permissive effect on β-adrenergic receptor function in vivo. Glucocorticoids enhance β-adrenergic receptor-mediated responses by regulating the coupling of β-adrenergic receptors to G proteins and the resulting activation of adenylate cyclase and by preventing downregulation of β-adrenergic receptors caused by chronic receptor stimulation (eg, by salmeterol). In simpler terms, salmetorol stimulates lipolysis through activation of β_2-adrenergic receptors on fat cells and fluticasone upregulates the cellular machinery/pathways turned on by salmeterol.

OTHER PC/DC FORMULATIONS IN USE WORLDWIDE

Amipharm's (Seoul, Korea) PC/DC formulation, Lipobean, is approved by the Korean FDA for use in treating hepatic coma, yet commonly used off-label in the country for localized fat reduction.[33] The brand name is based upon the source of phosphatidylcholine, the soybean. The formulation consists of PC 50 mg/mL and DC 24 mg/mL, similar to Lipostabil available in the United Kingdom. Standard practice in Korea is to dilute each 5 mL vial with 5 mL of normal saline, thus achieving a concentration of PC 25/DC 12. The solution is well tolerated, as swelling and postinjection discomfort is not as profound as with PC 50/DC 42, the United States standard compounding pharmacy ratio (with higher DC).

Charlatan use of any drug can cause widespread problems resulting in a bad reputation of an otherwise effective treatment. As long as there is unregulated availability of injectable lipolytics online, this will be a continuing problem and will cause damage to the reputation of any effective formulation. A recent report notes complications following self-injected Lipostabil,[34] which is easily available to any person wishing to purchase it online.[35–37] The target audience for many of these websites is bodybuilders who cannot achieve definition in diet-resistant and exercise-resistant areas. With no medical evaluation or supervised treatment, as well as in some cases, self-treatment by patients alone, abuse of these medication may continue.

REGIONAL GLOBAL EXPERIENCE

The routine use of targeted fat-reducing injections varies throughout the world. Viewpoints vary widely from country to country. The procedure remains banned in Brazil[38] and is forbidden in Turkey because of patient complications following charlatan use.[39] In Europe, injection lipolysis remains popular in Austria as well as in Germany,[40] and is quietly practiced in the United Kingdom.[41] According to Dr Mark Palmer, a UK physician, only German-produced Lipostabil is approved, but for the purposes of medical, intravenous use only. Although possible to use in an off-label manner, there are significant risks and a degree of medical-legal complexity in the importation and use of this product for aesthetic purposes.

Asian countries see much more use as Asian patients try to avoid a surgical approach if at all possible. The popularity of the procedure has declined dramatically in the United States after the collapse of several chains of providers in 2007 and 2008, but according to the Network Lipolysis, more than 12,000 treatments were performed in 2009.[23]

In Korea, injection adipolysis is reported to be more popular than Botox injections, although this is anecdotal. Amipharm sells approximately 115,000 vials of Lipobean per month, and this number has seen a dramatic recent increase despite the current recession or perhaps because of it. Korean practitioners attribute the popularity of injection adipolysis to its cost effectiveness, efficacy, and the Asian ethnic antipathy toward surgical incisions of any kind. There is a high cultural acceptance of cosmetic procedures in Korea, but the results must look natural and not extreme. Their product is approved by the Korean FDA for use in treating hepatic coma, so the use of PC/DC is therefore considered off-label.

Amipharm's largest customer is an obesity clinic that routinely administers these injections. After dilution of their 5.0% PC/2.4% DC formulation with 5 mL saline, the final injected ratio of PC/DC ratio is 2.5% PC/ 1.2% DC. Compounded medication is illegal in Korea, so the practice of PC/DC is limited to the use of Lipobean. According to the largest Korean obesity clinic chain, 365 MC, the most common treatment region is the abdomen. There is a marked difference in body mass index of the average Korean patient versus the average American patient. In most Koreans, the surface area and depth of fat pad is small, and therefore is more amenable to treatment with PC/DC. Patients at the obesity clinic report high satisfaction with treatment in the abdominal region, arms, thighs, and also the submental chin.

CLINICAL PRACTICE

The preface to this section is that there is no absolute standard of injection for injectable fat-reducing methods. The authors' guidelines are based on their experience only, not from registration study guidelines, which ultimately are the most appropriate guidelines to follow, should any of these medications be approved. Furthermore, the authors' experiences are based on medications legally available through compounding pharmacies. The authors suggest that clinicians interested in using fat reducing medications strongly consider waiting until an FDA approved pharmaceutical medication becomes available. State laws and local practices determine the indemnity risks associated with using compounding medications and 'standard of care,' respectively.

The best indication for treatment of a region with injection lipolysis or adipolysis is reduction of small, localized, regions of soft, not fibrous fat. Although broader regions of fat can be treated, results are not as dramatic after a single treatment. Multiple treatments of larger areas are often necessary. It is optimal to use a more dilute formulation in larger areas, both to reduce side effects and to minimize post-treatment swelling.

Experience from both authors has been generally positive. One author (DD) has performed several thousand patient treatments since 2004, and has observed it to be an excellent noninvasive treatment for the reduction of small focal areas of subcutaneous fat, especially associated with moderate skin tightening. It is particularly useful for facial contouring and volume reduction, especially for jowl reduction and jawline contouring. This procedure can have a hugely rejuvenating effect on patients' aging face and can delay or prevent the need for a more invasive intervention. The other author (AMR) has been using PC/DC and DC formulations since 2003, primarily in clinical trial and experimental laboratory settings, but has similarly found its benefits along the jawline and submental region gratifying.

Dr Duncan has used normal saline as the diluents, with the dilution with a dilution of PC 25 mg/mL, DC 12 mg/mL for the past 4 years; this ratio has minimized discomfort and produced a tolerable procedure. Similarly, Dr Rotunda uses a dilute formulation, approximately 0.75% DC (formulated with 3:1 ratio of 1% DC and 1% lidocaine without epinephrine). Most patients require 2 or 3 treatments for facial contouring. These formulations are particularly effective for defining the mandibular angle, jawline, and reducing submental fat. The results appear to be permanent and it is also highly useful for the reduction of small, localized subcutaneous areas of fat and volume in other body areas, including the chin, neck, inner knees, and inner and outer thighs where other more invasive treatment options may be unsuitable or avoidable. A volume of 0.5 mL (PC/DC) should be injected subcutaneously at a spacing of approximately 1.5-cm intervals into areas needing volume reduction or 0.2 mL per 1-cm space for the DC-only formulation. Areas where patients would not benefit from volume reduction or that need volume augmentation should be carefully avoided. A reduced volume of 0.2 to 0.3 mL (PC/DC) per injection should be used in areas close to areas of insufficient volume, such as nasolabial mounds lateral to the nasolabial fold, to avoid spread into the valley of the fold itself. With all adipolytic treatments, success outcome depends on success recovery; Dr Duncan treats every 8 weeks, Dr Rotunda treats every 4 to 6 weeks. For patients receiving jowls and marionette treatment, the wait period can be at least 10 weeks because overcorrection in these areas is difficult to repair.

In the upper face, small volumes of 0.05 to 0.1 mL per injection can be used, injected just subcutaneously, to successfully treat redundancy and skin laxity the malar areas, although these areas are prone to significant swelling, therefore the physician should proceed with caution and patients should be advised to expect that multiple treatments will be needed to obtain successful results.

In more than 6 to 7 years of clinical practice of these techniques and many thousands of patient treatments, the authors have not seen any adverse effect other than the expected temporary minor swelling and focal tenderness; therefore, it is one of the safest cosmetic medical interventions that the authors provide to their patients.

Basic Technique

Depth of injection is extremely important. The effect of these injections is a local one; the solution only diffuses in a 1- to 2-cm radius, depending on the volume and dose of the injection. Lower-face and neck injections are generally performed using a 6-mm depth meso needle and 13-mm BD needle (BD, Franklin Lakes, NJ, USA) injected halfway. It is not wise to use a longer needle as multiple injections are needed, and guesstimates of needle depth are often incorrect. One author (AR) uses a 30-gauge needle, although the other author (DD) prefers a 27-gauge needle, with the thought that high resistance to injection is encountered and therefore difficulty in determining whether dermis or fat is being injected. It is best to pinch the skin thereby lifting the fat from the deeper connective tissue, and thereafter inject the solution into the pinched tissue (pinch and prick).

The volume of each injection should be 0.1 to 0.6 mL to obtain the best dispersion with the fewest skip areas. Larger volumes have been shown to track up to the skin or deeper toward fascia. Smaller volumes are recommended as treatment regions become more superficial. The distance between injections is not recommended to exceed 1.5 cm. If injection sites are about 1 in, or 2.5 cm apart, skip areas are noted and the result can be lumpy.

COMPLICATIONS AND ADVERSE EVENTS

The rate of reported complications has dramatically decreased since the wane in popularity of

Lipodissolve. Safety issues persist, however, because of the lack of understanding of the physiologic basis of action of the injections, upper limits of dose (volume and concentration), lack of standardized formulation and pharmaceutical-grade preparations. Swelling can be profound and is an anticipated, unavoidable side effect. The anoxia caused by swelling is a trigger for oncotic induction of cell death. Cells not immediately killed by a direct chemical effect are affected by local swelling and external pressure on adipocyte circulation. Extracellular fluid accumulates and causes a jellylike consistency of treated tissue. Regions that already have poor circulation, such as distal extremities, and regions that have undergone previous surgery are at high risk for skin loss or extreme fat necrosis. Localized areas that have had aggressive liposuction may not be able to swell because of fibrosis of the subcutaneous compartment. In fact, a compartment syndrome can occur if swelling is prevented. Cases of skin loss and draining of liquefied necrotic fat have been reported in instances of previous inner-thigh liposuction, wearing of tight compression garments post-treatment, and even by patients wearing tight jeans following injection. Because of the marked temporary swelling deformity, many patients are reluctant to undergo more than 1 injection session, and may request that a large surface area or multiple regions be treated at one time. Published guidelines recommend limiting treatment to a region no larger than 12 × 15 cm if bilateral. Clinicians should not inject multiple regions (ie, abdomen, flanks, hips), unless quite small (ie, chin and jowls). The total dose of PC should not exceed 2500 mg, and further limiting this dose will reduce postinjection cholinergic side effects (nausea, vomiting, diarrhea), which can be accomplished by diluting the injected solution by as much as 50%. Further, dilution may markedly affect the efficacy of treatments. One author (AR) uses DC only and has not had patients experience cholinergic side effects; in fact, AR treats submental fat, jowls, and lipomas only.

Avoiding postinjection compression garments will decrease the risk of focal skin loss. Other more common causes of skin necrosis include intradermal or immediate subdermal injection, injecting the same site twice, and injection with a Mesorelle-type multiple needle device. Not commonly available in the United States, Mesorelle (BMA Biomedia, Italy) injection devices are widely used in Europe and Asia. The 3- to 5-needle attachment to a syringe theoretically reduces the number of times that patients feel a needle, and also reduces the number of times the physician makes an injection. However, safety of injections is greatly dependent on maintaining a uniform depth of injection. When tissue is injected, a curved surface rather than a flat surface is usually present. Therefore, the central tissue is injected at a deeper level than the peripheral tissue. A case report of focal skin loss in a male flank resulting from a Mesorelle-aided injection attests to the wisdom of avoiding their use.

A specific needle length is advised when performing injections. It is almost impossible to insert a long needle only part way into the tissue at a consistent depth. One author (DD) prefers 6-mm, 27-gauge meso needles for the face; whereas, 10-mm and 13-mm needles can be used when treating other body parts. Another author (AR) uses 13-mm BD, 30 gauge uniformly on the face and neck. It is unwise to use a needle too short (4 mm), or even a 13-mm needle in patients with thinner fat deposits. Again, the pinch-and-prick method (gently pinching the skin and injecting the pinched tissue) is recommended. Case reports of intramuscular injection with resultant fibrotic nodules and restriction of range of motion have been attributed to the use of a 13-mm needle for injections in a thin woman's thighs. A 4-mm needle has been reported to cause focal skin loss in a patient who received multiple superficial injections by a practitioner of mesotherapy.

Volume of injections also influences the safety profile. Dispersion studies show pooling and migration of fluid volumes more than 0.6 mL when injections are spaced 1.5 cm apart. On the other hand, injecting 1 mL of solution 2.5 cm apart is not encouraged, as a large volume of solution can migrate down to fascia, collect as a firm persistent subcutaneous nodule, or if placed too superficial, into the dermis. If the distance between injections is too great, skip areas are seen, and contour irregularities may result.

Other complications include hyperpigmentation, persistent nodules of focal fat necrosis, contour irregularities, and less-than-hoped-for fat reduction. Hyperpigmentation has been attributed to hemosiderin deposition, and is temporary in many cases. However, permanent discoloration of the treatment region can occur, and it typically does not respond to hydroquinone or kojic acid. Neovascularization of treatment regions can also occur, especially in areas with circulatory compromise. The formation of blood vessels under the skin of a treatment region does respond to intense pulsed light but damage to a previously unblemished skin surface generates significant unhappiness in these patients.

CONTRAINDICATIONS

No children under 18 years of age are treated. Patients who are breastfeeding are asked to wait to be treated for 6 weeks after they cease lactating. This procedure is not meant to be a rapid weight-loss program. Therefore, patients who are obese are not treated. No treatments should be performed for the purpose of breast reduction. Clearly, an allergy to soy products or other formula components, such as benzyl alcohol, is a contraindication to treatment with the injections when PC is incorporated in the formula. If in doubt, a small patch test can be done 1 week before the anticipated treatment. Most injectors do not treat patients who are diabetic, especially in the distal extremities. Microangiopathy and vascular insufficiency are also contraindications. Although Lipostabil is licensed in Germany for intravenous use in cases of coronary artery compromise, many physicians avoid treating patients who are hypertensive and cardiac. Patients with severe chronic illness should not be injected, especially those who are immunocompromised. It is not wise to treat patients with autoimmune disease, especially those with scleroderma. Two exceptions to this guideline are patients with Hashimoto's thyroiditis and rheumatoid arthritis. Many of these patients have been treated with good results and few post-injection problems. Although some physicians avoid treating patients who are HIV positive, many other patients get adequate results injecting the buffalo hump that frequently occurs with HIV medication. The majority of physicians avoid injecting patients on blood thinners, such as warfarin sodium (Coumadin) or clopidogrel bisulfate (Plavix). Although some avoid treating patients taking nonsteroidal antiinflammatory drugs, most do not see their use as an absolute contraindication. Patients on chemotherapy should not be treated until their immune system has recovered. Those on prednisone or another steroid regimen should also defer treatment with this technique. Local skin conditions may preclude treatments with any cutaneous injections. An ulcer or infection near the treatment region should negate treatment. Many respondents do not treat patients with active eczema or psoriasis.

Unrealistic expectations are also a relative contraindication to treatment. This treatment results in subtle improvement, not total elimination, of the localized fatty accumulation. An average of about 5% of patients do not respond to treatment, although with careful patient selection and proper dose, spacing, and injection depth, the great majority of treated patients will have some visible improvement. If patients are noncompliant or show up for only 1 treatment, they will not be satisfied with the outcome. Also, those patients who will not adhere to a diet and exercise plan and see the injections as a quick fix will be poor candidates for this treatment.

NEW USES AND CASE EXAMPLE

The new clinical use that has developed in the injectable fat loss arena is that of a redundant tissue and contour problem solver. When combined with collagenase, PC/DC injections or DC alone can be used to reduce contour irregularities following liposuction, and to reduce protrusions and adjacent depressed scars (**Fig. 6**).

Correction of a contour irregularity with these nonsurgical formulations can frequently produce a better result than revision surgery can (**Fig. 7**). By injecting the scar itself at multiple levels with collagenase 250 units/mL (Masterpharm, Richmond Hills, NY, USA), the tethering effect of the scar upon the surrounding tissue is reduced. Collagenase is enzymatically specific for collagen only; it has no effect on adipose tissue. The adjacent protrusions of fat are injected with PC/DC or DC, thereby serving as a combination technique. Tapering doses at the periphery of the protuberance will improve results; larger protrusions are injected with slightly more of the adipolytic agent, and minor protrusions with less. Some visible

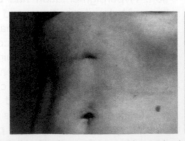 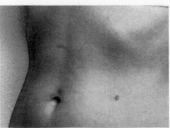

Fig. 6. (*Left*) Patient following liposuction with residual depressed laparoscopic cholecystectomy scar. (*Right*) Six weeks following injection at base of scar with 0.2 mL collagenase and PC/DC.

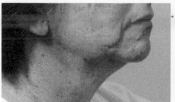
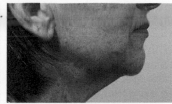

Fig. 7. A 53-year-old woman with dog bite scar along her right marionette line, with ptotic marionette fold. Improvement at 2 weeks following injection with 0.2 mL PC/DC centrally and 0.3 mL collagenase at base of scar. Ulthera microfocused ultrasound the same day.

effects can be seen as early as 3 days because of the rapidity with which collagenase works.

Another excellent use for adipolysis is nonsurgical contouring of small regions in combination with other treatments, such as microfocused-fractionated ultrasound (**Fig. 8**). The combination treatment resulted in good correction of the volume excess and redundancy in the lower face and neck region.

A third potential niche indication for injection adipolysis is focal skin tightening, although there is some unpublished data demonstrating DC alone as having minimal effect on submental skin laxity. An example of potential use for this treatment is residual periumbilical laxity following abdominoplasty. Many women who have had children have

the most extreme stretch and subsequent skin damage in the midline periumbilical region. This problem can be treated as a standalone process, or it can be combined with abdominoplasty. If combined, it is best to wait at least 3 months after abdominoplasty to allow most of the swelling resolve. A small amount of fat must be present underneath the lax skin in order for this process to be effective. The following case illustrates this point.

A 37-year-old woman underwent an abdominoplasty with initial good results. She returned 8 months postoperatively complaining of loose skin in the supraumbilical region and some periumbilical edema, a problem that is not uncommon, as many patients with postpartum deformities have striae

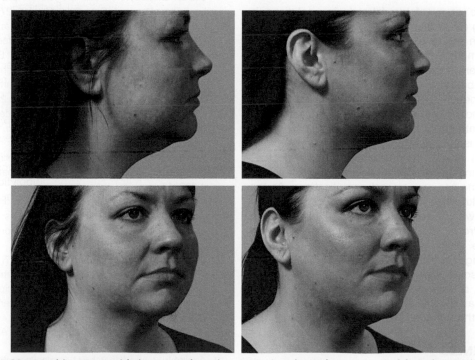

Fig. 8. A 38-year-old patient with heavy neck and a ptotic face beset by gravity and heredity. Eight weeks following combination treatment of adipolysis with PC/DC followed by Ulthera (Mesa, Arizona) microfocused ultrasound in the neck and lower face.

and damaged skin the periumbilical region. Women tend to develop a guitar-shaped region of lipodystrophy during and after childbearing. Unless liposuction accompanies the abdominoplasty, many patients are likely to have a mild postabdominoplasty residual of central lipodystrophy and loose, sometimes pendulous skin. Dermolipectomy and liposuction will not correct damaged skin that exists preoperatively. Even if patients understand this, patient may still express this postoperatively. It is difficult to surgically improve this situation, as a purse-string type suture around the umbilicus does not look aesthetically attractive. Excision of skin above the umbilicus can be done, but unless the problem is minimal, residual laxity or a vertical scar may result. A nonsurgical solution to this problem can be achieved with injection adipolysis. After the treatment region is delineated, a grid marking injection sites 1 cm apart is drawn. Injection depth is superficial, about 6 mm. Injection volume per site is 0.2 mL of PC 50/DC 42 is used. The region will profoundly swell immediately after injection, and may take 8 to 10 weeks for the early improvement to be seen. Care must be taken during the injection process to make sure the needle tip is in the subcutaneous layer and is not intradermal because skin loss can occur.

SUMMARY

The use of injectable fat-reducing solutions is evolving as we learn more about the mechanisms of action and more about the risks and limitations of treatment. When the process was first created, there were no apparent boundaries or limitations. Both laboratory research and clinical research and experience have contributed greatly to the compendium of knowledge regarding direct injectable treatment of fatty deposits.

Because of the initial lack of approved formulations in many countries, unscientific cocktail compounds were used, causing adverse sequelae and some serious regional complications. As the field of knowledge widens, and speculation is replaced with science, the industry is expected to grow. Proper research and development has led to safe and effective formulations that are emerging. After the sudden rise of popularity of Lipodissolve was followed by an equally rapid demise, a secondary slower growth phase is expected as lipolytic and adipolytic compounds are carried through the FDA regulatory process.

REFERENCES

1. Rotunda A, Suzuki H, Moy RL, et al. Detergent effects of sodium deoxycholate are a major feature of an injectable phosphatidylcholine formulation used for localized fat dissolution. Dermatol Surg 2004;30:1001–8.
2. Duncan DI, Rubin JP, Golitz L, et al. Refinement of techniques in injection lipolysis based on scientific studies and clinical evaluation. Clin Plast Surg 2009;36:195–209.
3. Peckitt N. Evidence-based practice. Yorkshire (UK): Jeremy Mills Publishing; 2005.
4. Hasengschwandtner F. Injection lipolysis for effective reduction of localized fat in the place of minor lipoplasty. Aesthet Surg J 2006;26:125–30.
5. LeCoz J. Traite de mesotherapie. Paris: Masson; 2004.
6. Majno G, Joris I. Cell death: oncosis and apoptosis. Cellular pathology. New York: Oxford University Press; 2004.
7. Duncan DI. Injection lipolysis as a problem solver. Presented at the Florida State Society of Plastic Surgery. Naples, December 5, 2007.
8. Duncan DI. Injection lipolysis for body contouring. Body contouring. Heidelberg: Springer; 2010.
9. Calhoun KH, Tan L, Seikaly H. An integrated theory of the no-reflow phenomenon and the beneficial effect of vascular washout on no-reflow. Laryngoscope 1999;109:528–35.
10. Klein Silvan M, Schreml Stephan, Nerlich Michael, et al. In vitro studies investigating the effect of subcutaneous phosphatidylcholine injections in the 3T3-L1 adipocyte model: lipolysis or lipid dissolution? Plast Reconstr Surg 2009;124:419–27.
11. Majno G, Joris I. Cell death with shrinkage: apoptosis. Cells, tissues, and disease. New York: Oxford; 2004.
12. Palumbo P, Melchiorre E, La Torre C, et al. Effects of phosphatidylcholine and sodium deoxycholate on human primary adipocytes and fresh human adipose tissue. Int J Immunopathol Pharmacol 2010;23:481–9.
13. Rittes P. The lipodissolve technique: clinical experience. Clin Plast Surg 2009;36:215–21, vi; [discussion: 223–7].
14. Hasengschwandtner F. Phosphatidylcholine treatment to induce lipolysis. J Cosmet Dermatol 2005; 4:308–13.
15. Duncan D, Rubin JP. Cytotoxicity and lipolytic activity of individual injection lipolysis formula components: a stem cell study. IFATS conference. Toulouse, France, October 18, 2008.
16. Laddy S. E-mail document. September 17, 2007.
17. Wang G. Liposomes as drug delivery vehicles. In: Rotunda A, editor. Drug Delivery Principles and Applications. New Jersey: Wiley Interscience; 2005. p. 411–34.
18. Available at: http://answers.ask.com/. Accessed August 18, 2010.
19. Available at: http://search.aol.com/aol/search?query= Wikipedia+micelle&s_it=keyword_rollover. Accessed September 22, 2010.

20. Duncan DI, Hasengschwandtner F. Lipodissolve for subcutaneous fat reduction and skin retraction. Aesthet Surg J 2005;25:530–43.

21. Thuangtong R, Bentow J, Knopp K, et al. Tissue specific effects of injected deoxycholate. Dermatol Surg 2010;36:899–908.

22. Uygur F, Evinc R, Duman H. Is phosphatidylcholine harmful to the peripheral neural tissue? An experimental study in rats. Aesthet Surg J 2008;28:663–7.

23. Duncan DI, Palmer M. Fat reduction using phosphatidylcholine/sodium deoxycholate injections: standard of practice. Aesthetic Plast Surg 2008;32:858–72.

24. Jancke J, Engeli S, Gorzelniak K, et al. Compounds used for "injection lipolysis" destroy adipocytes and other cells found in adipose tissue. Obes Facts 2009;2:36–9.

25. Schuller-Petrovic S, Wolkart G, Hofler G, et al. Tissue-toxic effects of phosphatidylcholine/ deoxycholate after subcutaneous injection for fat dissolution in rats and a human volunteer. Dermatol Surg 2008;34:529–42.

26. Duncan DI, Chubaty R. Clinical safety data and standards of practice for injection lipolysis: a retrospective study. Aesthet Surg J 2006;26:575–85.

27. Bechara F, Skygan M, Kreuter A, et al. Cytokine mRNA levels in human fat tissue after injection lipolysis with phosphatidylcholine and deoxycholate. Arch Dermatol Res 2008;300:455–9.

28. Majno G, Joris I. Cell injury and cell death. Cells, tissues, and disease. New York: Oxford Press; 2004. p. 234.

29. Available at: http://www.fda.gov. Accessed August 10, 2010.

30. Available at: http://www.mesotherapyonline.com. Accessed September 24, 2010.

31. Locke K. Lipo 102. E-mail document. September 17, 2010. Available at: http://www.lithera.com. Accessed December 20, 2011.

32. Jeoung, Eun Sook. Injection lipolysis; the Korean experience. MIPS conference. Seoul, Korea, September 11, 2010.

33. Ono S, Hyakusoku H. Complications after self-injection of hyaluronic acid and phosphatidylcholine for aesthetic purposes. Aesthet Surg J 2006;30:442–7.

34. Melt fat away: burn fat with injection. Available at: http://www.Lipostabil-diy.com/. Accessed August 18, 2010.

35. Available at: http://forum.bodybuilding.com/archive/index.php/t-640146.html. Accessed August 18, 2010.

36. Available at: www.consultdrminas.com/index.php?cnt=3&;sub=3. Accessed August 18, 2010.

37. Available at: www.weightlossresources.com/uk. Accessed August 18, 2010.

38. Available at: www.walesonline.co.uk/news. Accessed September 24, 2010.

39. Available at: www.drwelly.com. Accessed September 24, 2010.

40. Palmer M. E-mail document. 3 October 2010.

41. Available at: http://www.network-lipolysis.com/. Accessed September 24, 2010.

Noninvasive Body Contouring with Radiofrequency, Ultrasound, Cryolipolysis, and Low-Level Laser Therapy

R. Stephen Mulholland, MD, FRCS(C)[a],
Malcolm D. Paul, MD[b],*, Charbel Chalfoun, MD[c]

KEYWORDS

- Body contouring • Noninvasive body contouring
- Nonsurgical liposuction

Key Points

- Discuss current noninvasive body-contouring modalities, including suction massage devices, radiofrequency energy, high-frequency focused ultrasound, cryolipolysis, and low-level light laser therapy devices.
- Discuss imminent technologies awaiting approval by the Food and Drug Administration.
- Review the basic science and clinical effects behind each of these existing and emerging technologies.
- Address patient selection and clinical applications of each modality.
- Discuss the applicability and economics of providing noninvasive lipolysis services in office

---

Noninvasive body contouring is perhaps one of the most alluring areas of esthetic surgery today. Driven by strong public demand for safer procedures with quicker recovery, fewer side effects, and less discomfort, while supported by media attention and economic appeal, new modalities have been developed to address body contouring from a less-invasive perspective. Current surgical options carry the drawbacks of hospitalizations, anesthetics, pain, swelling, and long recovery, as well as inherent risks associated with surgery. Even standard surgical lipectomy methods have progressed from power-assisted liposuction, to ultrasound or laser-assisted modalities, to radiofrequency (RF) methods with a focus on gaining improved results, shorter postoperative recovery, and adjunctive benefits, such as less bruising and more skin tightening. Patients, however, are still seeking safer alternatives and are excited by the thought of losing fat quickly without having

---

Disclosure Statement: Dr Mulholland has received consulting fees from Syneron, Zerona, UltraShape, and Cynosure, all of which have body-contouring technology. He has received stock and stock options in Invasix, Inc, manufacturer of the TiteFX device. Dr Paul is a consultant to and receives stock options from Invasix, Inc.
a Private Plastic Surgery Practice, SpaMedica® Clinics, 66 Avenue Road, Suite 4, Toronto, ON M5R 3N8, Canada
b Aesthetic and Plastic Surgery Institute, University of California, Irvine, CA, USA
c The Plastic Surgery Group, 37 North Fullerton Avenue, Montclair, NJ 07042, USA
* Corresponding author. 1401 Avocado Avenue, Suite 810, Newport Beach, CA 92660.
E-mail address: mpaulmd@hotmail.com

Clin Plastic Surg 38 (2011) 503–520
doi:10.1016/j.cps.2011.05.002

to undergo surgery. Several technologies have emerged to attempt to address these concerns and propose a noninvasive, transcutaneous delivery of energy for lipolysis.

CELLULITE REDUCTION AND FAT CELL REDUCTION

Plastic surgeons have had a long and pioneering history in the art and science of body contouring. From the advent of liposuction in the late 1970s and early 1980s, the practice of body contouring has seen the growth of less-invasive and more-effective liposuction techniques. When one combines men and women together, liposuction is still the most common surgery performed by esthetic plastic surgeons in North America[1] and liposuction remains the number one esthetic procedure performed by plastic and cosmetic physicians worldwide. In 2009, it was estimated that there were 700,000 liposuction procedures performed in the United States (approximately 500,000 by board-certified plastic surgeons and the rest by cosmetic physicians) or 4% of all elective surgeries.[2] The number of liposuctions is anticipated to double over the next 4 years to 1.5 million procedures or 8% of all elective operations in United States.[3] This growth in body-contouring surgery is reflective in general of the expansion in the body mass index (BMI) of the average North American. The BMI and average weight of North Americans is increasing at an alarming rate; in fact, obesity is one of the most challenging epidemics facing North American health care. Fully 30% of Americans have a BMI higher than 30 and another 30% have a BMI between 27 and 30, making more than 200 million Americans candidates for weight loss programs and focal or generalized body-contouring procedures when weight loss has been achieved.[4] Some experts project that by 2015, 75% of adults will be overweight, with 41% obese.[5]

Increasing numbers of consumers desiring esthetic body-contouring changes are seeking less-invasive, less-traumatic, and more-effective procedures than traditional suction-assisted liposuction (SAL). Although, SAL is still perceived as the gold standard in nonexcisional body-contouring techniques by most plastic surgeons, recent developments in energy-based liposuction, including third-generation ultrasound (UAL), laser-assisted lipolysis (LAL), and RF-assisted liposuction (RFAL) may offer reduced ecchymosis, swelling, pain, and enhanced skin contraction when compared with SAL.[6–9]

However, as popular as the various forms of liposuction remain, the fastest growth market segment in esthetic medicine is in the area of noninvasive body contouring.[10] This reflects the underlying paradigm of many patients: that any surgery, no matter how "minimally invasive," is not what they want. As this timely issue in *Clinics in Plastic Surgery* is devoted to noninvasive and minimally invasive esthetic techniques, it is important that the modern plastic surgeon and the specialty of plastic surgery in general, be well versed in the various nonsurgical procedures and technologies that patients may use to enhance their figure and form, or, increasingly, offer these modalities in conjunction with their surgical body-contouring practice. In 2009, the global market for all body-shaping platforms was expected to reach $361.9 billion with more than 9 million procedures performed.[10] The annual growth in noninvasive body-contouring procedures is estimated to expand by 21% per year.[10]

This article focuses on the noninvasive body-contouring modalities that have become available in the US and North American markets over the past few years, as well as those that are imminent (selling worldwide but pending approval by the Food and Drug Administration [FDA]). We review the basic science and peer-reviewed articles on clinical outcomes. At the conclusion of the article, some basic business models on incorporating noninvasive body-contouring procedures into an esthetic plastic surgery practice are discussed.

It is an exciting time in esthetic plastic surgery and the growth in noninvasive plastic surgery techniques affords the forward-thinking plastic surgeon the opportunity to treat many more patients who either are not ready for invasive techniques or will never consider incisional plastic surgery. We hope this article provides a solid basis for understanding the noninvasive body-contouring options available in 2010.

CLASSIFICATION OF NONINVASIVE BODY-CONTOURING TECHNOLOGY

Over the past 5 to 10 years, there has been considerable growth in body size and patient BMI, both in North America and worldwide, which has coincided with market growth and advances in the technology devoted to the nonsurgical management of fat and body contouring. Just as liposuction is the number one cosmetic plastic surgery procedure performed worldwide, noninvasive body-contouring technology is the fastest growing segment of the esthetic capital equipment space.[10] In classifying the technologies related to noninvasive body contouring, we have decided to classify on the basis of the type of energy delivered by a particular technology in modifying the adipocyte. There are many exciting advances in body-contouring technology involving the transepidermal delivery of energy targeting the adipocyte.

Classification

1. Suction: Massage Devices
   a. Endermologie
2. Suction-Massage: Thermal Devices
   a. TriActive (Cynosure, Inc., Westford, MA, USA)
   b. Smoothshapes (Cynosure, Inc., Westford, MA, USA)
3. Radiofrequency Energy Devices
   a. VelaSmooth, VelaShape (Syneron, Inc., Irvine, CA, USA)
   b. Thermage™ (Solta Medical, Hayward, CA, USA)
   c. Accent (Alma Lasers Inc, Buffalo Grove, IL, USA)
   d. TiteFX (Invasix, Inc., Yokneam, Israel)
4. High-Frequency Focused Ultrasound Energy Devices
   a. UltraShape (UltraShape Ltd., Yoqneam, Israel)
   b. LipoSonix (Medicis, Scottsdale, AZ, USA)
5. Cryolipolysis Energy Devices
   a. Zeltiq (Zeltiq Aesthetics, Pleasanton, CA, USA)
6. Low-Level Light Laser Therapy Devices
   a. Zerona (Erchonia Medical, McKinney, TX, USA)

With the classification of noninvasive body contouring based on the kind of energy delivered to the adipocyte, we focus on the following: basic science, clinical results, and complications for those technologies that are the most relevant, peer reviewed, market proven, or exciting.

BASIC SCIENCE

The basic science of noninvasive body contouring is really the basic science of the adipocyte, its storage of triglyceride, and the aggregate number of adipocytes as they relate to the focal and generalized excess of adipose tissue, the convex distension that forms the focal "bulges," and more superficially, clinical cellulite topographically. The adipocyte is a very important cell involved in energy storage, hormonal regulation, and a host of other endocrinological functions. The adipocyte has a large amount of cytoplasm that serves as a storage depot for triglycerides, which are composed of glycerol and free fatty acids. The adipose cell is our intermediate and long-term energy storage depot. When caloric intake exceeds caloric output, adipocytes then swell with triglycerides. As adipocytes continue to enlarge within their intralobular and interlobular fascial compartments, they create "bulges" or convex distensions of soft tissue that then modify our contours. Typical convex distensions that one sees in the female

topography are "out-pouching," "bulges," or convex distensions of the hips, lower abdomen, outer thighs, inner thighs, inner knees, arms, and bra line. For men, the typical android distribution of subcutaneous adipose-derived convex distensions commonly include the flanks (love handles), lower abdomen, "spare tire," male fatty breast tissue, and the submentum.

Historically and currently, the gold standard for body contouring still remains the various techniques of liposuction. Great advances of liposuction have made this a much less invasive procedure, and this issue of *Clinics in Plastic Surgery* deals with some of the newer energy-based liposuction technologies such as RF-assisted liposuction and laser lipolysis. However, even though liposuction has become less invasive and more amenable to outpatient procedures, it is still a procedure that requires surgical instrumentation under the skin and has risk and morbidity in recovery. Many patients, no matter how less invasive liposuction may appear, will not submit, nor are they interested in a liposuction procedure. Many patients seek mild to moderate body contour improvements through diet and exercise and adjunctive noninvasive body-contouring procedures. We focus on the technologies that have the most peer-reviewed data and literature, and appear the most promising for long-term management of focal convex distension of adipose tissue, as well as for generalized figure and shape.

The basic science of the noninvasive modulation and modification of the adipocyte involves one of several mechanisms (which will be dealt with in more detail in the Clinical Results and Outcomes of Specific Technologies section). In one mechanism, the adipocyte experiences a periadipocyte thermal environment induced by transepidermal delivery of some energy and this heat increases the localized metabolic rate of the fat, evacuating, enhancing, and augmenting the natural egress of triglyceride out of the fat cell, resulting in a diminishment of the convex distension. Overlying this, there is also some thermal-related dermal tightening with these transepidermal body-contouring heating devices and a measurable circumferential reduction in fat. Most of these thermal technologies do not, in fact, kill the fat cell. Some technologies deploy energy, either a pulse of high-voltage RF current, or a focused high-frequency ultrasound energy experience that disables or destroys the adipocyte by permanently damaging the cell membrane, or coagulating or disrupting and releasing the adipocyte cell contents. And yet other technologies, such as low-level light laser therapy, create temporary disruptions in the cell membrane of the adipocyte allowing a temporary egress of the triglyceride from the cytoplasm, but the cell membrane then rights itself again. So, through these mechanisms, either thermal augmentation of normal metabolic pathways, thermal destruction, cavitational destruction, or an energy cascade and creation of a temporary adipocyte cell membrane pore, the final result is that the sizes of the adipocytes are either temporarily or permanently reduced and/or the number of adipocytes are reduced, which when translated over hundreds of thousands or millions of fat cells, will result in a measurable reduction of fat and a circumferential reduction of the body contour area in the treated area.

INDICATIONS AND CONTRAINDICATIONS OF NONINVASIVE BODY CONTOURING

In general, all the noninvasive body-contouring technologies share the same relative indications and contraindications for treatment.

Indications include realistic expectations of a modest reduction of localized fat, modest cellulite improvement, compliance with multiple visits, reasonable BMI and lifestyle, and are opposed to a surgical procedure, which would get a better result.

Contraindications include if the patient is pregnant, has a pacemaker, is medically unwell, has unrealistic expectations, or has a large BMI.

Proper Patient Preparation

With all body-contouring technologies, it is important to take consistent before-and-after photographs, make circumference measurements, and record weight change at each follow-up visit to document results and ensure the patient is not gaining weight because of a poor diet or lack of exercise. A proper consent should be executed.

The patient's target treatment areas are assessed and marked in a similar way as for patients undergoing liposuction. When assessing and marking the targeted treatment area, the patient should stand straight up and look forward. Soft tissue deformities (unwanted fat deposits) should be evaluated from multiple views for best assessment. Palpate the perimeter of the area to identify exactly where the deformity begins and mark the precise area for treatment with a single line. Only soft tissue deformities with at least 1.5 cm of fat thickness should be treated and not the adjacent flat or concave areas.

CLINICAL RESULTS AND OUTCOMES OF SPECIFIC TECHNOLOGIES
Suction/Massage Devices

The first class of body-contouring technology emerged approximately 15 to 20 years ago. Endermology is a suction/massage device manufactured in France. The device uses a mechanical suction and roller applicator used to pass over fatty areas of the body and cellulitic regions. There are peer-reviewed articles in the literature that show that in selected patients, particularly those with edematous type fatty tissue, endermology can result in measurable circumferential reduction. Endermology is often combined with increased exercise, caloric restriction, and increased water intake.[11] Although endermology is popular in the day spa environment, it has very mild, modest clinical effects and has had minimal penetration in the physician market. The indications are rather limited and more than 16 treatments are required, which last longer than 30 minutes, and thus it is not proven to be an optimal revenue generator nor successful in plastic surgery and physician offices.

Suction/Massage and Energy Devices

Augmenting the concepts of endermology are devices from several companies that use suction rollers in combination with transepidermal thermal energy. These devices will deploy diode arrays or diodes/nonfocused ultrasound around the applicator head that is then passed over the fatty areas of the body, such as TriActive and SmoothShapes (Cynosure, Inc., Westford, MA, USA) (Fig. 1). Again, results are mild to modest in effect and generally have not been incorporated into many practices for full-scale noninvasive body contouring.

Radiofrequency Energy Devices

The RF energy devices currently dominate the worldwide noninvasive body-contouring device market.[10] The first serious noninvasive body-contouring device that was widely incorporated in physicians' practices was the VelaSmooth (Syneron), followed 2 years later by the VelaShape. This was followed by other RF body-contouring devices, including Thermage™ (Solta Medical, Hayward, CA, USA), Accent (Alma Lasers), TriPollar (Pollogen, Tel Aviv, Israel), Freeze (Venus Concepts, Karmiel, Israel) and most recently TiteFX (Invasix).

VelaSmooth and VelaShape

In 2005, the VelaSmooth became the first energy-based medical device to be approved by the FDA for reducing the appearance of cellulite. In September 2007, VelaShape became the first FDA-approved noninvasive device for both cellulite and circumference reduction.

Device description Both VelaSmooth and VelaShape systems combine controlled 700-nm to 2000-nm infrared (IR) light and suction couple–

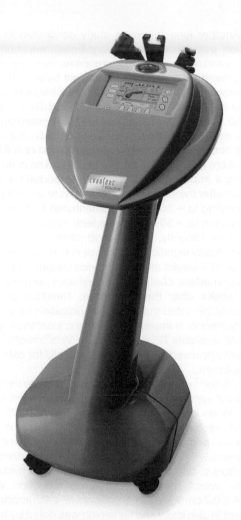

Fig. 1. TriActive device. (*From* Cynosure; with permission.)

conducted bipolar RF (1 MHz) energies with mechanical manipulation. Conductive RF energy is applied externally by suction coupling 2 electrodes to the skin surface. Both the geometry of the electrodes and the conductive RF pulse duration are optimized for safe heating of the skin. The use of conductive RF allows for a reduction in the necessary optical energy applied to the skin. Furthermore, this form of energy is not sensitive to skin pigmentation and therefore its use is advantageous in treating all skin types.

These systems are composed of a base unit to which 2 different applicators (large and small) may be connected (**Fig. 2**). The applicators are equivalent in their power density and each is fitted to the base unit via a replaceable cap. During treatment, the applied suction repeatedly pulls the skin into a chamber in the middle of the treatment cavity, where the skin is exposed to IR light and RF while its surface temperature is being monitored. The system enables the user to adjust the RF energy

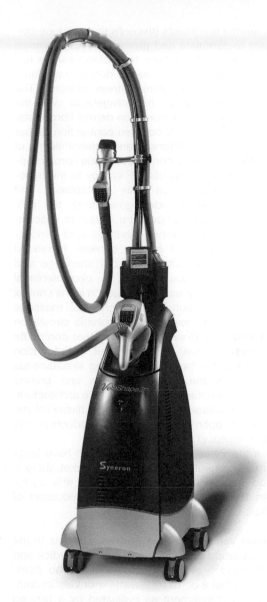

Fig. 2. VelaShape VSII device. (*From* Syneron and Candela Science; with permission.)

and optical energy levels, thereby using the optimal treatment parameters for each subject/anatomic area.

Mechanism of action The VelaSmooth and VelaShape mechanism of action is based on a novel combination of suction-coupled bipolar RF and optical energies delivered to the dermis/hypodermis zones. Optical IR energy targets mainly the dermal water, whereas the RF energy targets the hypodermis by controlled thermal stress. Applying thermal energy to the dermis causes dermal tightening and contraction but also activates a cascade of physiologic responses inside the dermal fibroblasts (the cells that produce collagen) to stimulate and promote neocollagenesis (new collagen formation). Neocollagenesis is further potentiated by increased dermal vascularity secondary to the thermal stress induced. The vacuum potentiates neocollagenesis via the mechanical stress imposed on dermal fibroblasts. Neocollagenesis and collagen contraction further contribute to enrichment and strengthening of the otherwise loose connective tissue fibrous septae. Applying the bipolar RF energy to the hypodermis increases fat cells' metabolism and accelerated triglyceride egress from the cell. Increased tissue temperature increases vascular perfusion, which further enhances lipid turnover owing to increased oxygen content. Increased lipid turnover results in fat cell shrinkage and reduced fat tissue volume, a circumferential reduction, and an esthetic reduction in the convex distension. Vacuum and mechanical massage increase blood vessel and lymphatic circulation and lymphatic drainage, which further contribute to lipid turnover and fat cell redistribution throughout the body. The resulting simultaneous increase in the dermal collagen and ground substance content, connective tissue architecture, and the decrease in subcutaneous fat tissue volume allow for optimal circumferential reduction and improvement in cellulite appearance.

As the VelaShape and VelaSmooth have long-term placements in the physician market, there is good peer-reviewed evidence of their efficacy for both the treatment and temporary reduction of cellulite and fat.

Clinical VelaSmooth and VelaShape results In the largest study of VelaSmooth to date, Sadick and Mulholland[12] evaluated 35 patients who completed either 8 or 16 treatments with VelaSmooth. Clinical improvement as evaluated by a blinded dermatologist revealed an average of 40% improvement in the appearance of cellulite and a measurable circumferential reduction in all.

Alster and Tanzi[13] conducted a self-control study, including 20 women patients who received 3 biweekly VelaSmooth treatments for thigh and buttock cellulite. Ninety percent of the patients noticed overall clinical improvement and side effects were limited to transient erythema in most patients.

A longer follow-up study performed by Kulick[14] evaluated the degree of improvement 3 and 6 months after the last session of treatment. According to the blinded physician evaluators, all patients were improved at both posttreatment periods with an average of 62% and 50% improvement at the 3-month and 6-month follow-up, respectively.

Another long follow-up study conducted in an Asian population found a significant reduction in thigh and abdomen circumferences up to 1 year after treatment. At 4 weeks after the last treatment, the average circumference reductions of the abdomen and thigh were sustained at 3.17 ± 2.75 cm and 3.50 ± 2.04 cm, respectively. At the 1-year follow-up visit, the average circumference reductions of the abdomen and thigh were maintained at 3.83 ± 0.76 cm and 3.13 ± 3.54, respectively. The average clinical improvement scores of the abdomen and thigh after the series of treatments were 0.75 (corresponding to ~25% improvement) and 1.75 (corresponding to ~50% improvement), respectively.[15]

More recently, Sadick and Magro[16] found a statistically significant decrease in thigh circumference at 4 weeks after VelaSmooth treatments, but no immediate change or a persistent decrease at 8 weeks after the procedure. Nevertheless, it should be noted that the main indication for using VelaSmooth is improving cellulite appearance, and of all available RF devices, only VelaSmooth has been approved by the FDA specifically for cellulite treatment.

Winter[17] evaluated the performance of the higher-power version of this technology (VelaShape with 50 W as opposed to VelaSmooth with 25 W) for body reshaping and improvement of skin texture/laxity in postpartum women. In this study, 20 women received 5 weekly treatments to the abdomen, buttocks, and thighs with the VelaShape system. The overall mean circumference reduction was 5.4 ± 0.7 cm (P < .001). Significant (P < .02) improvement in skin laxity and tightening was noted by both the physician and patients. Treatments were well tolerated with no major safety concerns (1 purpura, 1 mild burn).

In a recent study, Brightman and colleagues[18] revealed the clinical efficacy and the molecular mechanisms underlying treatments with VelaShape. Nineteen subjects underwent 5 weekly treatments of the upper arms, and 10 subjects underwent 4 weekly treatments of the abdomen and flanks. Change in arm circumference, at the fifth treatment was statistically significant with a mean loss of 0.625 cm. At 1-month and 3-month follow-ups, mean loss was 0.710 and 0.597 cm respectively. Reduction of abdominal circumference at the third treatment was statistically significant with a 1.25 cm mean loss. At 1-month and 3-month follow-ups, average loss was 1.43 and 1.82 cm respectively. Furthermore, the sustainable reduction in circumferences and the significant improvement in the appearance of the arms and abdomen correlated with significant morphologic and histologic changes observed in biopsies obtained in vivo from the treated areas.

In summary, there are many peer-reviewed articles to support the clinical efficacy and safety of using the combined bipolar RF, IR, and mechanical manipulation technology for cellulite improvement and circumference reduction in a wide variety of patient populations. The clinical and molecular data presented here further support the concept that the underlying mechanism of action for improved skin laxity and volume reduction is based on controlled RF and IR thermal modification of the dermal/hypodermal layers.

Thermage™ body and accent

There are 2 common monopolar RF devices sold in the marketing place, Thermage™ (Solta Medical, Hayward, CA, USA) and Accent (Alma Lasers). Both of these devices are discussed extensively in the RF for Skin Tightening article by Mulholland elsewhere in this issue. Thermage™ has had an FDA-cleared body tip since 2006 and Accent has had body clearance for more than 2 years. The monopolar RF in these systems is not suction coupled and there is no adjunctive optical energy source as in the VelaShape. Thermage™ RF body treatments have been shown in the animal and human biopsy model to result in lysis of the adipocyte membrane when high enough energies are deployed.[19] Thermage™ has been assessed in the treatment of cellulite with improvement scores of 30% to 70% and in treatment of stretch marks with improvement scores of 20% to 80%, when measured at least 6 months following treatment, depending on the study.[20–22] Thermage™ monopolar RF body treatment has also demonstrated moderate average circumferential reduction and fat-thickness reduction at 6 months following one or more treatments.[20] Accent is another monopolar RF system that operates at a high frequency and has shown improvement with noninvasive monopolar RF treatments of cellulite and fat reduction.[23,24] TriPollar (Pollogen, Tel Aviv, Israel) and Freeze (Venus Concepts) have 3 to 8 RF electrodes and show early promise for temporary adipocyte reduction and skin tightening.[25]

TiteFX: RF and high-voltage pulse electroporation

The TiteFX is an interesting emerging body-contouring technology that differentiates itself from other RF technologies, which (except in animal studies) use lower tissue levels of RF to metabolically enhance the triglyceride processing out of the adipocyte but not permanently kill or damage the fat cell and so the focal lipodystrophy or cellulite is more prone to recurrence. TiteFX uses suction-coupled RF to preheat the dermis and first 15 to 20 mm of fat and uses a precise thermistor built inside the suction cavity to monitor the uniform and even skin temperature and suction distribution. When the epidermal temperature reaches the desired level, usually 43 to 45°C, a high-voltage, electroporation pulse is generated through the adipose tissue resulting in an high voltage electroporation apoptocysis, or death of the fat cell over the following week.[26]

The device is very fast and the temperatures very uniform, making the treatment more tolerable than other RF systems that develop thermal "hot spots" and pain. With the TiteFX, like the high-intensity focused ultrasound (HIFU) family, a significant portion of the adipocyte population is targeted for cell death and thus the body-contouring circumferential reductions and cellulite improvements are more long term or permanent than other RF technologies.[26] TiteFX comes with a noninvasive fat-contouring and cellulite applicator, as well as a noninvasive face-tightening hand piece.

High-Frequency Focused Ultrasound Energy Devices

The HIFU noninvasive body-contouring devices, UltraShape and LipoSonix, have received a lot of media attention and both have been sold in many markets around the world, including Canada, but are awaiting FDA clearance. They are exciting technologies and, like Zeltiq and TiteFX, they both result in noninvasive adipocyte death, rather than just metabolic amplification of the fat cell metabolism and, as such, may offer long-term noninvasive body-contouring results. Many physicians around the world are achieving good body-contour results and have profitable body-contour programs using HIFU.

However, there are many noninvasive, nonfocused ultrasound devices on the market, such as Proslimelt (Medical Care Consulting, Murten, Switzerland), Medcontour (General Project, Florence, Italy), Ultracontour (Medixsysteme, Nimes, France), Novashape (Ultra Med, Milton, ON, Canada), Accent Ultra (Alma, Buffalo Grove, IL, USA), Vaser-Shape (Sound Surgical Technologies, Louisville, CO, USA), or the so-called "Ultracavitors," that claim to have an effect on the fat cell, but there is no known published scientific, preclinical, or clinical data to support such claims. Most of these devices use a variation of standard physiotherapy ultrasound technology indicated for diathermy, combined with some type of massage or vacuum. The nonfocused ultrasound simply heats the underlying skin and tissue just as any standard physiotherapy ultrasound device. These devices do not meet the requirements to produce focused ultrasound; therefore, they cannot increase maximal pressure deep without causing skin damage. The likelihood for cavitation is characterized by the mechanical index (MI), and based on the ultrasound specifications of these devices, they do not meet the minimum MI and pressure threshold for cavitation in fat; therefore, they do not disrupt fat cells. These physiotherapeutic ultrasound devices are not new to plastic surgeons, as they are similar to the external-assist UAL technologies of the early 1990s. These devices may create a temporary effect but there is no known scientific or preclinical evidence (histology or gross pathology) of fat cell disruption. Most of these devices are sold in Europe or Asia to beauty spa markets where there are fewer regulations and/or enforcement of unsubstantiated or nonapproved marketing claims, but they are also finding their way into US markets. We focus our attention on the HIFU technologies with peer-reviewed evidence of fat disruption.

UltraShape

The UltraShape Contour I system (UltraShape Ltd.) was the first HIFU system launched commercially in the world and UltraShape has the most basic science, peer-reviewed articles, and worldwide clinical experience of the HIFU systems. It uses nonthermal selective focused ultrasound to produce localized, mechanical motion within fat tissues and cells for the purpose of producing mechanical cellular membrane disruption.[27] The Contour I operating parameters are designed to deliver concentrated pulsed energy through the skin into a focal volume at a precise depth to disrupt subcutaneous fat cells without harming neighboring tissues (eg, nerves, blood vessels, and connective tissue).

Peer-reviewed published preclinical research demonstrates that fat tissues and cells are disrupted and surrounding structures exposed to these effects are not damaged.[28] Tissue selectivity is achieved by using a pulsed ultrasound wave, limiting temperature increases in the target tissue and differential susceptibility to mechanical (nonthermal) stresses induced by the ultrasound energy in these tissues and the ultrasound focal distance. Precision and safety are further reinforced by an integrated acoustic contact sensor, which provides real-time feedback on acoustic contact, thus ensuring proper transducer-to-skin contact and efficient energy delivery to the treatment area. The Contour I device is composed of the following subsystem components: the system console, the therapeutic ultrasound transducer, and a real-time video-tracking and guidance system. The video-tracking and guidance system ensures that the treatment is performed homogeneously only within the designated area. Peer-reviewed published clinical studies show that UltraShape is safe and effective for circumference reduction and reduction of localized fat deposits on the abdomen, flanks, and thighs.[27,29]

Experimental and clinical studies have been performed to demonstrate significant reduction in subcutaneous fat. Brown and colleagues[28] studied the physics of focused external ultrasound using the UltraShape Contour I device and attempted to validate its efficacy in a porcine model. Gross and histologic evaluations of porcine adipose tissue after treatment with the device confirmed cavitation induced zones of injury in the adipose tissue with sparing of nervous and vascular structures as well as skin.

Several studies have extrapolated these results to the clinical setting. A prospective study conducted in Spain by Moreno-Moraga and colleagues[29] involved 30 patients. Each patient underwent 3 treatments at 1-month intervals. Areas treated were the abdomen, inner and outer thighs, flanks, inner knees, and male breasts. Ultrasound measurements and circumference measurements were used to assess changes in fat thickness. They found that the mean reduction in fat thickness after 3 treatments was 2.28 ± 0.80 cm, whereas the circumference was reduced by a mean of 3.95 ± 1.99 cm. No significant changes in weight were identified to suggest changes as secondary to weight loss. Serum triglyceride levels and liver ultrasound evaluations for steatosis were also performed for safety profiles, all of which showed no significant abnormalities.[29] The group reports treating more than 400 patients outside of the clinical study with successful reduction in localized adiposity and great patient satisfaction.

Teitelbaum and colleagues[27] performed a multicenter study (2 centers in the United States, 1 in the United Kingdom, 2 in Japan) involving 164 patients, 137 of whom had undergone a single treatment of focused external ultrasound lipolysis, whereas 27 served as controls. Follow-up was performed on days 1, 3, 7, 14, 28, 56, and 84. They reported a single contour treatment produced a mean reduction of approximately 2 cm in treatment area circumference and approximately 2.9 mm in skin fat thickness. No adverse effect was noted on lipid profiles or liver sonography. Complications were mild and included erythema, mild blistering in 2 patients, and mild dermal erosion in 1 patient that resolved by the end of the follow-up period.

Shek and colleagues[30] attempted to validate the results of prior studies in the Asian population, but found strikingly different results. Fifty-three patients had up to 3 treatments 1 month apart. Efficacy was assessed by changes in abdominal circumference, ultrasound fat thickness, and caliper fat thickness. A patient questionnaire was also used to assess satisfaction. Weight loss–induced measurements were also monitored. Shek and colleagues[30] found that there were no significant changes in any of the measurements before and after treatment. Patient satisfaction was also poor, because results were suboptimal. Shek and colleagues[30] attribute the discrepancy in results to body frame size of Southern Asians compared with Caucasians, suggesting that a modification in the transducer may alleviate the difficulties in delivery of ultrasonic energy on a smaller body habitus.

The UltraShape procedure is guided by a proprietary real-time tracking and guidance system designed to deliver smooth, uniform body-contouring results. The tracking and guidance system consists of a video camera, frame grabber, and software package all together capturing, processing, and displaying in real time, the location of the treatment area with an overlay dictating to the operator where to place the transducer for each pulse of energy. The software calculates and maps the treatment area in 3 dimensions, which guarantees adherence to a predetermined computer-controlled treatment algorithm.

Key parameters of the computer-controlled treatment algorithm include the following:

1. Treatment is performed only within the marked treatment area.
2. Each point (node) is treated only once.
3. Each pulse of energy is delivered immediately adjacent to the prior pulse, ensuring complete uniform coverage over the entire treatment area.

This algorithm ensures complete and uniform energy delivery over the entire treatment area, minimizing the risk of contour irregularities, a common side effect of liposuction.

The tracking system also addresses the dynamic nature of the treatment area, as it monitors and synchronizes patient position in real time, enabling the patient to move freely without affecting the treatment.

Second-generation UltraShape technology After 3 years of clinical experience outside the United States, UltraShape launched its new, improved, and faster system in January of 2008. This advanced-generation system includes upgraded software and an improved transducer that offers reduced treatment time, lower treatment cost, and an enhanced operator and patient experience. A summary of the Contour II upgrades includes the following:

1. Reduced the average treatment time to between 40 and 60 minutes, depending on

the treatment area, a reduction of more than 35% over the prior version.
2. The transducer emits 50% more ultrasonic pulses for the same price as the previous one, thus reducing treatment cost by 35%.
3. Clinical studies conducted in France, Canada, and Israel demonstrated that 3 successive UltraShape treatments at 2-week intervals are safe and effective, and show significant treatment area reduction—3 treatment series can be completed within 1 month without compromising results.[31,32]

Third-generation UltraShape technology The newest UltraShape model, the Contour I Ver3 multiapplication platform was launched in January 2010, includes an advanced focused ultrasound technology and vacuum-assisted radio frequency, all in an upright mobile-upgradeable device (**Fig. 3**).

Some of the new features of the UltraShape Ver3 include the following:

1. New software featuring an intuitive "TOUCH" graphic user-interface for shorter treatment set-up and treatment time; 3-dimensional treatment mapping for improved treatment area coverage; and advanced proprietary tracking and guidance software for enhanced treatment efficiency.
2. Digital ultrasound pulsar designed to deliver higher energy more consistently to target tissue, further improving efficacy and reproducibility.
3. Two complementary energy-based technologies: advanced nonthermal selective focused ultrasound and vacuum-assisted RF combined in one platform. These 2 technologies support same-session combination therapy, allowing for a synergistic treatment effect for a complete body-contouring solution.[32,33]

Step 1: Tightening and tissue preparation with suction-coupled RF. The theory is that preheating the tissue increases local blood circulation and creates mild edema producing a more "wet environment" in the target tissue, which may enhance the cavitational mechanical effects of focused ultrasound treatment.

Step 2: Immediate fat cell destruction to reduce localized fatty areas with the focused ultrasound.

Step 3: Tightening and expedited fat clearance with the focused ultrasound. The theory is that treating with vacuum-assisted RF after the focused ultrasound treatment can increase blood circulation and stimulate localized lymphatic drainage and accelerate fat clearance for even better and more consistent results.

4. Planned 2010 upgrades include a patent-pending Vertical Dynamic Focus (VDF)

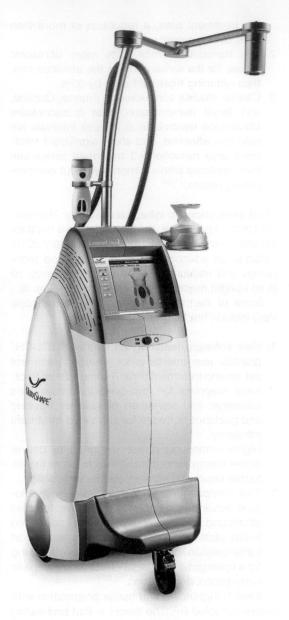

Fig. 3. UltraShape Contour v3 device. (*From* Ultra-Shape NA Inc., and Global Sales; with permission.)

ultrasound technology. VDF is designed to treat multiple depths in a single pulse, allowing the flexibility to treat focal depths from superficial to deep. This new technology will deliver higher acoustic peak pressure and treat more fat volume per pulse, which should increase the amount of fat reduction achieved with each patient session.

The UltraShape Contour I System is designed to target and selectively disrupt (lyse) fat cells so that any released triglycerides can be processed by the body's natural physiologic and metabolic pathways that handle fat during weight loss. Ultra-Shape's published multicenter-controlled clinical study and other independent clinical trials have shown that triglycerides do not accumulate to any clinically significant extent in the blood or liver.[28]

The safety and effectiveness of the UltraShape Contour I is backed by scientifically demonstrated results from clinical trials performed on hundreds of patients worldwide. Since UltraShape received the CE (European Conformity) Mark from the European Commission and a Medical Device License from Health Canada, more than 200,000 commercial patient treatments have been performed through August 2010 with no reported treatment-related serious adverse events.

The clinical and histologic effects of UltraShape have been reported in peer-reviewed articles and national meetings. The highly selective, focused, nonthermal high-frequency UltraShape energy leaves nonadipose tissue undamaged, so the patient has no pain or swelling postoperatively and, with no edema, patients can start to see results in several weeks.[27–33] In general, an average of 2 to 4 cm of circumferential fat reduction[30–33] can be achieved over 3 sessions and 6 weeks from the abdominal and hip regions and about 2 to 3 cm from the inner and outer thighs.[30–33] With the VDF and combined suction-coupled RF, it is anticipated that this can occur after a single treatment.[33]

UltraShape treatment protocol Palpate the perimeter of the area to identify exactly where the deformity begins and mark the precise area for treatment with a single line. Only soft tissue deformities with at least 1.5 cm of fat thickness should be treated and not the adjacent flat or concave areas.

Proper patient positioning is a critical factor for a successful treatment. It is important to position the patient so that the treatment area is as flat as possible, enabling complete transducer-to-skin contact and preventing adjacent anatomy from interfering with the transducer movement throughout the treatment. Once the patient is positioned on the treatment bed with a flat area marked for treatment, it is important to lift and reposition the soft tissue around the treatment area with soft positioning blocks and medical tape to maintain maximum fat thickness in the zone of treatment. These positioning and taping techniques have been shown to increase efficacy and reproducibility of results.

After proper positioning, the treatment drapes and marker areas are applied. The intuitive graphic user interface will walk the operator through the final set-up. Once the treatment area and markers have been acquired, the real-time tracking and guidance system will guide the operator through the treatment per a preprogrammed treatment algorithm. To optimize results, patients should undergo a series of 3 UltraShape treatments spaced 14 days apart. Maximum fat thickness and circumference reduction should be seen by 15 to 30 days after the final treatment.

The UltraShape procedure is performed during a convenient, "walk-in, walk-out" session performed in an office-based environment; it requires no anesthesia or sedation, and the vast majority of patients report no pain or discomfort. There is no bruising, swelling, or downtime associated with the UltraShape procedure. After treatment, patients immediately resume their daily routines with no need for maintenance treatments.

LipoSonix
The LipoSonix system delivers HIFU energy that can disrupt subcutaneous adipose tissue to provide a noninvasive approach to body sculpting, such as a reduction in waist, abdomen, and thigh circumference.

HIFU mechanism of action LipoSonix HIFU, is highly convergent energy that is tightly focused in a manner analogous to focusing sunlight with a magnifying glass. Whereas UltraShape is focused, nonthermal, and cavitates only the adipose tissue, LipoSonix core HIFU technology enables its HIFU to be directed with very high intensity and in a very small volume at a specific location. At high energy levels, HIFU energy absorption within the focal zone induces high temperatures at the focal point, causing coagulative necrosis and almost instantaneous cell death.[34,35] The volume of destroyed cells is referred to as a "lesion". Importantly, the intensity levels above and below the focal zone remain relatively low, keeping temperatures at levels that are not cytotoxic to the untreated, or nontargeted tissue.[34,35] An important feature of HIFU lesions is that the damage is spatially confined with no surrounding cellular damage in areas outside the focal zone. In summary, thermal tissue damage occurs at the focal point without causing injury to the skin and intervening tissues beyond the focal point.

After the treated adipose tissue has been thermally coagulated and destroyed, chemotactic signals activate the body's normal inflammatory response mechanisms. Macrophage cells are attracted to the treated area where they engulf and transport the lipids and cellular debris. The lipids released from disrupted adipose tissue are ultimately metabolized and the lesion gradually heals in a normal fashion. This results in a volumetric collapse of the treated tissues and an overall reduction in local adipose tissue volume.[34,35]

The LipoSonix system is equipped with a programmable system pattern generator that consistently and automatically directs HIFU energy over the entire treatment area. The preprogrammed movement of the transducer creates a continuous lesion. The amount of HIFU energy delivered by the LipoSonix system may be adjusted by changing the peak power and by changing the duration of each energy dose. In addition, the system has a user-adjustable focal depth of 1.1 to 1.8 cm. The LipoSonix system must be used with distilled water as a coupling agent to prevent the occurrence of significant acoustical reflections from air pockets at the HIFU treatment head/skin interface.

LipoSonix preclinical trial results Preclinical studies were conducted in a porcine model because their skin and subcutaneous adipose tissue closely resembles that of humans. During these studies, the placement of thermocouples in the skin and tissues surrounding the focal zone consistently demonstrated that the application of HIFU results in rapid increases in temperature exceeding 56°C (133°F).[34,35] These temperatures were confined to the focal zone and did not extend outside of the targeted subcutaneous adipose tissue. These results were confirmed by histologic analyses demonstrating that coagulative necrosis was confined to the targeted adipose tissue with no injury to nerves and arterioles outside the treatment area.

Clinical trial results Results from the preclinical studies were confirmed in human subjects during an early clinical study. This nonblinded trial enrolled 19 healthy female subjects who were scheduled to undergo elective abdominoplasty. Three patients were treated with 1 of 5 different HIFU energy levels (n = 16) or 2 treatments using 1 to 2 HIFU energy levels performed 4 weeks apart (n = 3). Patients were evaluated after 1, 2, 3, 4, 7, 28, and 56 days. Abdominoplasty was performed 1 to 18 weeks following treatment. Histologic examination of excised tissue showed well-demarcated adipocyte disruption. A normal inflammatory response with the presence of macrophages was observed and phagocytosis of released lipids occurred after 14 to 28 days. Healing progressed normally. Adverse events include swelling, ecchymosis, dysesthesia, and pain on treatment.[35]

Peer-reviewed studies published recently reveal that circumferential reductions of 2 to 5 cm can still be achieved after a single treatment session, but fluence and parameters used to achieve this may result in patient discomfort. Multiple treatments at modified settings are being studied.[35–37]

Cryolipolysis

Cryolipolyis refers to a novel noninvasive technology of using cold exposure to selectively and gradually lead to the reduction of subcutaneous fat. Although the mechanism of action is not fully understood, there is evidence to suggest the onset of an inflammatory reaction within the adipose tissue in response to cold exposure.[38] The mechanism for this phenomenon is a cold-induced apoptotic adipocyte cell death for those fat cells that have been exposed to a cold stimulus that is above freezing but below body temperatures for a defined duration.[39] Results also suggest that fat cells may be more sensitive to cold than other tissues. Manstein and colleagues[40] performed porcine experiments to evaluate the effect of controlled application of cold to skin and subcutaneous fat. Three complementary pig studies were completed: an initial exploratory study, a dosimetry study, and a follow-up safety study to assess the impact of such selective lipolysis on lipid levels. They used a copper plate that was cooled and regulated to −7°C by an attached heat-exchanger chamber, and applied the plate to multiple sites on the animals. Exposures varied between 5 and 21 minutes and the pigs were observed for 3.5 months. No significant skin changes had manifested during the observation period, but selective fat absorption had occurred at treatment sites, as evidenced by contour indentations. On gross tissue observation, a 40% reduction in fat thickness had occurred, which was confirmed by histology to demonstrate reduction in distance between fat septae.

Originally, both Zeltiq and Zerona had both received limited FDA clearances for skin cooling and blood flow enhancement respectively, are now both FDA cleared for long reduction of subcutaneous fat (love handles for Zeltiq and multiple areas for Zerona). The success in the porcine studies led to human applications. The device consists of a control console and an umbilical cable connecting the cooling applicator cup or paddles to the console. The tissue to be treated, most commonly love handles and lower abdominal tissue, is drawn up with mild suction and the tissue is held between the panels of the treatment cup for 30 to 60 minutes. The amount of cooling (selected energy extraction rate) is controlled by the thermoelectric cooling cells powered by DC current and controlled by thermisters that monitor the skin temperature.

Clinical results from an early report show that consistent fat thickness and circumferential reductions occur that are competitive with other focal reduction technologies.[41,42] Dover and colleagues[43] demonstrated the use of cryolipolysis for reduction of lateral flank and back adiposities. Thirty-two subjects underwent cryolipolysis with one side serving as the treatment side and the other as the control. Efficacy was determined by ultrasound measurements of fat-layer reduction, photograph comparisons, and physician evaluations. At 4 months, 22% fat reduction was demonstrated in 10 patients undergoing ultrasound evaluation. Visible contour changes were noted in the others, with the most pronounced in those with modest and discrete adiposities.

Coleman and colleagues[42] treated 10 patients to determine the effect of cold exposure on fat loss and sensory nerve function. At 6 months after treatment, there was a fat layer reduction of 25.5% with no long-term sensory disturbances. Six of 9 patients had mild transient reduction in sensation that returned spontaneously with 7 weeks of treatment. One patient underwent a nerve biopsy, which showed no significant changes. Klein and colleagues[44] evaluated the effect of cryolipolysis on serum lipid levels and liver function tests in 40 patients. No appreciable changes were noted in either test after a 12-week follow-up, suggesting the technology has unlikely adverse effects over lipid profiles and liver function.

There is a significant risk of temporary sensory nerve dysesthesia, which resolves over 2 to 3 months.[41,42] The disadvantages of the current device are its slow speed, ergonomics of cup application, and disposable cost, but these can be offset, as the device does not require a technician to operate.

Low-Level Laser Therapy (Zerona)

Although lasers are often used in various aspects of medicine with success, their role in lipolysis is only starting to be delineated. Low-level laser therapy (LLLT) is defined as treatment with a dose rate that causes no immediate detectable temperature rise of the treated tissue and no macroscopically visible changes in tissue structure.[45,46] Laser dosage is a magnitude used to define the laser beam energy applied to the tissue. Units are expressed as joules per centimeter squared, and the dosage is calculated as the laser power measured in milliwatts, multiplied by treatment time in seconds, and divided by the area of the laser spot directed toward the tissue.[46]

The Zerona (Erchonia Medical) is a low-level laser device emitting a wavelength at 635 nm with an output power that distinguishes Zerona as a class IIIB laser. In recent years, LLLT has emerged as an efficacious adjunct therapy for numerous cosmetic procedures, including breast augmentation and lipoplasty.[47] However, the completion of numerous histologic investigations and a placebo-controlled, randomized, double-blind, multisite study resulted in Zerona emerging, on its own, as a viable, independent, therapeutic strategy for the circumferential reduction of the waist, hips, and thighs.

The histologic and basic science research behind LLLT is very solid, perhaps more so than most technologies in the noninvasive body-contouring market. Multiple histologic examinations were performed to assess how laser light, with well-defined parameters, was able to modulate adipocyte function. Neira and colleagues[45] in 2002 reported on the effect of low-level laser energy on adipose tissue, demonstrating that a 6-minute exposure of 635-nm 10-mW laser diode energy created a 99% release of fat from adipose tissue taken from abdominoplasty samples. These samples were evaluated by transmission electron microscopy after irradiation, which revealed a transitory pore in the cell membrane opening, which thereby permitted the fat content to leak out of the cell into the interstitium. The laser does not destroy or lyse the adipocyte completely, which is a differentiation from the proposed mechanism for ultrasound-induced changes. Brown and colleagues,[46] in 2004, reported a completely opposite conclusion from previous findings using a similar laser. Histologic and electron microscopy data from their porcine model and human subjects revealed no significant difference between laser-treated and nonexposed treatment sites, nor could they demonstrate disruption to adipocyte membranes.

Despite this dichotomy, a few small clinical series have demonstrated promising results. Jackson and colleagues[47] demonstrated in a 35-patient double-blind, placebo-controlled trial, a significant reduction in treatment area circumference after 2 weeks, at 3 sessions per week. Patients underwent treatment of their hips, thighs, and waist. After completing all sessions, there was an overall reduction of 3.51 inches in all 3 sites collectively. Participants had a 0.98-inch reduction at the waist, 1.05 inch at the hip, and 0.85 inch in the thighs. Similarly, Caruso-Davis and colleagues[48] demonstrated a 2.15-cm cumulative reduction in waist circumference over a 4-week treatment course in 44 patients.

The membrane invagination or transitory "pore" was found to be unique to those adipocytes receiving laser therapy at 635 nm and is believed to serve as the primary passage by which the stored triglyceride and fatty debris are removed from the cell. The wealth of basic science research and histologic evidence certainly points to the concept that adipocyte membrane disruption is secondary to light stimulation at 635 nm and is responsible for the egress of triglyceride, evacuation of cells, and the ultimate slimming event observed following a Zerona treatment series.[45,49]

Photobiomodulation via an external light delivery system represents a unique and misunderstood sector of medicine; yet, studies continually affirm that light has the capacity to penetrate the skin barrier and trigger real and measurable photochemical responses within the targeted tissue.[45,49]

Early utility of LLLT was found as an adjunct therapy to liposuction improving the ease of extraction and reducing postsurgical pain. A 700-patient report was published documenting improved contour and skin retraction, with an overall improved postoperative recovery when lipoplasty was coupled with LLLT.[47]

Mechanism of action

The 635-nm LLLT Zerona laser penetrates the first few millimeters of fat and, through a cytochrome oxidize enzyme interaction, results in the creation of a temporary pore in the adipocyte lipid belayed. Liberation of intracellular fat transitions into the interstitial space that is regulated by the lymphatic system and possesses the capacity to hydrolyze triglycerides into nonesterified free fatty acids (NEFAs), which is important for fat catabolism. As the fluid passes along the anastamosing network of lymphatic vessels, it ultimately arrives at lymph nodes where the extraneous materials are filtered out via macrophages that contain enzymes capable of degrading triglycerides and cholesterol. It is postulated that the fatty debris released after laser therapy is transported to lymph nodes where lysosomal acid lipase (LAL) hydrolyzes the released triglycerides to generate NEFAs.[45,49]

Clinical results

A placebo-controlled, randomized, double-blind, multicentered clinical study was conducted to evaluate the efficacy of the Zerona for noninvasive body slimming.[47] There were 67 participating subjects, of which 35 were randomized to the active treatment group and 32 were randomized to the sham-treatment group. Subject randomization was performed by a third party and was computer generated. Subjects assigned to the test group were treated with a multiple-head low-level diode laser consisting of 5 independent diode laser heads, each with a scanner emitting 635-nm (red) laser light with each diode generating 17 mW output (Zerona, manufactured by Erchonia Medical). Sham-treatment group participants were treated with a multiple-head nonlaser red light-emitting diode (LED) consisting of 5 independent red diode light heads each with a scanner emitting 635-nm (red) light with each diode generating

2.5 mW power. Both the sham-treatment light and real-laser devices were designed to have the same physical appearances, including the appearance of any visible light output. The primary success criterion was established by the FDA, which was defined as at least a 35% difference between treatment groups, comparing the proportion of individual successes in each group. Further, it was determined by the FDA that a reduction of at least 3 inches was clinically meaningful and patients were determined successful if that reduction was revealed in 2 weeks.

Comparison of the 2 independent-group means for the continuous variables of mean change in total combined circumference (total number of inches) from study baseline to end point demonstrated a mean difference of −2.837, a deviation found to be statistically significant ($t = -7.30$; $df = 65$; $P<.0001$). Treatment participants produced a reduction of 3 inches or greater in 2 weeks, compared with 2 subjects within the sham light group revealing a similar outcome. The difference was determined to be significant at $P< .0001$ (**Table 1**).

Compared with baseline, the changes in total circumference measurements between groups were statistically significant at all 3 subsequent evaluation points: −1.794 inches at week 1 ($t = -3.83$; $df = 65$; $P = .00029$ [$P<.0005$]), −2.838 inches at week 2 ($t = -7.30$; $df = 65$; $P<.0001$), and −2.593 inches at 2 weeks after the procedure ($t = -6.66$; $df = 65$; $P< .0001$). Zerona test subjects responded to the satisfaction survey. Thirty of the 35 test subjects and 31 of the 32 sham light–treated subjects recorded their satisfaction level subsequent to the treatment administration phase. Twenty-one test group participants (70%) and 8 sham-light group participants (26%) recorded a "satisfied" rating (see **Table 1**).

Moreover, 1 test group participant and 11 control group participants recorded a "dissatisfied" rating (see **Table 1**). The difference of the rating score between the 2 treatment groups was found to be statistically significant ($P<.0005$).

The commercial Zerona unit has an array of 6 × 635-nm diodes, each with a source fluence of 15 W and all 6 are adjusted to within 6 inches of the patient's body (**Fig. 4**). The patient is treated for 20 minutes on the front and then 20 minutes on the back. It is important that the treatments are conducted 48 hours apart to optimize the transitory pore. Between treatments, patients are asked to walk 30 minutes per day, drink 1 L of water, and take a supplement called Curva that contains niacin and some homeopathic substances, all of which is designed to increase lymphatic flow and "wash out" the interstitial triglyceride. Minimization of inflammatory processes like alcohol and smoking should be attempted. The current Zerona protocol calls for 6 to 12 treatments, depending on the adipose make up on the patient. The "average" Zerona patient undergoes a treatment every 48 hours for a total of 9 treatments over 2 weeks. The lead author (RSM) has deployed Zerona in his practice for 10 months. A review of 110 consecutive, well-selected patients shows that the minimum

Table 1	
Noninvasive body slimming subject ratings	
	Respondents • 35 Total test subjects • 32 Total control subjects
"Satisfied" Rating	
Test group subjects	70% (21/30)
Control group subjects	26% (8/31)
"Unsatisfied" Rating	
Test group subjects	3% (1/30)
Control group subjects	35% (11/31)

Thirty of the 35 test subjects and 31 of the 32 sham light-treated subjects recorded their satisfaction level subsequent to the treatment administration phase. Twenty-one test group participants (70%) and 8 sham light group participants (26%) recorded a "satisfied" rating.

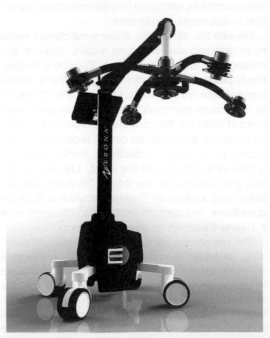

Fig. 4. Zerona device. (*From* Zerona Science and Media Images; with permission.)

"guarantee" of 3-inch to 9-inch reduction measured over 10 pinch locations occurred in 80% of patients. The company stands by their "guarantee" of 3 to 9 inches and we offer a second complimentary set of treatments (6 treatments over 2 weeks) to nonresponders. In the 20% of initial nonresponders, we salvaged 50% and were left with 10% of patients who did not hit the minimum guaranteed of 3-inch pinch reduction. Our patient happiness index remains very high, as we under promote and guarantee our minimum. It is possible to combine Zerona with other more focal, ablative, fat-reduction technologies to gain a generalized slimming and enhanced focal fat reduction.

Zerona truly occupies a unique position in the noninvasive body-contouring space, as it is the only generalized laser-slimming technology. Further, the departure from adipocyte ablation positions, the Zerona is in a unique and beneficial category as it exemplifies a truly noninvasive approach inducing slimming without cell death or upregulation of inflammation. Well-selected patients are generally very satisfied with their treatment.

CELLULITE

As cellulite is such a common presenting complaint of our body-contouring patients, it is important to mention some of the exciting new frontiers in the management of this pathology. Cellulite is the phenotypic description of lumpy, bumpy, irregular "peau d'orange "or "cottage cheese"–like skin. The etiology and pathophysiology in the basic science of cellulite are still poorly understood and debated, but various hypoxic, ischemic, hereditary, hormonal, and multifactorial theories are postulated. Over time, the cellulitic skin progresses from lymphedema to a lipidema, then to mild fibrous retraction bands and exacerbated hypoxia and matrix sclerosis. Herniated edematous fat lobules move up into the reticular dermis, creating lumpy, bumpy, irregular skin.

Of the noninvasive body-contouring technologies that are used to treat convex and focal distension of fat, some can also be used for the treatment of cellulite. The VelaSmooth and VelaShape have perhaps the greatest reported experience in the treatment of cellulite and improvements of 60% after multiple sessions have been reported.[16] Thermage™ and the Accent monopolar RF devices have also shown some success with multiple treatments for cellulite.[19–23]

Because cellulite is so ubiquitous, it can affect patients with higher and lower BMI. It is going to be a continued area of growth. New minimally invasive technologies that have been developed by Invasix that use a bipolar RF device with 1 electrode on the skin and 1 RF electrode under the skin immediately in the subdermal and hypodermal areas are used to treat cellulite. This application of RF energy results in adipocyte destruction and the external electrode moves smoothly along the surface of the skin delivering a monopolar, gentle dermal tightening effect. Recent BodyTite (Invasix, Inc., Yokneam, Israel) studies on cellulite show that increased collagen at the subdermal hypodermal junction may act as a barrier, which, together with the adipocyte RF coagulation and dermal tightening, accounts for the RFAL cellulite improvement with the RF Cellutite™ applicator. This minimally invasive technology has shown tremendous long-term improvement in cellulite in early studies with 70% to 80% improvement with Grade 3 cellulite followed for greater than a year.[8]

LLLT is also being investigated for the treatment of cellulite. Although various creams, mechanical manipulation of tissues, mesotherapy, and others have been attempted, treatment of cellulite remains a challenge.[50] Low-level laser energy may have a role. Lach[51] reported the use of a vacuum/massage and dual-wavelength (650 and 915 nm), low-level laser energy device to improve the appearance of cellulite. One thigh was treated circumferentially with massage alone, whereas the other circumferential thigh was treated with dual-beam laser energy. Sixty-five patients received an average of 14 treatments, 1 to 3 per week over 4 to 6 weeks, and were followed with magnetic resonance imaging measurements, which were obtained before and after the last treatment. The fat thickness decreased over time by 1.19 cm^2 in the leg treated with laser and massage, whereas the leg treated with massage alone increased by 3.82 cm^2.

Kulick[52] demonstrated the efficacy of a noninvasive laser-suction device using a low-level dual-energy laser in the treatment of cellulite. Twenty women with mild to moderate cellulite underwent treatment of their lateral thighs and were evaluated with body weight measurements, digital photographs, 3-dimensional images, and questionnaires. Two treatments per week for 4 weeks were performed using a commercially available machine emitting a 1-W, 650-nm and 10-W, 915-nm dual-laser combined with suction. The treatments resulted in 76% improvement in cellulite reduction based on 3-dimensional imaging and patient satisfaction surveys.

Management and treatment of cellulite is a very common problem in North America and Europe, and less common in the Asian skin type. The complications in the management of cellulite can include thermal skin injury and safety and efficacy protocols need to be followed. The complications, however, are rare. The biggest complication again is patient dissatisfaction from unrealistic expectations. With the ability to pass RF heat across and now under the skin, cellulite may become a surgically manageable process with good long-term improvements.

NONINVASIVE BODY-CONTOURING COMPLICATIONS

All of the noninvasive body-contouring technologies described in this article are extremely safe. Rare reports of focused ultrasound thermal injuries over thin bony prominences can be avoided by following the recommended techniques and protocol set out by the companies. The thermal injuries from the RF devices can occur but, again, are very rare with instances far less than 1%.[18] With the cryolipolysis technology, a reported temporary, but annoying, dysethesia can happen in up to 20% of patients, but there are no reports of permanent sensory loss.[42]

Although the safety and efficacy of these noninvasive body-contouring devices have been proven and documented in peer-reviewed literature, by far the most common complication is patient dissatisfaction. Patients who present to the plastic surgeon's office for noninvasive body contouring are often thinking they will receive "liposuction"-like results and it is critical to educate patients on the modest significance of 2 to 4 cm of circumferential improvement in body contour. With noninvasive and minimally invasive facial rejuvenative procedures, we can achieve remarkable results with a combination of Botox, soft tissue fillers, subdermal RF, laser heating, and fractional resurfacing. Such results are comparable with more aggressive surgical interventions. However, the same cannot be said of noninvasive or minimally invasive body-contouring technologies. Although it is impressive that we can achieve 4-cm or more reductions with most of the technologies in the truncal region, those patients who present for noninvasive body contouring with large BMIs, or individuals with large focal fatty deposits, will see limited benefit. Reductions of 4, 5, or 6 cm still leave behind most of the fatty tissue causing the convex distention. Patients wanting noninvasive body contouring need to be judiciously selected and the procedures should not be overpromoted. The best candidates and indications for noninvasive body contouring are those patients who are very accepting of a mild to moderate result; in fact, the best candidates are those who state they will be happy with any measurable reduction in fat. These well-selected patients are not willing to undergo any form of liposuction or body-contouring surgery, as these will invariably give the best results.

With proven safety and efficacy, the future of noninvasive body contouring looks bright. Plastic surgeons who incorporate these technologies into their practices will be able to offer noninvasive as well as invasive body contouring and offer synchronous programs that can move patients from noninvasive to invasive and back again. Again, like purchasing expensive facial skin–tightening and rejuvenation technologies, a business model and an appreciation of the marketing behind the business model for patients wanting noninvasive body contouring is an important part of this emerging area of noninvasive plastic surgery.

REFERENCES

1. American Society of Aesthetic Plastic Surgery. Quick facts: 2009 ASAPS Statistics. Available at: http://www.surgery.org/media/statistics. Accessed July 12, 2011.
2. American Society of Aesthetic Plastic Surgery, 2009 ASAPS statistics: complete charts (including percent change, gender distribution, age distribution, national average fees, practice profile). Available at: http://www.surgery.org/media/statistics. Accessed July 12, 2011.
3. Global aesthetic medicine VIII: the global aesthetic market study. Aliso Viejo (CA): Medical Insight Inc; 2010.
4. Heart Disease News. "Waist size predicts heat disease risk better than BMI." 2008. Available at: www.healthhubs.net. Accessed July 12, 2011.
5. Wang Y, Beydoun MA. The obesity epidemic in the U.S.—gender, age, socioeconomic, racial/ethnic, and geographic characteristics: a systematic review & meta-regression analysis. Epidemiol Rev 2007;29: 6–28.
6. Goldman A. Submental Nd:YAG laser assisted liposuction. Lasers Surg Med 2006;38(3):181–4.
7. Rohrich RJ, Beran SJ, Kenkel JM, et al. Extending the role of liposuction in body contouring with ultrasound-assisted liposuction. Plast Reconstr Surg 1998; 101(4):1090–102 [discussion: 1117–9].
8. Paul MD, Mulholland RS. A new approach for adipose tissue treatment and body contouring using radiofrequency-assisted liposuction. Aesthetic Plast Surg 2009;33(5):687–94.
9. Blugerman G, Schalvezon D, Paul MD. A safety and feasibility study of a novel radiofrequency-assisted liposuction technique. Plast Reconstr Surg 2010;125(3): 998–1006.
10. Body shaping and cellulite reduction: technology proliferation driven by demand. Medical Insight Inc; 2009.
11. Güleç AT. Treatment of cellulite with LPG endermologie. Int J Dermatol 2009;48(3):265–70.

12. Sadick NS, Mulholland RS. A prospective clinical study to evaluate the efficacy and safety of cellulite treatment using the combination of optical and RF energies for subcutaneous tissue heating. J Cosmet Laser Ther 2004;6:187–90.

13. Alster TS, Tanzi E. Cellulite treatment using a novel combination radiofrequency, infrared light, and mechanical tissue manipulation device. J Cosmet Laser Ther 2005;7:81–5.

14. Kulick M. Evaluation of the combination of radio frequency, infrared energy and mechanical rollers with suction to improve skin surface irregularities (cellulite) in a limited treated area. J Cosmet Laser Ther 2006;8:185–90.

15. Wanitphakdeedecha R, Manuskiatti W. Treatment of cellulite with a bipolar radiofrequency, infrared heat, and pulsatile suction device: a pilot study. J Cosmet Dermatol 2006;5:284–8.

16. Sadick N, Magro C. A study evaluating the safety and efficacy of the Velasmooth system in the treatment of cellulite. J Cosmet Laser Ther 2007;9:15–20.

17. Winter ML. Post-pregnancy body contouring using a combined radiofrequency, infrared light and tissue manipulation device. J Cosmet Laser Ther 2009; 11(4):229–35.

18. Brightman L, Weiss E, Chapas AM, et al. Improvement in arm and post partum abdominal and flank sub cutaneous fat deposits and skin laxity using a bipolar radiofrequency, infrared, vacuum and mechanical massage device. Lasers Surg Med 2009;41:791–8.

19. Zachary CB, Mian A, England LJ. Effects of monopolar radiofrequency on the subcutaneous fat layer in an animal model [abstracts]. American Society for Laser Medicine and Surgery 2009;38:105.

20. Anolik R, Chapas AM, Brightman LA, et al. Radiofrequency devices for body shaping: a review and study of 12 patients. Semin Cutan Med Surg 2009; 28:236–43.

21. Rubbani S. Advances in monopolar radiofrequency for the treatment of stretch marks in the arms, thighs and abdomen [abstracts]. American Society for Laser Medicine and Surgery 2008;370:111.

22. Rubbani S. The immediate effect of a new monopolar radiofrequency treatment tip on cellulite [abstract]. American Society for Laser Medicine and Surgery 2008;369:110.

23. Goldberg DJ, Fazeli A, Berlin AL. Clinical, laboratory, and MRI analysis of cellulite treatment with a unipolar radiofrequency device. Dermatol Surg 2008; 34:204–9.

24. Pino ME, Rosado RH, Azuela A, et al. Effect of controlled volumetric tissue heating with radiofrequency on cellulite and subcutaneous tissues of the buttocks and thighs. J Drugs Dermatol 2006;5:714–22.

25. Kaplan H, Gat A. Clinical and histopathological results following tripolar radiofrequency skin treatments. J Cosmet Laser Ther 2009;11:78–84.

26. Mulholland RF, Kriendel M. The use of bipolar radiofrequency combined with high voltage electroporation pulses for non-invasive body contouring treatment [abstract]. IMCAS Asia, Hong Kong, July 2010.

27. Teitelbaum SA, Burns JL, Kubota J, et al. Noninvasive body contouring by focused ultrasound: safety and efficacy of the Contour I device in a multicentered, controlled clinical study. Plast Reconstr Surg 2007;120(3):779–89.

28. Brown SA, Greenbaum L, Shtukmaster S, et al. Characterization of nonthermal focused ultrasound for non-invasive selective fat cell disruption (lysis): technical and preclinical assessment. Plast Reconstr Surg 2009;24(1):92–101.

29. Moreno-Moraga J, Valero-Altes T, Riquelme AM, et al. Body contouring by non-invasive transdermal focused ultrasound. Lasers Surg Med 2007;39:315–23.

30. Shek S, Yu C, Yeung CK, et al. The use of focused ultrasound for non-invasive body contouring in Asians. Lasers Surg Med 2009;41:751–9.

31. Ascher B. Safety and efficacy of UltraShape contour 1 treatments to improve the appearance of body contours: multiples treatments in shorter intervals. Aesthet Surg J 2010;30(2):217–24.

32. Mulholland RS. Body contouring results combining focused, high frequency non thermal ultrasound (Ultrashape Contour V3) with suction couple radiofrequency energy in an accelerated program: updated efficacy. Presented at IMCAS Asia Hong Kong, July 12, 2010.

33. Leal H. Combined modality of focused ultrasound and radiofrequency for non-invasive fat disruption and body contouring—results of a single treatment session. Presented at IMCAS Paris, January 9, 2010.

34. Ter Haar G, Coussios C. High intensity focused ultrasound: physical principle and devices. Int J Hyperthermia 2007;23:89–104.

35. Garcia-Murray E, Rivas OA, Stecco KA, et al. The use and mechanism of action of high intensity focused ultrasound for adipose tissue removal and non-invasive body sculpting. Presented at the American Society of Plastic Surgery Annual Meeting. Chicago (IL), September 28, 2005.

36. Fatemi A, Kane MAC. High-intensity focused ultrasound effectively reduces waist circumference by ablating adipose tissue from the abdomen and flanks: a retrospective case series. Aesthetic Plast Surg 2010;34(5):577–82.

37. Fatemi A. High-intensity focused ultrasound effectively reduces adipose tissue. Semin Cutan Med Surg 2009;28:257–62.

38. Avram MM, Harry RS. Cryolipolysis for subcutaneous fat layer reduction. Lasers Surg Med 2009; 41(10):703–8.

39. Zelickson B, Egbert BM, Preciado J, et al. Cryolipolysis for noninvasive fat cell destruction: initial

results from a pig model. Dermatol Surg 2009; 35(10):1462–70.

40. Manstein D, Laubach H, Watanabe K, et al. Selective cryolysis: a novel method of non-invasive fat removal. Lasers Surg Med 2009;40:595–604.

41. Manstein D, Laubach H, Watanabe K, et al. A novel cryotherapy method of non-invasive, selective lipolysis. Lasers Surg Med 2008;40(S20):104.

42. Coleman SR, Sachdeva K, Egbert BM, et al. Clinical efficacy of noninvasive cryolipolysis and its effects on peripheral nerves. Aesthetic Plast Surg 2009; 33(4):482–8.

43. Dover J, Burns J, Coleman S, et al. A prospective clinical study of noninvasive cryolypolysis for subcutaneous fat layer reduction—interim report of available subject data. Lasers Surg Med 2009; S21:45.

44. Klein KB, Zelickson B, Riopelle JG, et al. Noninvasive cryolipolysis for subcutaneous fat reduction does not affect serum lipid levels or liver function tests. Lasers Surg Med 2009;41(10): 785–90.

45. Neira R, Arroyave J, Ramirez H, et al. Fat liquefaction: effect of low-level laser energy on adipose tissue. Plast Reconstr Surg 2002;110(3):912–22.

46. Brown SA, Rohrich RJ, Kenkel J, et al. Effect of low-level laser therapy on abdominal adipocytes before

lipoplasty procedures. Plast Reconstr Surg 2004; 113(6):1796–804.

47. Jackson R, Roche G, Butterwick KJ, et al. Low level laser-assisted liposuction: a 2004 clinical trial of its effectiveness for enhancing ease of liposuction procedures and facilitating the recover process for patients undergoing thigh, hip and stomach contouring. Am J Cosmet Surg 2004;21(4):191–8.

48. Caruso-Davis MK, Guillot TS, Podichetty VK, et al. Efficacy of low-level laser therapy for body contouring and spot fat reduction. Obes Surg 2011;21:722–9.

49. Neira R, Jackson R, Dedo D, et al. Low-level-laser assisted lipoplasty: appearance of fat demonstrated by MRI on abdominal tissue. Am J Cosmet Surg 2001; 18(3):133–40.

50. van der Lugt C, Romero C, Ancona D, et al. A multicenter study of cellulite treatment with a variable emission radio frequency system. Dermatol Ther 2009; 22:74–84.

51. Lach E. Reduction of subcutaneous fat and improvement in cellulite by dual-wavelength, low-level laser energy combined with vacuum and massage. J Cosmet Laser Ther 2008;10:202–9.

52. Kulick MI. Evaluation of a noninvasive, dual-wavelength laser-suction and massage device for the regional treatment of cellulite. Plast Reconstr Surg 2010;125(6):1788–96.

Lifting and Wound Closure with Barbed Sutures

R. Stephen Mulholland, MD, FRCS(C)[a],
Malcolm D. Paul, MD[b],*

KEYWORDS

- Suture lifting • Barbed suture brow lifting
- Barbed suture neck lifting • Barbed suture midface lifting
- Threadlift • Barbed suture abdominoplasty closure
- Barbed suture mastopexy closure
- Barbed suture brachioplasty and armlift closure

The expansion of aesthetic plastic surgery in the last 2 decades has been a combination of invasive and noninvasive procedures. In the past 10 years, invasive procedures have grown approximately 100%, whereas noninvasive procedures have grown almost 1000%.[1] Although consumers of cosmetic plastic surgery seek to look and feel their best, most potential patients also generally desire procedures that are affordable and have minimal pain, recovery, and downtime. The mobilization and repositioning of soft tissue, whether of the brow, midface, neck, breast, or body contouring, is often a significant and important goal in an aesthetic plastic surgery procedure. The use of sutures to suspend soft tissues is not new. Suture suspension techniques have been used in medicine to treat several functional and aesthetic problems including congenital ptosis, sleep apnea, and bladder suspension for urinary incontinence.[2–5] In aesthetic plastic surgery, nonbarb suture suspension techniques have been used alone or in combination with other surgical maneuvers to elevate soft tissue of the midface, brow, and cervical mental angle.[6–10] The reported problems with simple 2-point suture fixation techniques are principally the phenomenon of cheese wiring of either

end of the suture fixation and/or stress relaxation of the skin under tension, both of which compromise the suture suspended elevation and repositioning.[11,12] Cheese wiring occurs when suspended tissues are under tension and, with constant movement, the sutures migrate through the soft tissue fixation points, even if fascial tissue sutures are deployed, resulting in the loss of part, or all, of the elevation or repositioning.[11] The stress relaxation occurs when soft tissue, particularly skin, is held under tension in 2 points, and the tensile relaxation properties of the dermis reorganize the collagen, elastin, and ground substances to lengthen the distance between the fixation points. Like tissue expansion, the body's ability to recruit tissue to reduce tension loading compromises the elevation when the repositioning is supported in only 2 points. Multiple-point fixation techniques and technologies, like the Endotine device or barbed sutures, can minimize stress relaxation and cheese wiring (Coapt Systems, Inc., Palo Alto, CA, USA). Without multiple fixation points, there is often limited long-term efficacy of pure suture suspension techniques.[6–10]

The advent of barbed sutures has been a novel and useful adjunct for the aesthetic plastic

Conflicts of interest and financial disclosures: none for Dr Stephen Mulholland; Dr Paul serves as a consultant to, and receives a stipend from, Angiotech, Pharm., the parent company of Surgical Specialties and the manufacturer of QuillSRS barbed sutures.
^a Private Practice Plastic Surgery, SpaMedica® Clinics, 66 Avenue Road, Suite 4, Toronto, ON M5R 3N8, Canada
^b Aesthetic and Plastic Surgery Institute, University of California, Irvine, Newport Beach, CA, USA
* Corresponding author. 1401 Avocado Avenue, Suite 810, Newport Beach, CA 92660.
E-mail address: malcolmpaulmd@gmail.com

surgeon in properly selected patients. The deployment of a barbed suture minimizes the risks of cheese wiring and stress relaxation, facilitating the minimally invasive repositioning of soft tissue in the head and neck, as well as optimizing and enhancing traditionally long and potentially tedious procedures in body contouring.[11,12] This article highlights the advances, advantages, and efficacy associated with the use of barbed sutures in lifting and wound closure.

SCIENCE OF BARBED SUTURES

The advent of the barbed suture for lifting began with the antiptosis procedure using APTOS sutures.[13] The APTOS suture, called Feather Lift, deployed a 15-cm segment length of dyed polypropylene suture with barbs cut at an angle in the suture and organized facing toward the midline in a bidirectional fashion. Both halves of the sutures had barbs pointed toward the middle. The Feather Lift approximated tissue but was not fixed to any stable craniofacial structures. APTOS sutures and the Feather Lift procedure were introduced into the worldwide market in the late 1990s, for nonfixed soft tissue repositioning of lax, soft tissue elements. Because APTOS sutures were not fixed to the cranial fascial skeleton, they were prone to migration, relapse, and long-term lack of efficacy.[14] Because the sutures were dyed, there was a significant risk that, in time, they would become visible and palpable.[14] Short-term results in the midface in early reports were acceptable; however, because of the lack of fixation and lack of long-term efficacy, the APTOS suture did not achieve US Food and Drug Administration (FDA) approval and they did not experience widespread popularity in the United States.

Surgical Specialties (Reading, PA, USA) and Dr Gregory Ruff introduced a clear, barbed polypropylene suture called the Contour Threadlift, which was FDA-cleared for soft tissue elevation of the midface in 2005. The Contour Threadlift suture was used and promoted principally for the closed soft tissue elevation of facial tissues. The purely closed Threadlift technique was designed to be delivered percutaneously with minimal to no undermining.[11] Although there were some reasonably good results with repositioned soft tissue of the brow, midface, and neck, the Threadlift procedures were prone to unpredictability in efficacy, palpability of sutures, tenderness, extrusion of knots, fracture of the suture, and migration.[11,15]

Angiotech Pharmaceuticals, Inc. (Vancouver, Canada) acquired Surgical Specialties and launched the Quill SRS (Suture Retained Suspension). The Quill suture has been available since January, 2007, and represents the evolution of the original contour thread. The Quill SRS suture is the most widely used barbed suture in the United States and worldwide. Its use continues to evolve into many applications of plastic surgery (as well as in general surgery, vascular surgery, gynecologic laparoscopic surgery, robotic surgery, and orthopedic surgery), and most of this article focuses on the Quill suture and its growing array of peer-reviewed applications.

The Quill SRS suture is a bidirectional barbed suture. It incorporates small barbs (which are back cuts in the suture performed in an automated computer-generated fashion). Approximately 30% of the diameter of the suture makes up the barb. The barbs are spaced evenly in helical array, like a DNA helix, along its length. The barbs face in opposite directions from the midpoint, the midpoint segment being approximately 2 cm in length, in the double-armed suture and toward the fixation end (entry end) on the single-armed suture. On either end of the Quill SRS suture are fixation needles, and the Quill barb suture comes in different lengths, absorbable and nonabsorbable, different diameters, and with different attached needles. The Quill SRS suture is available in a blue polypropylene and a clear polypropylene as well as a violet polydioxone and an absorbable superficial skin closure called Monoderm.[11,12]

The science of the Quill fixation technology is based on multiple barbs engaging in the soft tissue at multiple points along a tensile loaded tissue and dispersing this tensile load along the length of the suture, rather than placing a maximal amount of tension at the knot and fixation point. In addition to spreading a tensile load along the length of the barbed segment, the Quill allows the surgeon to suture without the use of knots. The advantages of multiple barbs along the length of a closure are greatly reduced stress relaxation and cheese wiring effects with potentially more efficacious long-term closure of wounds under tension, such as midline abdominoplasty plications, dermal lipectomies, brachioplasties, mastopexy, and breast reduction procedures, in which the biomechanically efficient distribution of tensile load and high pull-out forces and breaking strengths of the barbed Quill SRS suture may optimize the short-term and long-term behavior of these scars.[11] The use of multiple ischemia-inducing, 2-point fixation sutures (traditional wound closures with interrupted sutures), as opposed to a barbed suture and a no-knot tension balanced closure, has been shown to increase the risk of tissue ischemia, compromised wound strength, increased incidence of suture abscesses, wound dehiscence, and decreased scar cosmesis.[11,12,16–19] Wounds closed under tension with even tension loading and diminished stress relaxation may have fewer hypertrophic scars and spread scars from wound ischemia and stress relaxation. Thus, the science of barb sutures may improve high-tension wound closure, facilitate more rapid closure, and result in superior scar cosmesis. In nonplastic surgery arenas such as laparoscopic and endoscopic endocorporal surgery, the advent of the Quill barbed suture has allowed endoscopic surgeons to perform anastomosis of delicate structures with reduced tissue ischemia, stronger anastomoses, and improved operative efficiency without the need to tie endoscopic knots.[20,21]

The biomechanical in vivo characteristics of a barbed 0, 2-0 and 3-0 Monoderm (a bidirectional barbed, absorbable polyglycolide-poly-e-caprolictone copolymer) was compared with the nonbarbed equivalent Monocryl (a poliglecaprone 25, a copolymer of glycolide and e-caprolictone 1 size smaller, because of the barbs) In vitro tensile strength and break strengths were studied. Comparative studies of barbed and nonbarbed were also performed with polydiaxone and polypropylene. In all of these in vitro studies, the bidirectional, barbed, nonknotted, self-retaining sutures were significantly stronger than the conventional sutures of the same polymer of 1 size smaller (because of the barbs compromising 30% of the suture diameter) at each of days 7, 14, and 21. In most cases, the break strength for tension was nearly double that seen for the nonbarbed suture.[11,12,16–19] Between days 28 and 45, the strength remaining was zero or minimal for all suture types and sizes regardless of barbed or nonbarbed configuration. These studies confirm that barbed sutures exhibit superior breaking strengths, tensile strengths, and pull-out strengths compared with their nonbarbed suture equivalents and that the tension loading of the barbed closure of the entire wound minimizes stress relaxation and cheese wiring, which may greatly aid in the long-term results of soft tissue repositioning and high-tension wound closure.[11,12,16–19]

Although the Quill suture is FDA approved and by far the most commonly used barbed suture in aesthetic plastic surgery, there is another modified suture, called the Silhouette Suture (Kolster Methods, Inc. [KMI], Corona, CA, USA), which is also used internationally. The Silhouette Suture, instead of containing barbs within the polypropylene suture, has intermittent knots organized along both halves of the suture and the knots house, in a bidirectional fashion from each midpoint, little caps or cones of polyglactic acid. These polyglactic acid caps provide the tension loading for elevated soft tissue and, similar to the barb-

modified sutures, are placed intermittently in helical fashion along each half of the suture. The cones are a copolymer of glycolic acid and lactic acid. Between the cones are knots that control the position of the cone, and the cone anchors the suture and allows in-growth of soft tissue. Unlike a barb, the cone grasps tissue in 360 degrees, whereas the barb only grasps the soft tissue at 1 fixed point, thus enhancing the tensile loading capability of a cone, not just across the length of the suture but in 360 degrees around the cone and the cone length of the suture. The Silhouette Suture is used principally for lifting and repositioning soft tissue of the midface and not for wound closure. The Silhouette Suture received its US FDA approval for midface suspension in November, 2006. The initial reports for this suture have been favorable for midface repositioning.[22]

CLASSIFICATION OF BARBED SUTURES

The Quill SRS barb-modified suture, the most prevalent barbed suture used in plastic surgery worldwide, may be classified according to the suture polymer incorporated, the diameter, or barb technique, and the procedure in which they are used.

Classification of barbed sutures

1. Tissue behavior and polymer content
   a. Absorbable
      i. Monoderm
      ii. Polydioxanone (PDO)
   b. Nonabsorbable
      i. Polypropylene
2. United States Pharmacopeia (USP) diameter size
   a. 2,1,0, 2-0, 3-0
3. Clinical procedure
   a Facial soft tissue repositioning
      i. Closed soft tissue repositioning
      ii. Semiclosed, composite lifting
      iii. Open face suspension
   b. Body high-tension closure
      i. Abdominoplasty (plication and/or wound closure)
      ii. Brachioplasty
      iii. Mastopexy or breast reduction closure
      iv. Body lift.

BARBED SUTURES FOR LIFTING
Closed Barbed Suture Lift of the Brow, Midface, and Neck

A closed, percutaneous barbed suture lift of the midface, brow, or neck requires little or no undermining. The barbed suture is used both as the lifting vehicle and fixation support mechanism, taking advantage of the antistress relaxation and even tension loading provided by the Quill SRS and the former Contour Threadlift suture. Although, in selected patients, the initial results can be impressive, there is unpredictability as to which patients will do well, and a high relapse rate, especially in the brow and neck.[11,15] Contraindications for a closed barbed suture lift are patients with high body mass index (BMI), round heavy faces, excessive age and laxity, or those who are not opposed to an excisional procedure and more significant results. In selected patients, with thinner soft tissue envelopes with moderate midface ptosis who are opposed to an open procedure, the closed barbed closed skin lift may be a viable opportunity for short-term tightening.[23] This is especially true with the advent of an absorbable, Monoderm suture, in which knot or fixation palpability, migration, and sensitivity are no longer postoperative concerns. The author has previously reported his experiences with 25 closed, percutaneous, polypropylene barbed suture lifts of midface.[24] The results of this procedure in properly selected patients can be good, with long-term maintenance of midface position in more than 50% of patients at 12 months. The closed, absorbable barbed suture skin lift of the midface may be combined with soft tissue fillers, fractional and nonfractional lasers, and neurotoxins. This combination therapy, performed under local anesthesia with a recovery period of 3 to 4 days, has a definite place in modest facial aesthetic plastic surgery options, especially for patients seeking nonexcisional options.[24,25]

Closed, Percutaneous, Composite, Widely Undermined Barbed Lift to the Brow, Midface, and Neck

The composite nonexcisional, percutaneous lift technique incorporates the concept of a wide surgically undermined tissue flap and then deploying the barbed suture as a passive fixation system, with the stress relaxation and tension load sharing of the barbed configuration.[24,25] Like the closed barbed skin lift, the closed composite barbed suture lift does not involve excision of tissue and can be performed through small percutaneous stab incisions that do not need to be closed. Indications for a closed, composite barbed suture lift of the brow and/or midface lift are a patient with low BMI with moderate to thin facial soft tissue, reasonable expectations of a facial rejuvenation that is less than 50% of an open, excisional facelift (discussed later) and a patient not amenable to an open, excisional procedure (however, it should be offered).

Composite percutaneous barbed suture–supported midface lift

Under local anesthesia and oral sedation, 2 entrance points are chosen in the temporal hair-bearing scalp approximately 2 cm behind the hairline (**Fig. 1**A). One is 2 to 3 cm superior to the zygomatic arch. A 3-mm dermatologic punch is used to remove a portion of the scalp and dissection with a Stephens tenotomy scissor is carried down to the superficial layer of the deep temporal fascia. Through this small incision a small periosteal dissector is used to elevate the temporal parietal fascia down to the superior aspect of the zygomatic arch. No dissection is performed over the zygomatic arch, to minimize inadvertent neuropraxia of the frontal branch of the facial nerve (see **Fig. 1**B). An intraoral transbuccal sulcus stab incision with a small 11 blade is made and the scissors are used in a closed fashion to dissect the soft tissue down to the maxillary buttress. A small periosteal elevator is then used to blindly dissect the inferior 70% of the malar fat pad, subperiosteally, over the malar eminence and up to the zygomatic process of the zygomatic arch (see **Fig. 1**C). Again, a small composite amount of tissue is left intact over the zygomatic arch to preserve the frontal temporal branch. With the division and release of the periosteum through the blind buccal sulcus incision and elevation of the subperiosteal tissues, the mobile malar fat pad and the overlying soft tissue including the suborbicularis oculi fat (SOOF) and subcutaneous malar fat should be well mobilized. With the malar soft tissue fat pad adequately mobilized, using a long Keith needle, a barbed Quill suture is passed through the temporal dermatologic punch port over the superficial layer of the deep temporal fascia, care being taken not to engage this tissue layer, passing the Keith needle through to the zygomatic arch, then extending subcutaneously over the zygomatic arch, pinching the malar fat pad, and passing the Quill suture through the entire soft tissue mobile fat pad of the malar eminence and exiting approximately 1 to 2 cm lateral and posterior to the nasolabial fold, just above the lateral commissure (see **Fig. 1**D). The second arm is passed a little more superiorly through and across the same planes but exiting approximately 3 to 4 cm superior to the previous suture, just lateral to the nasal base, and lateral to and posterior to the nasolabial fold. By pulling on the barbed sutures, the composite malar fat pad and periosteal tissue can be mobilized. The mobile malar fat pad should move significantly superiorly and laterally, creating a revolumization of the midface. An adequately mobilized composite malar fat pad barbed suture lift should result in an immediate and obvious

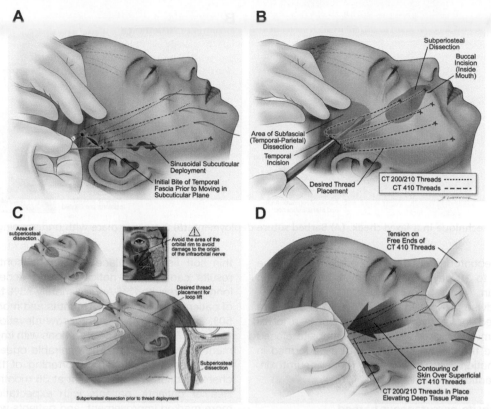

Fig. 1. Composite percutaneous barbed suture–supported midface lift. (*A*) Entrance points behind the hair-bearing scalp. (*B*) Elevation of the fascia down to the superior aspect of the zygomatic arch. (*C*) Intraoral subperiosteal dissection. (*D*) Passage of Quill barbed suture.

correction with an improvement of the lower lid–malar junction and some amelioration of the nasolabial fold. The 2 proximal limbs of the barbed suture are then passed through the temporal parietal fascia, cephalad and out through a second dermatologic punch incision proximally where a knot is tied over the temporal parietal fascia, minimizing the risks of cheese wiring.

In patients with laxity of the cheek skin, when the first suture does not provide adequate correction, further cheek skin and jowl elevation can be performed. A widely undermined subcutaneous flap can be created and suspended by barbed sutures. A dermatologic punch is used to create an entry port, just inferior to the previous access point for the malar fat pad elevation (**Fig. 2**A). One limb of the barbed suture is passed inferiorly and obliquely, exiting just lateral to the labial-mental fold and just superior to the jowl. I leave the Keith needle in the soft tissue, as a second limb is passed inferiorly and obliquely exiting just inferior to the jowl and lateral and posterior to the labial-mental fold. Once the Keith needles and sutures are in place, leaving the Keith needles in situ, an extensive undermining of the soft tissue leaving

a 1-cm width around each Keith needle suture is performed (see **Fig. 2**B). Wide subcutaneous undermining above this malar soft tissue allows superior mobilization of the subcutaneous envelope. The Keith needles are then removed and the barbed sutures are engaged. These sutures are similarly fixated by passing the proximal limbs of the barbed suture posteriorly and superiorly through a second dermatologic punch and sutured down to the temporal parietal fascia. Attention is directed to ensuring that these sutures are passed deep, especially if a nonabsorbable suture is used. If there is still a palpable knot, which can be sensitive, the absorbable suture provides the benefit for patients in that it will dissolve in time. The distal limbs of all 4 sutures can be left 2 cm long and, in the first week to 10 days, remobilization of soft tissue can occur along the subcutaneous tunnels and the patient can be seen every second day. A soft wrap can be used during the first week and patients are advised to sleep on their occiput. The use of an airplane pillow often helps prevent sleeping on the face. Avoiding sleeping on the face is advised for 3 to 4 weeks until adequate initial soft tissue coagulum and prefibrosis occur.

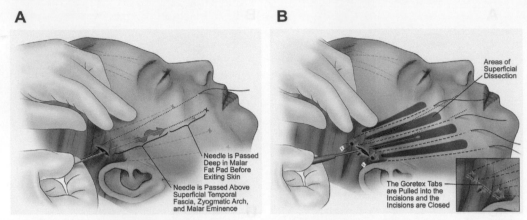

A

Needle is Passed
Deep in Malar
Fat Pad Before
Exiting Skin

Needle is Passed Above
Superficial Temporal
Fascia, Zyogmatic Arch,
and Malar Eminence

B

Areas of
Superficial
Dissection

The Goretex Tabs
are Pulled into the
Incisions and the
Incisions are Closed

Fig. 2. Technique in a laxed cheek. (*A*) Barbed suture deployment. (*B*) Sutures in place with undermining.

After recontouring of the cheek and jowl during the first 7 to 10 days, the sutures are cut flush with the skin.

I advise all patients that 7 to 14 days are required for recovery, because there is a lot of ecchymosis and swelling. The composite closed lift, like the closed skin lift, can be performed in conjunction with soft tissue fillers, neurotoxin, and fractional ablative lasers.

Composite percutaneous barbed suture–supported brow lift

The same dermatologic punch is used for port entry, just behind the hair line. Subperiosteal elevation is prepared down to the superior orbital rim and lateral to the midpupillary line (and presumptive supraorbital nerve) (**Fig. 3**A). A stab incision in the brow hair line and an 18-gauge needle can be used to incise the periosteum around and down the lateral canthus. The inferior 50% of the conjoint fascia along the temporal line is divided blindly. A long v-dissector is then used to elevate the subcutaneous envelope, creating a biplanar elevated flap (subperiosteal and subcutaneous dissections) (see **Fig. 3**B). Two absorbable barbed Quill SRS Monoderm sutures are used, 1 deep in the periosteal flap and 1 in the subcutaneous flap. The composite brow flap is then elevated superiorly and fixed as high as possible on the barbed suture. Ensure that the skin and its glide plane over the periosteal flap are completely stable after fixation. As with the midface lift, the brow soft tissue can be elevated and repositioned every second day by leaving the distal limbs of the barbed suture long (see **Fig. 3**C).

Results of the closed, wide undermining composite suture lift

The long-term results observed for 36 months are reasonable. When patients have moderate to thin soft tissue, midface and jowl recontouring results can lead to noticeable and acceptable long-term results.[24,25] Approximately 75% to 80% of patients are happy at 12 months and more than 50% of patients have some brow elevation at 1 year and 70% of midface elevations with improvement of the convexity. The desirable ogee curve of the cheek mound and shortening of the lid-cheek junction are still present at 36 months.[24,25] Heavier patients, patients with expectations of more marked improvement, and patients who are willing to have more invasive procedures may be better candidates for traditional open, extended procedures with soft tissue excision, contouring, and more secure fixation techniques.

One of the principle advantages of this composite, closed barbed suture–supported procedure of the brow and the midface is that it can be performed quickly under local anesthesia. The brow procedure can be performed in approximately 10 minutes and the midface procedure takes less than 10 minutes on each side. The entire closed, nonexcisional, composite wide undermining barbed lift procedure of the brow midface can take 30 to 45 minutes.[24,25] The composite, closed lift can be performed synchronously with neurotoxins, volumization, either hyaluronic acid gel, Radiesse (Merz Aesthetics, San Mateo, CA, USA) or Sculptra (Sanofi-Aventis U.S. LLC) injections of the midface and nasojugular groove, chin, and nasolabial folds, with combined resurfacing techniques using intense pulse light and carbon dioxide or erbium fractional resurfacing of the epidermal dermal junction. The entire composite procedure with adjunctive techniques, including fillers and laser, can take 60 minutes or less and can provide acceptable, if modest, facial rejuvenative goals for most patients. These procedures can be performed inexpensively compared with the more extensive open procedures and it generally

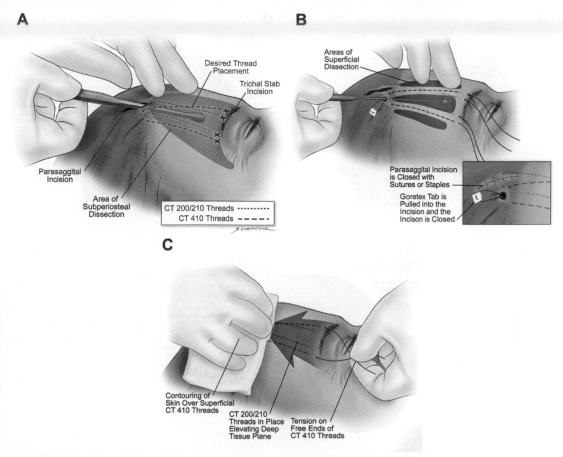

A

Desired Thread Placement

Trichal Stab Incision

Parasaggital Incision

Area of Subperiosteal Dissection

CT 200/210 Threads ·········
CT 410 Threads ― ― ― ―

B

Areas of Superficial Dissection

Parasaggital Incision is Closed with Sutures or Staples

Goretex Tab is Pulled into the Incision and the Incison is Closed

C

Contouring of Skin Over Superficial CT 410 Threads

CT 200/210 Threads in Place Elevating Deep Tissue Plane

Tension on Free Ends of CT 410 Threads

Fig. 3. Composite percutaneous barbed suture–supported brow lift. (*A*) Subperiosteal dissection down to the superior orbital rim. (*B*) Subcutaneous dissection. (*C*) Barbed sutures in place.

takes 7 to 14 days before patients can look presentable.[24,25]

The Use of Barbed Sutures in Open Lifting of the Brow, Face, and Neck

In a series of papers, Paul[26] outlined his approach to elevating a subperiosteal composite flap either through a paramedian or temporal incision and fixation support using barbed Quill SRS suture. In this technique, a classic endoscopic lateral or full brow lift is performed and then the Quill SRS is used for barbed suture fixation (**Fig. 4**A, B). He reported reasonable long-term results and brow position and soft tissue control, comparable with those that might be achieved with endoscopic procedures supported by a bone tunnel or a single-screw fixation, or multiprong Endotine fixation systems. The advantages of this technique compared with a closed composite lift are endoscopic visualization and complete release of the pericranial soft tissues in the periorbita, as well as the ease of the barbed suture placement and

stable fixation. Again, similar to the closed, wide composite technique, the end of the sutures may be left long for adjustment for a 2-week period (see **Fig. 4**C).

OPEN MIDFACE BARBED SUTURE–SUPPORTED MIDFACE LIFT

Paul[27] also describes a transtemporal, along with a transoral, approach for minimally invasive midface elevation. The transtemporal incision is 3 to 4 cm in length, positioned posterior to the temporal hairline in the vector of malar/midface elevation (**Fig. 5**A). Undermining to the superficial layer of the deep temporal fascia, blind dissection to the lateral orbital rim and over the body of the zygoma (see **Fig. 5**B). The technique may also be combined with a transbuccal mobilization of the SOOF and the malar fat pad (see **Fig. 5**C). Once adequate mobilization of the malar fat pad is performed, the Quill sutures are used to pass transtemporally and then exiting from the subperiosteal tissue through the SOOF and malar fat pad

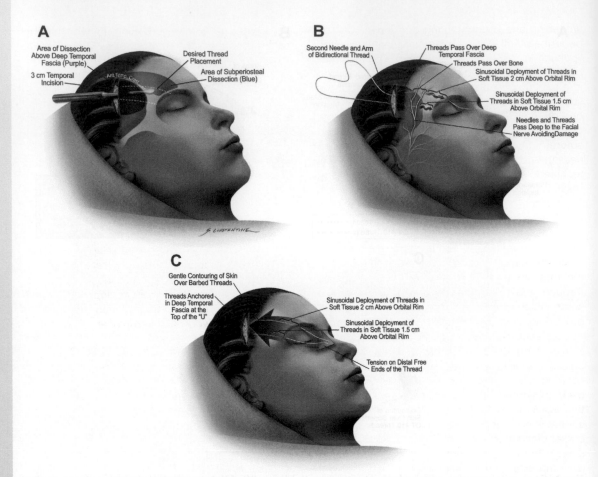

Fig. 4. Open lifting of the brow. (*A*) Dissection to orbital rim. (*B*) Passage of barbed sutures. (*C*) Sutures exit below brow.

and the subcutaneous envelope. This shish kebab of soft tissue is then reelevated, improving the lower lid-cheek junction and increasing the interzygomatic distance (see **Fig. 5**D). Barbed sutures may be left long again distally lateral to the nasolabial fold at their exit point and used to recontour the midface over the subsequent 2 to 3 days in the clinic. This simple technique for barbed suture support of the midface can be performed in conjunction with the standard face and neck lift or in conjunction with a minimal access cranial suspension (MACS)[28] type lift, a superficial musculoaponeurotic system (SMAS) plication type facelift, or a lateral SMASectomy.[29]

SMAS APPLICATION TECHNIQUES AND SMASECTOMY TECHNIQUES

The barbed suture can also be an adjunct in closing a SMAS imbrication procedure, a SMASectomy defect (**Fig. 6**), or a SMAS rotation flap.[26] In the traditional MACS lift, a nonbarbed suture is used in a large purse string fashion, which can

result in some bunching and excessive tension with cheese wiring of the suture, or stress relaxation of the SMAS and platysma support in the long-term.[28] The use of the Monoderm or PDO absorbable barb sutures during a MACS lift can negate the need for a knot and provide even tension loading over the entire mobilization of the SMAS flap, perhaps leading to greater longevity and less relapse, cheese wiring, or loss of SMAS soft tissue support (**Fig. 7**).[27] In addition, with use of the double-armed barbed sutures, there is a less frequent need to address the bunching of the soft tissue that can occur with a purse string suture.

BARBED SUTURE USE IN NECK AND CERVICAL MENTAL REJUVENATION

A new and exciting area of the versatile use of the barbed suture in minimally invasive plastic surgery involves use of the Quill SRS barbed suture in submental and cervical mental angle contouring. Either traditional suction-assisted lipectomy (SAL) or, more recently, radiofrequency–assisted tightening and lipocontouring of the neck can be performed. Following the radiofrequency-assisted liposuction (RFAL), a bimastoid, bidirectional barbed suture Monoderm, 3-O or 2-O, is passed in a subcutaneous space, and is brought out the submental area in the region of the hyoid. Pulling on both mastoid areas tightens and improves the cervical mental angle. The position of the barbed sutures during the scarification phase of wound healing improves the contour of the jawline. This technique has been presented and the short-term results seem promising.[25] During open cervical mental contouring, barbs sutures have become indispensable and are used to close the platysmal diastasis (**Fig. 8**). When a lateral approach seems most appropriate to improve the cervical mental angle, the Quill SRS barbed suture is anchored to the mastoid fascia and then each limb passes through the platysma muscle to tighten the submandibular tissues, especially in the case of ptotic submandibular glands, exiting in the paramedian submental area (**Fig. 9**).

In addition, the SMASectomy can be closed and one of the distal ends of barbed sutures can be secured down over the mandibular angle and used to tighten and plicate centrally, or tighten the platysma laterally (see **Fig. 8**). This barbed suture lateral lift supports the classic Feldman corset platysmaplasty (see **Fig. 9**),[30] and helps to sustain the cervical mental contour until there is a composite soft tissue healing between the muscle and the overlying skin.[26] The barbed suture has been used for elevation of the SMAS to support the ear complex and help prevent post-facelift inferior migration (pixie deformity), and rotatory defects of the pinna.[31]

BARBED SUTURE TECHNIQUE IN WOUND CLOSURE AND BODY SURGERY

The Quill SRS suture has been reported to significantly enhance the speed and efficacy of many commonly performed body-contouring procedures. Both the larger 0 and 2-0 polydioxone and the 3-0 and 2-0 Monoderm sutures have found a significant place in body contour surgery. Recent reports of closure of midline abdominoplasty rectus diastasis plications show good long-term results and no recurrent diastasis herniation has been reported.[32,33] In addition, the technique of advancing sequential tension closure and using the Quill suture to close the dead space in an abdominoplasty flap can obviate the need for drains.[32,33] The advantages of the barbed sutures in high-tension body-contouring closures are even tension loading along with minimization of cheese wiring, 2-point suture

ischemia, and stress relaxation to which non-barbed sutures are more prone. Comparative studies have shown that the barbed suture, although more expensive than a nonbarbed suture, can save significantly in operative time and hence operative costs.[13,14,16–19,32,33] The authors have found that, in situations in which drains are deployed, the barbed suture is used for rectus plication, deep polydioxone barbed suture is used for Scarpa fascia closure, and Monoderm barbed sutures are used for subdermal closure, total operative time for a standard abdominoplasty can be reduced to 60 to 70 minutes. In addition, it is the experience of both authors that the long-term (more than 1 year) midline rectus plication results do not show a relapse rate any higher that traditional rectus fascia closure. Furthermore, the early high-tension scar results seen in abdominoplasty and brachioplasty barbed suture closures seem favorable when polydioxone barbed sutures were deployed in Scarpa fascia and Monoderm barbed sutures were placed for the subdermal closure. Having observed that the early scar results at 6 months seem favorable, further objective work needs to be conducted. There is a minimal amount of suture spitting and tissue reaction in wounds closed with high-tension barbed sutures and this may provide for better scars in tension-loaded wounds such as abdominoplasty and extended abdominoplasties.[11,12] The barbed suture closure technique is valuable in brachioplasty, where deep polydioxone suture fascial closure is followed by Monoderm for deep dermal skin closure. Up to an hour can be saved on a brachioplasty procedure and through stress relaxation avoidance and tension loading may prove to enhance the brachial scar. In total body lifting with large excisions, complete inner thigh lift, back lifting, and large flank reductions, the barbed suture is proving invaluable in savings of time. Breast contouring, short-scar breast reduction, formal Wise pattern breast reduction, and periareolar breast reduction all benefit from the tensile loading, antistress relaxation, rapid closure, and lack of knots. The usual high-tension areas in a typical Wise pattern can be minimized with the use of barbed sutures and short-scar techniques for breast mastopexy can also be performed quickly and efficiently with good intermediate-term and long-term scar results.

COMPLICATIONS OF BARBED SUTURES IN LIFTING AND WOUND CLOSURE

The evolution in barbed suture technology in the past 4 to 5 years has resulted in the development of a significant tool for the plastic surgeon to

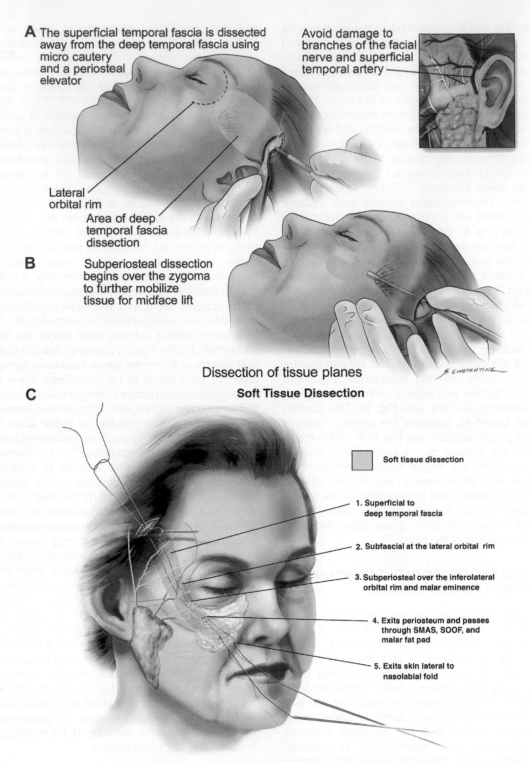

A The superficial temporal fascia is dissected away from the deep temporal fascia using micro cautery and a periosteal elevator

Avoid damage to branches of the facial nerve and superficial temporal artery

Lateral orbital rim

Area of deep temporal fascia dissection

B Subperiosteal dissection begins over the zygoma to further mobilize tissue for midface lift

Dissection of tissue planes

S. CONSTANTINE

Soft Tissue Dissection

C

Soft tissue dissection

1. Superficial to deep temporal fascia

2. Subfascial at the lateral orbital rim

3. Subperiosteal over the inferolateral orbital rim and malar eminence

4. Exits periosteum and passes through SMAS, SOOF, and malar fat pad

5. Exits skin lateral to nasolabial fold

Fig. 5. Open barbed suture–supported midface lift. (*A*) Temporal access incision. (*B*) Undermining over deep temporal fascia to zygoma. (*C*) Suture deployment. (*D*) Shish kebab stacking of soft tissue.

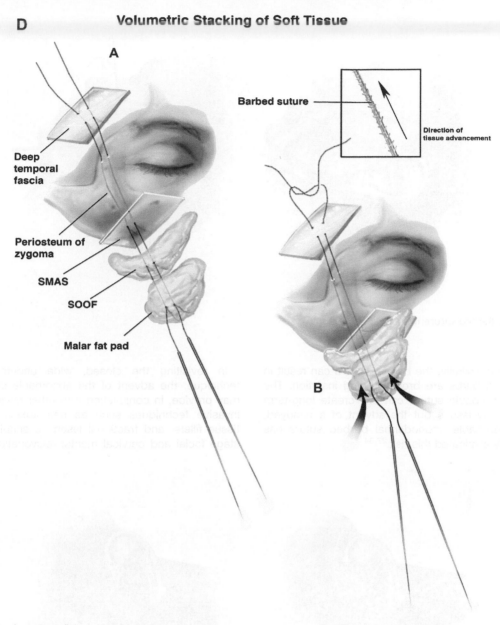

D

Volumetric Stacking of Soft Tissue

A

Barbed suture

Direction of
tissue advancement

Deep
temporal
fascia

Periosteum of
zygoma

SMAS

SOOF

Malar fat pad

B

Fig. 5. (*continued*)

deploy in selected cases of facial rejuvenation and as a closure device for many of the body-contouring and aesthetic and reconstructive breast surgical procedures. The addition of absorbable Quill SRS sutures and a more consistent helical array of barbs has afforded the plastic surgeon more rapid closure techniques, the ability to optimize tension-loading and tension-sharing technology along the entire aspect of a high-tension closure, and to minimize the risk of stress relaxation in significant elevations of soft tissue.

The enhanced wound healing characteristics and the increased strength of the suture in the first 1 to 3 months may result in improved scar characteristics, although further studies assessing the long-term scar outcomes in barb-supported high-tension closures need to be conducted.[16–19] Complications with barbed sutures still persist, including palpability of the knot if a nonabsorbable device that requires the tying of a knot is used in the temporal and brow region. Palpability of the knot in the mastoid region can be sensitive. If not

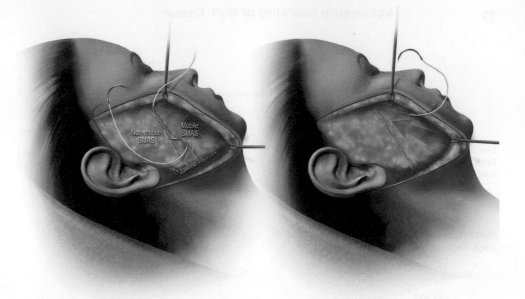

Fig. 6. Barbed suture in lateral SMASectomy.

handled skillfully, the barbed suture can result in failure if barbs are broken during insertion. The nonabsorbable suture can still create long-term sensitivity issues but the advent of a nondyed, bioabsorbable, monodermal barbed suture has greatly eliminated this risk.[27,34]

In revisiting the closed, wide undermined technique, the advent of the absorbable suture may provide, in conjunction with other minimally invasive techniques such as neurotoxins, soft tissue fillers, and fractional lasers, a simple, 1-stage facial and cervical mental rejuvenation. In

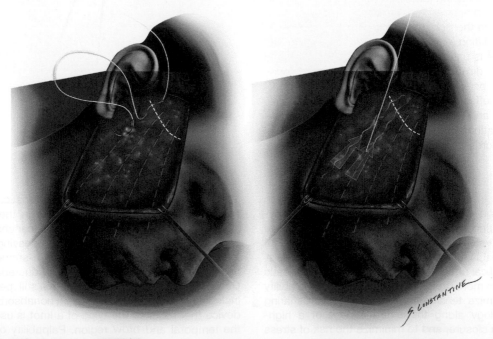

Fig. 7. Barbed suture in MACS lift.

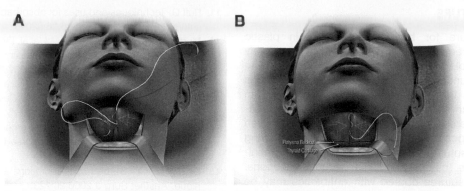

Fig. 8. Barbed suture in midline (corset) platysmaplasty (A) and platysma backcut (B).

combination with SAL, laser-assisted liposuction or RFAL may be enough for patients who are not seeking more extensive and more effective open techniques. The biggest risk of these nonexcisional barb-supported suture lifts of the face is a dissatisfied patient whose expectations were unrealistic.[11,15,24–27] The absorbable and nonabsorbable polyethylene and polypropylene barbed sutures are rarely associated with soft tissue infection. Risks of neurogenic injury on suture insertion are rare in the hands of a plastic surgeon who is skilled in the placement of these devices and best served by those who also perform open surgery. Suture failure leading to relapse of soft tissue or dehiscence of high-tension closures is unusual; it is less common than with nonbarbed wound closure or suture suspension techniques.[11,15]

One of the most common barbed suture complications in the percutaneous, closed, wide undermining lifting techniques of the brow and the midface is unreasonable patient expectation and patient dissatisfaction.[15] These nonexcisional, closed barbed lifting techniques are generally not as effective as full open, extensively undermined, and securely fixed surgery, and patients' expectations, as in all aesthetic plastic surgery procedures, need to be managed to avoid

disappointment. In the early days of the Contour Threadlift, the closed technique with minimal to no undermining resulted in many unhappy patients. With wide undermining, closed percutaneous surgery, or open surgery, the barbed suture becomes more of a passive fixation system. With antistress relaxation and tension unloading properties, the results of these procedures can be acceptable in patients who are properly selected. When patients are properly selected, with mild to moderate ptosis, reasonable BMIs, and without corpulent cervical facial morphologies, the closed and open wide undermined brow and midface techniques are rapid, effectively maintained, and generally result in happy patients with good long-term results.

SUMMARY OF BARBED SUTURE LIFTING AND WOUND CLOSURE

This article outlines the updated uses and clinical results of barbed suture lifts, both open and closed, of the soft tissue of the face and neck. Long-term results make this barbed suture lift a predictable alternative for those seeking modest, nonexcisional facial rejuvenation of the midface and brow. For open face and necklifts, including the MACS lift, the barbed suture has emerged as an excellent fixation option. The Quill SRS barbed sutures can also be used in body-contouring procedures to significantly increase the speed of abdominoplasty, brachioplasty, mastopexy, and breast reduction surgery. The use of the Quill suture in sequential tension reduction by suturing Scarpa fascia to the rectus sheath is a quick technique that potentially eliminates the use of drains without increasing the risk of seroma. In addition to significantly increasing the speed of these body-contouring procedures, the Quill SRS suture, by more effective tension unloading, may also improve the long-term quality of these high-tension scars.

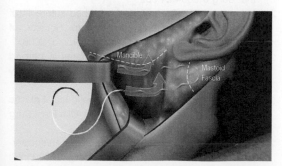

Fig. 9. Barbed suture for lateral platysmaplasty.

THE FUTURE

The future for barbed technology in plastic surgery remains bright. The advent of completely absorbable sutures, combined with undermining and adjunctive therapy, gives plastic surgeons adept in the technique, or willing to revisit the option, another nonexcisional procedure in treating patients receiving facial rejuvenation. Even though postoperative infection is rare, coating barbed sutures with antibiotics may further minimize the risk of bacterial wound infections. Barbed sutures coated with antibiotics may be used in operative cancer fields. The barbed suture will prove to be a valuable asset in all body-contouring techniques in which large incisions, plication, support, and tension unloading are beneficial. New applications for these devices will emerge and plastics surgeons will continue to be innovative in their uses.

REFERENCES

1. Cosmetic Industry Update. Medical Insights. Biotech Week May 12, 2010.
2. Webster RC, Davidson TM, Reardon EJ, et al. Suspending sutures in blepharoplasty. Arch Otolaryngol 1979;105:601.
3. Wagner RS, Mauriello JA, Nelson LB, et al. Treatment of congenital ptosis with frontalis suspension: a comparison of suspensory materials. Ophthalmology 1984;91:245.
4. Matarasso A, Pfeifer TM. The use of modified sutures in plastic surgery. Plast Reconstr Surg 2008;122:652–8.
5. Coleman J, Bick PA. Suspension sutures for the treatment of obstructive sleep apnea and snoring. Otolaryngol Clin North Am 1999;32:277–81.
6. Giampapa VC, Dibernardo BE. Neck recontouring with suture suspension and liposuction. Aesthetic Plast Surg 1995;19:217.
7. Hobar PC, Flood J. Subperiosteal rejuvenation of the midface and periorbital area: a simplified approach. Plast Reconstr Surg 1996;97:836.
8. Anderson RD, Lo MW. Endoscopic malar/midface suspension procedure. Plast Reconstr Surg 1998;102:2196.
9. Sasaki GH, Cohen AT. Meloplication of the malar fat pads by percutaneous cable –suture technique for midface rejuvenation: outcome stud (392 cases, 6 years experience). Plast Reconstr Surg 2002;109:2074–86.
10. La Ferriere KA, Castellano RD. Experience with percutaneous suspension of the malar fat pad for midface rejuvenation. Facial Plast Surg Clin North Am 2005;13:393.
11. Ruff G. Techniques and uses for absorbable barbed sutures. Aesthet Surg J 2006;26:620–8.
12. Murtha AP, Kaplan AL, Paglia MJ, et al. Evaluation of a novel technique for wound closure using a barbed suture. Plast Reconstr Surg 2006;117:1769–80.
13. Sulamanidze MA, Shiffman MA, Paikidze TG, et al. Facelifting with APTOS threads. Int J Cosmet Surg Aesthetic Dermatol 2001;4:275–80.
14. Lyka B, Bazan C, Poletti E, et al. The emerging technique of the antiptosis subdermal thread. Dermatol Surg 2004;30:241.
15. DeLorenzi CL. Barbed sutures: rationale and technique. Aesthet Surg J 2006;26:223.
16. Dattilo PP, King MW, Leung JC. Tissue holding performance of knotless absorbable sutures. In: Programs and abstract in the Society for Biomaterials 29th Annual Meeting Transactions. 2003. p. 101.
17. Dattilo PP, King MW, Cassill NL, et al. Medical textiles: an application of an absorbable, barbed, bi-directional surgical suture. Journal of Textile and Apparel, Technology and Management 2002;2:1–5.
18. Leung JC, Pritt S. Barbed bi-directional surgical sutures: in vivo strength and histopathology evaluations. In: Programs and abstracts in the Society for Biomaterials 29th Annual Meeting Transactions. 2003. p. 100.
19. Leung JC. Barbed suture technology: recent advances. In: Proceedings Medical Textiles 2004. Advances in biomedical textiles and healthcare products conference. Pittsburg; 2004. p. 62–80.
20. Greenberg JA, Einarsson JI. The use of bidirectional barbed suture in laparoscopic myomectomy and total laparoscopic hysterectomy. J Minim Invasive Gynecol 2008;15:621–3.
21. Moran ME, Marsh C, Perrotti M. Bidirectional barbed sutured knotless running anastomosis v classic van Velthoven in a model system. J Endourol 2007;21:1175–7.
22. Gamboa GM, Vasconez LO. Suture suspension technique for midface and neck rejuvenation. Ann Plast Surg 2009;62:478–81.
23. Wu WT. Barbed sutures in facial rejuvenation. Aesthet Surg J 2004;24:582.
24. Mulholland RS. The composite barbed suture lift of the brow and midface. Canadian Society of Aesthetic Plastic Surgery Meeting. Toronto, 2006.
25. Mulholland RS. Advances and updates in barbed suture composite facelifts. IMCAS. Paris, January 2008.
26. Paul MD. Barbed sutures for aesthetic facial plastic surgery: indications and techniques. Clin Plast Surg 2008;35:451–61.
27. Paul MD. Using barbed sutures in open/subperiosteal midface lifting. Aesthet Surg J 2006;26:725–32.

28. Tonnard P, Verpaele A, Monstrey S, et al. Minimal access cranial suspension lift: a modified s-lift. Plast Reconstr Surg 2002;109:2074–86.

29. Baker DC. Lateral SMASectomy. Plast Reconstr Surg 1997;100:509–13.

30. Feldman J. Necklift. St Louis (MO): Quality Medical Publishing; 2006.

31. Man D. Reducing the incidence of ear deformity in facelift. Aesthet Surg J 2009;29:264–71.

32. Warner JP, Gutowski KA. Abdominoplasty with progressive tension closure using barbed suture technique. Aesthet Surg J 2009;29:221–5.

33. Rosen AD. Use of absorbable running barbed suture and progressive tension technique in abdominoplasty: a novel approach. Plast Reconstr Surg 2010;125:1024–7.

34. Paul MD. Complications of barbed sutures. Aesthetic Plast Surg 2008;32:149.

Index

Note: Page numbers of article titles are in **boldface** type.

Clin Plastic Surg 38 (2011) 537–541
doi:10.1016/S0094-1298(11)00082-4

Moving?

Make sure your subscription moves with you!

To notify us of your new address, find your **Clinics Account Number** (located on your mailing label above your name), and contact customer service at:

Email: journalscustomerservice-usa@elsevier.com

800-654-2452 (subscribers in the U.S. & Canada)
314-447-8871 (subscribers outside of the U.S. & Canada)

Fax number: 314-447-8029

Elsevier Health Sciences Division
Subscription Customer Service
3251 Riverport Lane
Maryland Heights, MO 63043

*To ensure uninterrupted delivery of your subscription, please notify us at least 4 weeks in advance of move.

ELSEVIER